D0098800

Treating Personality Disorders in Children and Adolescents

A Relational Approach

EFRAIN BLEIBERG

THE GUILFORD PRESS
New York London

© 2001 The Guilford Press
A Division of Guilford Publications, Inc.
72 Spring Street, New York, NY 10012
www.guilford.com

All rights reserved

No part of this book may be reproduced, translated, stored in a
retrieval system, or transmitted, in any form or by any means,
electronic, mechanical, photocopying, microfilming, recording,
or otherwise, without written permission from the Publisher.

Printed in the United States of America

This book is printed on acid-free paper.

Last digit is print number: 9 8 7 6 5 4 3 2 1

Library of Congress Cataloging-in-Publication Data

Bleiberg, Efrain, 1951–
    Treating personality disorders in children and adolescents : a
relational approach / by Efrain Bleiberg.
        p.   cm.
    Includes bibliographical references and index.
    ISBN 1-57230-698-X
    1. Personality disorders in children. 2. Personality disorders
in adolescence. 3. Personality disorders in children—Treatment.
4. Personality disorders in adolescence—Treatment. I. Title.

RJ506.P32 B54 2001
618.92′858—dc21
                                                    2001033661

About the Author

Efrain Bleiberg, MD, was born in Monterrey, Mexico. He is a graduate of the School of Medicine of the University of Nuevo Leon, the School of Psychology of the University of Monterrey, the Psychiatry and Child Psychiatry residency programs of the Karl Menninger School of Psychiatry and Mental Health Sciences, and the Topeka Institute for Psychoanalysis (adult and child psychoanalysis). He has served as Unit Director, Director of the Child Psychiatry Training Program, Director of the General Psychiatry Residency Program, Dean of the Karl Menninger School of Psychiatry and Mental Health Sciences, Vice President for Education and Research, Vice President and Director of the Children's Division, and Chief of Staff and President of The Menninger Clinic in Topeka, Kansas. He is currently Senior Executive Vice President of The Menninger Clinic, the Alice Friedman Professor of Psychiatry and Developmental Psychopathology in the Karl Menninger School of Psychiatry and Mental Health Sciences, and a Training and Supervising Psychoanalyst at the Topeka Institute for Psychoanalysis.

Preface

This book represents an effort to make sense of the plight of children and adolescents who are in the process of structuring a severe personality disorder. My interest in this area grew out of many encounters with children whose troubling behaviors effectively conceal their pain and anguish. While they are often strikingly arrogant, defiant, and manipulative, they also convey a touching determination to survive and connect with others. Yet they excel at defeating the efforts to help them break the grip that anxiety, anger, and vulnerability have fastened on their loneliness.

Some of these children's minds and bodies have suffered the destructive intrusions of sexual or physical abuse or the more insidious damage of neglect and insensitivity. Others are burdened by an array of constitutional vulnerabilities, ranging from handicaps in attention and mood regulation to developmental reading disorders and deficits in executive functions. Yet, regardless of the degree of environmental assault or biological misfortune that they experienced, they often display an uncanny sensitivity to other people's mental states. This sensitivity incongruously coexists with striking self-centeredness and callous disregard for the feelings of others. One moment they can be thoughtful and appealing; the next moment, however, their rage, demandingness, destructiveness, and self-destructiveness become overwhelming,

This bewildering behavior places considerable strain on caregivers, teachers, and therapists. For many therapists, the demands of carrying on a treatment relationship become difficult to bear as they find themselves falling into a dark despair not unlike that experienced by their young patients.

The paradoxical coexistence of mysterious sensitivity and brutal lack of concern also offers clues about the processes by which these children generate and organize their subjective experiences, coping mechanisms, and relationship patterns. These clues open a pathway into their inner world, but exploring this world is fraught with disturbing feelings and unnamed terrors. Most striking indeed is how often these children's experiences seem to resist naming or comprehension. Instead, they and their interactive partners—including their therapists—find themselves compelled by powerful forces of raw affect to enact rigid patterns of interpretation and response that are not amenable to reflection or modulation.

The groundbreaking work of Peter Fonagy and his collaborators, particularly Mary Target and George Gergely in Europe, and Jon Allen and Helen Stein in the United States, provided me with a conceptual framework on which to anchor a formulation of the development of severe personality disorders and of a treatment model tailored to the developmental and contextual issues underlying and perpetuating the misery and maladjustment of these children and their families.

At the heart of this framework is the concept of reflective function—more recently referred to by Fonagy (2000) as the "interpersonal interpretive mechanism." Reflective function is the biologically prepared capacity to develop a mind that can interpret and respond to the world—the world of our own selves and the world of other people—in human, meaningful terms. As Fonagy's research demonstrates, this capacity emerges in the interactive processes of the attachment system. Arguably, reflective function becomes the key mechanism to appraise, moderate, and shape the psychosocial environment that modulates gene expression.

Reflective function enables children to read other people's minds and grasp the feelings, beliefs, thoughts, and intentions underlying human behavior—their own and that of others. The developmental trajectory leading to severe personality disorders reaches a critical milestone when children buffeted by genetic vulnerabilities, unusual sensitivities, traumatic intrusions, and intermittent misattunement develop protective coping strategies that rely on the active inhibition of reflective function in response to specific internal and interpersonal cues. These are the cues that normally trigger an intensification of the needs for proximity and human connection. But these same signals of distress and desire for closeness often evoke a parallel protective inhibition of reflective function in the caregivers. As a consequence, children and caregivers become entrapped in coercive cycles of relatedness that, while allowing for a semblance of human connection and a sense of control—a pattern of disorganized attachment—also fuel anger, hopelessness, and despair, and reinforce maladjustment in the child and in the family.

The first part of this book is a discussion of how severe personality disorders become organized and structured in childhood and adolescence. My aim is to be able to conceptualize personality disorders as the outgrowth of disorganized attachments and the subsequent efforts of children and caregivers to stay connected and attain self-agency by actively and intermittently inhibiting reflective function.

The second half of the book discusses a systematic treatment approach that seeks to create the conditions, both in the child and in the family, under which disorganized attachments, coercive cycles, and inhibited reflective function can evolve into healing and sustaining connections supported by an enhanced capacity for reflective function.

In describing this approach to treatment, I tried to sort out the theoretical baggage that was impeding my work with children with severe personality disorders and their families. My belief in the therapeutic power of insight had to be tempered by an appreciation that these children seemed to feel less helped by my remarkable revelations about *what* they had in mind than by a deliberate focus on *how*, on a moment-to-moment basis, they organize their experience of themselves and others. Keeping this focus is particularly difficult with children who have largely given up hope and have withdrawn to a point where they are almost beyond reach. These children call for a capacity to feel and think *for them* until they are able to do it for themselves. This is a capacity that requires using the disturbance these children engender in us to appreciate the extent of their terror, particularly the terror they experience at being able to truly grasp the mental states of those close to them. Therapists who can withstand their own reactions and survive the attempts of these children—and their caregivers—to oppose change and sabotage the efforts made on their behalf are better able to establish a true therapeutic alliance with both the patients and their caregivers. Such an alliance grows from an understanding of the courage children and caregivers require in order to relinquish a painstakingly achieved adaptation and face instead the terror and pain of becoming alive in a fully human way.

Acknowledgments

I could not have written this book without the help and support of many people and our exceptional organization. I have worked for almost 25 years at the Menninger Clinic, where I first came as a psychiatric resident and as a candidate at the Topeka Institute for Psychoanalysis. Thus, I grew up as a clinician nurtured by Menninger's rich tradition of respect and appreciation for the forces promoting and opposing development. Unlike any other place, at Menninger I had the opportunity to observe and participate in the careful design of treatment programs seeking to heal the wounds and remove the blocks that impede the development of individuals and families. It is an approach to treatment founded on the conviction that therapeutic relationships offer troubled people the best opportunity to rekindle hope and find the courage to move in the direction of their own evolution. To that tradition of care, I owe much of the spirit that animates this book.

This spirit is embodied in many people at Menninger: colleagues, mentors, supervisors, administrative staff, and the patients and families who give us the privilege of sharing their struggles. Many made helpful and important suggestions, and I hope for forgiveness from those whose names I omit. I am particularly grateful to Jerry Katz, who taught me firsthand the healing power of human relationships and nurtured in me the hope that it was possible to make sense from and come to terms with one's unacknowledged fears and vulnerabilities. My teachers and supervisors at the Topeka Institute for Psychoanalysis contributed immensely to my personal and professional growth. I would like to express my gratitude to Len Horwitz and Irv Rosen and to the memory of

Stu Averill, Ishak Ramzy, and Jack Ross. All shared generously with me the wealth of their clinical experience and their sense of wonder at the unique dramas of our patients' lives, and taught me to listen and help children find their own voices. In the process of teaching and supervising me, they became mentors and then colleagues and friends.

Cotter Hirschberg provided me with a generation of child psychiatrists and child psychoanalysts at Menninger with a vision and a model of the child and adolescent clinician who blends technical skill and theoretical sophistication with human decency, sensitivity, integrity, and compassion. The acute insights of Don Rinsley provided the seed that initially propelled me to write this book. Marty Leichtman supervised my early writings on borderline children and helped me ground my ideas in a developmental framework. His seminal ideas on the nature of reality contact in borderline youngsters confer on him a substantial share of the intellectual paternity of this book. His work with Maria Luisa Leichtman on residential treatment of troubled youngsters contributed critical aspects to the model of treatment I discuss.

I cannot adequately acknowledge my debt to the Menninger Children's Hospital. I worked for 10 years there under the leadership of JoAnn Myers. It was an exhilarating opportunity to work in depth with children and their families alongside a remarkable group of professionals who shared freely their warmth, humor, courage, and wisdom.

Many of the ideas presented here were shaped and enriched by more than 10 years of discussions at a symposium on narcissistic and borderline disorders in children and adolescents organized by the late Joe Noshpitz, which was part of the meetings of the American Academy of Child and Adolescent Psychiatry. The discussions with Dr. Noshpitz and my fellow panelist, Paulina Kernberg, provided me with a unique forum to focus, clarify, and amend my evolving concepts.

My interest in understanding how the mind of the clinician "works" to grasp and find meaning in one's own experience and the experiences constructed jointly with our patients came to life and gained substance in a spirited partnership of ideas with two dear friends, Joe Hyland and Becquer Benalcazar. Dr. Hyland's untimely death robbed us all of his wit, his generosity of spirit, and his immense capacity to probe the nuances of human understanding. In honor of Joe's memory, Becquer and I presented "How the Mind of the Analyst Works" at meetings of the International Psychoanalytic Association and the American Psychoanalytic Association, where he continues to challenge himself and the participants at a twice-yearly symposium to bare their humanity with nothing to cloak it but searing honesty and unfailing passion for the struggle to make sense of the intensity and richness of the psychoanalytic and psychotherapeutic encounter.

Glen Gabbard's brilliant integration of psychoanalysis with the neurosciences and developmental and psychosocial research provided me with an inspiration and a model of the potential for creating a coherent formulation that benefits from the layering of multiple perspectives held together by the conceptual glue of a developmental–psychodynamic point of view. His important contributions to the understanding and treatment of severe personality disorders greatly influenced my own thinking. His clear and straightforward writing style prompted me to seek clarity, focus, and restraint when my own inclinations led in the direction of meaning-obscuring muddiness.

And now, my acknowledgment of Peter Fonagy's contributions. I feel enormously grateful for a chance encounter, at a hotel lobby in Tokyo, between two lonely and jet-lagged individuals, that has grown into a rare occurrence of genuine love and friendship largely devoid of envy and competition. Peter's brilliant conceptualization and original research is pushing the boundaries of psychoanalysis and developmental psychology and is ushering a true revolution in our own understanding of the development of psychopathology in children and adults, particularly those with severe personality disorders.

The ideas that I described here were shaped by many hours of discussion with Peter that highlighted the necessity to anchor my enthusiasm for conceptualization in the hard evidence derived from rigorous research. I could learn this lesson only because of Peter's unsparing—mostly of his own foibles—humor and lovely irony, the excellent single-malt scotch he invariably brings with him, and the true reading of each other's minds that mysteriously happens between soulmates.

A special thanks to what I would argue is the most extraordinary psychiatric, psychological, and psychoanalytic library in the world, the library of The Menninger Clinic and its staff, under the direction of Alice Brand Bartlett. In the Division of Scientific Publications, Mary Ann Clifft and Phil Beard edited meticulously to bring greater clarity to my manuscript. The residents and students of the Karl Menninger School of Psychiatry and Mental Health Sciences and the candidates of the Topeka Institute for Psychoanalysis discussed most of the material presented in this book. They challenged me to clarify my concepts and stimulated me with the freshness of their views and their hunger for understanding. Kitty Moore, Senior Editor at The Guilford Press, helped me organize the material and ably set apart the wheat from the chaff. With gentleness and firmness, Kitty prompted me to complete this project while nevertheless enduring my delays with utter grace. Nancy Adair, a most competent secretary, patiently typed many of the early drafts. The finished manuscript was completed thanks to the thorough word processing and editing, and the caring and moral support of Nancy Gordon. I am also indebted to Walt Menninger for his encouragement and unfailing support.

Last, but most significant, my thanks and my love to Ellen Safier and our sons. Ellen is the loving heart of our family, in addition to being my closest friend and colleague. She tolerated my theorizing about attachment, which she turns into living and loving reality, while I neglected the shared responsibilities of parenting. Ellen has taught me much, not the least of which is to view families—ours included—with respect and compassion. And I thank our sons, Alex, Daniel, and Benjamin, for making clear to me what is truly meaningful and lasting in life.

Contents

TREATING PERSONALITY DISORDERS IN CHILDREN AND ADOLESCENTS

1

Introduction

The anguish and rage of children with severe personality disorders assail clinicians with uncanny power. Like no other patients, these children challenge the clinician's skill and sensitivity. Although they strain the resources of schools and caregivers, their remarkable determination to survive can be both touching and endearing. Yet they excel at defeating the efforts to help them.

The means these children use to ensure their emotional survival can inflict enormous pain on themselves and their families, and can evoke responses from others that reinforce their maladaptation. Indeed, treatment often fails as clinicians succumb to their own inability to manage the emotional reactions elicited by these children.

On closer examination, these children's disruptive behavior appears to be the manifestation of severe personality disorders that surface in the process of becoming organized and structured. Such patterns of maladjustment span a cluster of conditions encompassing the borderline, histrionic, narcissistic, and antisocial personality disorders, which the fourth edition of the *Diagnostic and Statistical Manual of Mental Disorders* (DSM-IV; American Psychiatric Association, 1994) groups together as the Cluster B, or the "dramatic," personality disorders. I refer to this cluster of disorders as the severe personality disorders because of the enormous personal, social, and financial cost associated with them.

In this book, I examine the processes by which youngsters affected by various combinations of constitutional vulnerability, maltreatment, and specific developmental difficulties generate and organize "dramatic" or severe personality disorders. These personality organizations ensure these youngsters a semblance of identity, human connection, and sense of control. The harrowing consequences of these efforts at adaptation and the price paid by these children, their families, and society for such precarious adjustment build the rationale for a systematic effort to create more effective therapeutic and preventive approaches. The central premise of this book is that disruptions in the development of the biologically prepared capacity for reflective function (i.e., the moment-to-moment ability to grasp the meaningfulness and intentionality of human behavior, both the child's own and that of others) are the key to understanding personality disorders in children and adolescents. This understanding provides the basis of an effective treatment model.

CAN CHILDREN HAVE A PERSONALITY DISORDER?

"Personality disorders" are defined in DSM-IV (American Psychiatric Association, 1994) as relatively enduring and pervasively maladaptive patterns of experiencing, coping, and relating. Such a definition raises the question: How can children and adolescents, immersed as they are in extraordinarily fluid developmental processes, qualify for such designation? Every aspect of children's bodies and personalities is constantly changing, and at different rates, creating a constantly shifting equilibrium and disequilibrium within themselves and in their relationship with the environment. Maturation and experience provide children with ever-changing tools to cope, perceive, organize their subjective experience, and relate to others, making it difficult, if not impossible, to speak of "rigid and enduring patterns."

Until recently, the question of whether child and even adolescent patterns of experiencing, coping, and relating can indeed become rigidly and maladaptively fixed was largely argued in the arena of theoretical dispute. Over the past 20 years, however, a growing body of developmental research and prospective studies has provided an empirically supported basis for understanding the interactions of genetic and psychosocial factors that create the risk factors and protective influences shaping how children generate, organize, and structure their subjective experiences, coping mechanisms, and relationship patterns (Beeghly & Cicchetti, 1994; Cicchetti & Rogosch, 1997; Cicchetti & Toth, 1995; Fonagy, 2000a; Fonagy & Target, 1997; Perry & Pollard, 1998; Rutter, 1987, 1999; Sroufe, 1997; Wyman et al., 1999).

Such studies support the contention of Paulina Kernberg (1990) and Kernberg, Weiner, and Bardenstein (2000), among others, that children exhibit distinctive traits and patterns of perceiving, relating, and thinking about the environment and themselves, including traits such as impulsivity, introversion, egocentricity, novelty seeking, inhibition, sociability, activity, and many others. Kernberg added that these traits and patterns endure across time and situation, and warrant the designation of personality disorder regardless of the children's age, when they (1) become inflexible, maladaptive, and chronic; (2) cause significant functional impairment; and (3) produce severe subjective distress. Building on this work, I propose that the defining feature of children with a dramatic or severe personality disorder is their "loss" or inhibition of the capacity to maintain a reflective stance, thus replacing the normal grasping and conveying of meaningful mental states, which is the basis of flexible adaptation, with a rigid, nonreflective mode of organizing experience and relating to others. This rigid mode of organization, in turn, evokes interpersonal responses that further reinforce and validate these children's inner organization. Joe, for example (whom I describe in more detail in Chapter 5), responded to feelings of vulnerability and desires for attachment with a rigid and ruthlessly threatening stance, which almost inevitably triggered retaliation by others. In the subsequent chapters, I examine the developmental trajectories that lead to specific patterns of maladjustment in the cluster of the dramatic or severe personality disorders.

Undoubtedly, as Shapiro (1990) cautions, only rigorous research can establish the validity of the construct of "personality disorder" in children and adolescents. Today there is relatively scant empirical evidence documenting the clinical and developmental continuities between children labeled as antisocial, narcissistic, borderline, or histrionic, and adults with similar diagnoses. Furthermore, the high prevalence observed in these children of Axis I diagnoses, such as attention-deficit/hyperactivity disorder, developmental reading disorder, eating disorder, somatoform disorder, substance abuse, separation anxiety, mood disorder, and posttraumatic stress disorder, raises the question of whether "dramatic personality disorders" are really atypical, complicated, or severe forms of Axis I diagnoses. In particular, a history of maltreatment—most significantly physical and sexual abuse—in the backgrounds of many of these children prompted some authors (e.g., Herman, 1992a, 1992b; Herman, Perry, & van der Kolk, 1989) to state that terms such as "borderline" are little more than pejorative designations for people suffering a complex posttraumatic condition as a consequence of protracted abuse and victimization.

ANTISOCIAL, NARCISSISTIC, HISTRIONIC, AND BORDERLINE PERSONALITY DISORDERS IN CHILDHOOD AND ADOLESCENCE

Children appear unfazed by the arguments denying them the capability of creating enduring patterns of maladjustment. Clinicians' awareness that personality disorders do not appear suddenly at age 18 has led to widespread use of the diagnosis of personality disorder—particularly borderline personality disorder—to characterize the difficulties of some children and adolescents. Thus, by 1983, Pine reported that the flow of children given the diagnosis of borderline had reached flood proportions. Eighteen years later, the "flood" has not receded, yet the concept of dramatic personality disorders in childhood and adolescence remains mired in unclarity and controversy.

The effort to make sense of these children's clinical and developmental problems can be traced at least to the late 1940s and early 1950s, when clinicians such as Mahler, Ross, and Defries (1949) and Weil (1954) identified a group of "atypical" children whose disturbance in ego functions and object relations was less severe than that presented by psychotic children, yet more serious than that displayed by neurotic children. Mahler and her colleagues placed these children at the mild end of a clinical and developmental continuum that extends to the most severe and primitive psychotic conditions—the autistic and symbiotic psychoses of childhood. Thus, Mahler and colleagues (1949) articulated the notion of "benign" or "borderline" psychosis, a precursor to the idea of a schizophrenic spectrum in which borderline conditions would represent an attenuated, incipient, or less severe variant.

Ekstein and Wallerstein (1954) proposed the term "borderline" to designate children who were *not* on the way to becoming psychotic but who, instead, presented a "characteristic pattern of unpredictability which is paradoxically one of [their] most predictable aspects" (p. 345), constantly fluctuating between a neurotic and a psychotic level of contact with reality, object relations, and defensive organization. Ekstein and Wallerstein thus advanced the concept of borderline children as a stable clinical entity defined precisely by ongoing and very rapid shifts in ego functioning.

These pioneer efforts generated a great deal of interest, particularly among psychoanalytically oriented clinicians, leading to a number of attempts to delineate more systematically the developmental and clinical features characteristic of borderline children. Frijling-Schreuder (1969), Geleerd (1958), Marcus (1963), and Rosenfeld and Sprince (1963), among others, described children who presented a wide and fluctuating constellation of problems, including impulsivity; low frustration tolerance; uneven development; proneness to withdraw into fantasy or to regress into primary process in response to stress, lack of structure, or separation from caretakers; pervasive, intense anxiety; multiple neurotic symptoms, such as phobias, compulsions, or ritualistic behaviors; somatic complaints; and sleep problems.

After reviewing the literature, Bemporad, Smith, Hanson, and Cicchetti (1982) and Vela, Gottlieb, and Gottlieb (1983) reported substantial consensus among clinicians on the diagnostic criteria for borderline children. Bemporad and colleagues (1982) spelled out the following diagnostic criteria: (1) a paradigmatic fluctuation of functioning, with rapid shifts between psychotic-like and neurotic levels of reality testing; (2) a lack of "signal anxiety" (Freud, 1926/1959) and a proneness to states of panic, dominated by concerns of body dissolution, annihilation, or abandonment; (3) a disruption in thought processes and content consisting of rapid shifts between normal and loose, idiosyncratic thinking; (4) an impairment in relationships, with much difficulty, when under stress, in distinguishing self from others, in appreciating other people's needs, or in integrating disparate emotional experiences into a coherent relationship; and (5) a lack of impulse control, comprising an inability to contain intense affects, delay gratification, control rage, or modulate destructive and self-destructive tendencies. Along similar lines, Vela and colleagues (1983) described six features: (1) disturbances in interpersonal relationships; (2) disturbances in the sense of reality; (3) excessive anxiety; (4) severe impulse problems; (5) "neurotic-like" symptoms; and (6) uneven or distorted development.

These clinical criteria closely parallel the adult criteria for borderline personality disorder, as defined in the successive editions of the *Diagnostic and Statistical Manual of Mental Disorders* (American Psychiatric Association, 1980, 1987, 1994). The DSM classifications, striving for an empirically based, atheoretical system, shied away from Kernberg's (1975, 1976) notion of a developmental level of personality organization. Instead, borderline, designated as one of the specific personality disorders—the borderline personality disorder—is one of the Cluster B, or "dramatic," personalities, a group that also includes the histrionic, the antisocial, and the narcissistic personality disorders.

Such differentiation has led to greater diagnostic specificity with borderline children. Petti and Vela (1990) identified the confusion in the literature between children with borderline personality/borderline spectrum disorders and children who, while often referred to as "borderline," are more appropriately described as falling within the schizotypal personality/schizoid spectrum disorders. Both groups of youngsters present transient psychotic episodes, magical thinking, idiosyncratic fantasies, suspiciousness, and a disturbed sense of reality. Yet only schizotypal children have a family history of schizophrenia spectrum disorder or present constricted or inappropriate affect, oddness of speech, and extreme discomfort in social situations, which contrasts with the intense, dramatic affect and hunger for social response of borderline, histrionic, and narcissistic youngsters. Petti and Vela's conclusions are supported by the findings of genetic, epidemiological, and follow-up studies of adult borderline personality disorder that differentiate the borderline spectrum from the schizophrenic–schizotypal spectrum.

Studies such as Petti and Vela's paved the way for more systematic efforts to test empirically the validity and reliability of the borderline personality disorder construct in childhood and adolescence. Although the results of such investigations are far from definitive, several studies (e.g., Goldman, D'Angelo, & Demaso, 1993; Ludolph et al., 1990) conclude that semistructured interviews, such as the Diagnostic Interview for Borderlines (DIB; Gunderson, Kolb, & Austin, 1981), and DSM-III-R criteria (American Psychiatric Association, 1987) can be applied to borderline youngsters. Based on this research, Goldman and colleagues (1993) propose that, with very slight modification, DSM-III-R adult criteria can be applied to youngsters with borderline personality disorder.

In contrast, however, to the lively literature on borderline personality in childhood, there has been a striking paucity of discussion of the other dramatic personality disorders—histrionic, narcissistic, and antisocial—as they develop and crystallize during childhood and adolescence. The relative absence of debate is all the more remarkable considering the interest in the psychiatric and psychoanalytic literature on these disorders, particularly on the narcissistic personality disorder. Such interest, of course, reflects the prominence of narcissistic features in contemporary life and the frequency with which the complaints heard in clinical practice bear the hallmark of narcissistic disorders: pervasive feelings of unhappiness, inner emptiness, and boredom; dependence on external approval and admiration; fears of closeness and intimacy; exploitativeness and manipulation in interpersonal relationships; intense fears of death and aging; and inability to experience love or meaning in life.

But only a few authors have examined narcissistic traits and narcissistic disorders as they emerge in children (Beren, 1992; Bleiberg, 1984, 1988, 1994; Cohen, 1991; Egan & Kernberg, 1984; Kernberg, 1989; Ornstein, 1981; Rinsley, 1984, 1989), building on models to explain narcissistic psychopathology (i.e., Kernberg, 1975, 1976; Kohut, 1971, 1972, 1977) and focusing on distortions or arrests in early development. Yet support for these models comes largely from the retrospective accounts collected in the treatment of adult patients.

From a different perspective, an extensive literature has examined delinquent youth. A tremendous catalyst to explore the development of delinquents was August Aichhorn's (1935) bold proposal to apply psychoanalytic principles to create a human relationship as a vehicle for understanding and caring for "wayward," hateful, impulsive youngsters and for helping them resume their thwarted development.

Rutter and Giller (1983) and Rutter, Giller, and Hagel (1998), attempting to make sense of the various combinations of biological and psychosocial vulnerabilities displayed by delinquent youngsters, concluded that the most meaningful dimension determining outcome is the children's capacity to form enduring affectionate bonds and to experience concern for others. Almost in passing, Rutter and Giller wondered whether the truly significant differentiation is between *degrees or types of personality disturbance.*

This line of thinking is supported by the factor-analytic studies of delinquent youth carried out by Marohn, Offer, Ostrov, and Truillo (1979), which revealed four psychological subtypes: (1) the impulsive, (2) the narcissistic, (3) the empty-borderline, and (4) the depressed-borderline. Each of these types of delinquency encompasses specific but overlapping maladaptive patterns of experiencing, coping, and relating, whose features seem strikingly similar to the personality disorders in the dramatic cluster. These dramatic personality disorders represent overlapping developmental paths, leading to a cluster of enduring patterns of maladjustment that reflect various combinations of constitutional vulnerability and psychosocial misfortune.

CLINICAL PRESENTATION OF CHILDREN
WITH DRAMATIC PERSONALITY DISORDER

"Dramatic" children indeed create drama and stir up turmoil around them, but they vary greatly in their adjustment and behavior at any given moment. Specific triggers—changes in children's subjective experience linked to interpersonal or internal cues—bring about prototypical modes of rigidly organizing their subjective experience, coping mechanisms, and relationship patterns.

By school age, most children with a dramatic personality disorder meet diagnostic criteria for one or more Axis I diagnoses, more commonly a disruptive behavior disorder, an anxiety disorder, or a mood disorder. I propose that the two modal types within this cluster are the narcissistic and the borderline. Some narcissistic youngsters present a more malignant ruthlessness linked to the antisocial disorders, while others are more dramatic in their communication, impressionistic in their cognitive style, and hungry for attention, shading into the histrionic personality. Some children—predominantly those who are narcissistic or narcissistic–histrionic—are cool and canny far beyond their age. They appear well controlled and capable, and they impress people with their remarkable strength, charm, and charisma, their ability to place themselves at the center of everyone's attention, and their shrewd awareness of how to elicit specific responses from the environment. Other narcissistic or narcissistic–antisocial youngsters can be relentlessly destructive, defiant, and apparently lacking in remorse, concern, or constraints.

THE PROTOTYPE OF THE NARCISSISTIC
PERSONALITY DISORDER

The prototypical response of narcissistic children—whether "malignant" or histrionic—to threats of vulnerability, humiliation, or lack of attention is first to organize their sense of self around an illusory conviction of perfection, power, or control. Arguably, the developmental antecedent of this response is the dismissive/avoidant attachment pattern, which, as I discuss later, is a coping strategy against attachment disorganization.

These children disown those aspects of themselves that fail to measure up to such standards of perfection or simply to their expectation to be "cool," "tough," and self-sufficient. In particular, they reject experiences of helplessness, vulnerability, pain, dependency, and—for narcissistic–histrionic children—the dreaded experience of being ignored. Subsequently, they project these unbearable aspects of the self onto others, who they then perceive as helpless, worthless, or insignificant, mere tools to manipulate or props to help them achieve acclaim, power, or satisfaction. At the same time, they require from others an ongoing confirmation of their perfection, magnificence, and power. Yet no matter how much adulation or confirmation, or how much success they achieve, they are haunted by the possibility that their shortcomings will be exposed. Shame and the fear of ridicule and humiliation loom as ever-present threats throughout their lives. For example, Elliot, a 10-year-old boy whom I describe in more detail in Chapter 6, shared, with just a hint of condescension, his plans to become a Nobel Prize–winning nuclear physicist, the best neurosurgeon in the world, and a future President of the United States. Yet when I—mistakenly—inquired about his feelings of uncertainty or bafflement, the very feelings that may underlie the behavior that brought him to treatment, he became anxious, provocative, and even more determined to make me feel stupid and helpless.

As Egan and Kernberg (1984) pointed out, narcissistic youngsters contrast with normal children, who "do not need to be unusually admired as sole owners of everything enviable and valuable" (p. 42) and who make demands that are related to real—and realistic—needs. The demands of children with a narcissistic personality are "excessive, can never be fulfilled, and are in fact secondary to an ongoing angry denigration" (p. 42) of those who attempt to care for them. Whereas small children can be warmly grateful, narcissistic youngsters are cool and aloof, and show disregard for others, except for momentary idealization.

The hallmarks of the prototypical narcissistic personality in childhood are grandiose fantasies, excessive demands, intense self-absorption, grandiosity that defensively reverses overwhelming feelings of inadequacy and helplessness, and inability to experience genuine attachment, trust, and interest in others.

THE PROTOTYPE OF THE
BORDERLINE PERSONALITY DISORDER

As infants, borderline children often burden their caregivers with their high activity level, poor adaptability, negative mood, and problems settling into predictable sleep–wake and feeding patterns. They are, in short, temperamentally "difficult" babies. *Some* of these children, as I discuss later, will form attachment bonds that foster the selective inhibition of reflective function, a developmental feature that appears to be signaled by the presence of a disorganized pattern of attachment (Main & Solomon, 1990). Infants with a disorganized attachment respond to the presence of their caregivers with a chaotic mix of approach–avoidance and "trance-like" behaviors. Clinginess, vulnerability to separations or hyperactivity, and proneness to tantrums are also common features of their early development.

Many of these youngsters appear hyperactive, moody, irritable, and explosive. Minor upsets or frustrations trigger intense affective storms, episodes of uncontrolled emotion that are wholly out of proportion to the apparent precipitant. Other youngsters are anxious, hypersensitive to the comings and goings of their caregivers, impossible to comfort after separations, and demanding of constant attention and reassurance against abandonment. One moment they may feel elated and expansive, blissfully connected with a protective caregiver. But the next moment they plunge into bitter disappointment and rage, coupled with self-loathing and despair.

As with narcissistic youngsters, self-centeredness is a striking characteristic of these children, who also crave attention and respond with rage or despair to rejection or indifference. But in prototypical borderline youngsters, such events trigger profound feelings of subjective dyscontrol, hyperarousal, loneliness, and a fragmented sense of self and others. These feelings bring about rigid patterns of coping, experiencing, and relating. As a result, borderline children seductively strive to coerce others into providing them with emotional "supplies" because they are unable, under specific stressors, to evoke images of other people as soothing and comforting. Instead, they find themselves swept away by the feelings and needs of the moment, and they experience utter chaos, both in their inner world and in the world around them.

By adolescence, they often find that they can modulate their vulnerability to hyperarousal and subjective dyscontrol by deliberately seeking thrills, by desperately attempting to numb themselves, by actively pursuing self-victimization, and by manipulatively striving to prevent abandonment. Food binges, promiscuous sex, or drug abuse become key strategies to achieve these aims. Self-mutilation and suicidal gestures are more common among girls, whereas aggression covering hidden fears of vulnerability is more typical of boys. Unstable relationships with peers and adults become more prominent as transient idealization and clingy overdependence alternate with rage, devaluation, and feelings of abandonment and betrayal. Although they can derive some feelings of nurturance from food, drugs, or sex, they are soon left with only shame, guilt, and a sense of inner deadness.

INTEGRATING POINTS OF VIEW: THE PERSPECTIVE OF DEVELOPMENTAL PSYCHOPATHOLOGY

Faced with the bewildering challenges posed by children with dramatic or severe personality disorders, clinicians have searched through a variety of theoretical roadmaps for signposts to guide their interventions. In this book, I seek to demonstrate that in the development of children with severe personality disorders, specific genetic vulnerabilities find expression in the context of attachment relationships that predispose children to inhibit selectively a key processing mechanism, that of reflective function. This perspective is embedded in the contemporary framework of developmental psychopathology. That framework is built on the assumption that the relationship environment equips children with psychological mechanisms of appraisal and processing, in turn regulating gene expression and having an impact on the environment (Elman et al., 1996; Emde, 1989; Fonagy, 2000a; Rutter, 1999). The central point of these perspectives is that developmental outcomes are generated by the action of psychological, mediating functions that determine whether specific environmental factors, such as trauma, trigger the expression of genetic vulnerabilities.

This perspective is based on multiple contributions from various viewpoints. The early efforts to make sense of these children were rooted in the soil of psychoanalytic theory, including Aichhorn's previously mentioned efforts to understand and treat young delinquents. Aichhorn's ideas were based on the underlying premises of psychoanalytic theory: an appreciation of the power and significance of unconscious motivation, and a belief in the centrality of early development and early relationships in shaping psychic experience.

By the early 1950s, Aichhorn's seminal work had inspired a number of important contributions to the psychoanalytic understanding of delinquency. Redl and Wineman (1951, 1957) described the failure of ego controls underlying the difficulties of "children who hate." Johnson and Szurek (1952) examined adolescents' enactments of their parents' unconscious delinquent tendencies. Winnicott (1958) interpreted the antisocial tendency as an effort to test and establish relationships.

Two decades later, Mahler, Pine, and Bergman (1975) and Otto Kernberg (1975) produced a set of key concepts that were to become the fundamental framework for the psychoanalytic understanding of how severe personality disorders are generated.

According to Mahler's concept of *separation–individuation*, during the first 3 years of life, children normally go through a series of developmental stages in which they (1) internalize some of the soothing, equilibrium-maintaining functions initially performed exclusively by caregivers—what Winnicott (1965) called "the holding environment"—and acquire the capacity to carry out these functions with some degree of autonomy; (2) practice ego skills and use them to expand their knowledge of themselves and the world, while figuring out how to evoke desired responses from the environment; and (3) integrate the "good"—pleasurable and safe—and the "bad"—unpleasant and unsafe— representations of the self and others. These achievements subsequently permit children to accept the reality of their existence as separate individuals and to develop object constancy, which is the ability to maintain relationships and evoke loving and comforting images of their caregivers even when absent or when the children are upset with them.

Otto Kernberg (1967, 1975), through his influential contributions, sought to define "borderline" as a level of development in personality organization. The developmental markers of the borderline level of organization, according to Kernberg, are the differentiation of the self-representation from the representation of the object—which he believes is the basis of the capacity for reality testing—but without integration of the "good" and the "bad" aspects of the self and the object. For Kernberg, the crux of the borderline personality is the ongoing defensive need to retain an internal split between two sets of self–object units: a "good" self-representation linked to a "good" object-representation by

libidinal affects of pleasure, safety, and satisfaction on the one hand, and a "bad" self-representation linked to a "bad" object-representation by affects of tension, distress, pain, anger, and frustration on the other.

According to Kernberg, the defensive need for splitting derives from the burden of excessive aggression that children carry as a result of either genetic loading or inordinate frustration. Heightened aggression, in turn leading to a predominance of "bad" introjects, fosters the defensive need to protect the "good" sense about the self and the object from the unremitting attacks from the bad introject. Splitting, however, precludes a real integration of the self- and the object-representation, and thus interferes with the achievement of both cohesive identity and object constancy.

For Kernberg, a number of personality disorders, including the narcissistic, the schizoid, the paranoid, and the antisocial, generally function at this borderline level of personality organization. This broad use of the term "borderline" resonated with clinicians working with children. Pine (1974), for example, defined the "borderline" condition of children and adolescents as a group of disorders with common developmental and structural features, although substantially different clinical manifestations.

Psychoanalytic clinicians seeking to understand the developmental and clinical problems of youngsters with dramatic and severe personality disorders conceptualized these problems in terms of splitting and the derailment of Mahler's separation–individuation. The psychoanalytic literature soon came to ascribe such developmental problems to parental—particularly maternal—failure. Adler (1985), for example, postulated that the central feature of borderline psychopathology is the patient's inability to evoke the memory of a soothing, comforting object when faced with separation or distress. He attributed this defect of internalization to a parental failure in providing an adequate "holding environment." The consequence of such failure for the child is an inner state of emptiness, reliance on angry, manipulative efforts to secure involvement and attention from others, and use of drugs or food to soothe and comfort. This dependence on external supplies is similar to the reliance of young children on transitional objects and experiences described by Winnicott (1953).

Along similar lines, Masterson (1981), Masterson and Rinsley (1975), and Rinsley (1980a, 1984, 1989) claimed that specific patterns of mother–infant interaction thwart the separation–individuation process and lead to borderline or narcissistic psychopathology. In their view, the mothers of future borderline individuals take pride in, and find gratification in, their children's dependency. These mothers, claim Rinsley and Masterson, reward children's passive–dependent, clinging behavior while withdrawing or otherwise punishing them when they strive for autonomy. These mothers are sensitively attuned to and exquisitely responsive to their children's pain, helplessness, and proximity-seeking behavior, but they subtly or overtly rebuff their children when they exhibit activity, mastery, or independence. According to these authors, the central message that mothers of future borderline individuals communicate to their children is, as Rinsley (1984) said, that to grow up is to face "the loss or withdrawal of maternal supplies, coupled with the related injunction that to avoid that calamity the child must remain dependent, inadequate, symbiotic" (p. 5).

Future *narcissistic* individuals, according to Rinsley (1984), receive a different message. Their mothers communicate to them that they are loved and cherished, maybe more than anyone is or ever has been, *because* they are special people. It is as if they are told: "I love you, but to keep my love, you *must* grow up and be wonderful, so that everything you accomplish is a reflection of me, your mother." This selectivity of maternal attunement and response is not, as in the case of mothers of borderline individuals, to the child's deflated and pained states, but to the child's competent, attention-getting aspects that best enhance the mother's self-esteem and prevent her narcissistic collapse.

This focus on maternal responsibility in conceptualizing the development of both borderline and narcissistic personality disorders, however, served mostly to expose the limitations of prevailing psychoanalytic formulations. The emphasis on the mother's failure ignored the growing evidence about the critical role of maltreatment—particularly sexual abuse—often perpetrated by fathers and other caregivers in the pathogenesis of severe personality disorders.

As Gabbard (1994) points out, psychoanalytic formulations overemphasize *early* development, notably the separation–individuation process, at the expense of other sensitive developmental stages—times when critical events such as sexual abuse may occur. But perhaps more significantly, these formulations focus largely on only *one* developmental stage and assume an *arrest* in development at that stage. Last, but certainly not least, psychoanalytic formulations—with the exception of those by Kernberg—move away from consideration of the significance of constitutional factors. This neglect made it difficult for these perspectives to explain why *some* children exposed to, for example, dependency-rewarding and autonomy-punishing mothers did *not* grow up to become borderline, while other children, clearly *not* exposed to such an environment, did develop a borderline personality.

A similar wave of criticism turned the early enthusiasm for psychoanalytic models of delinquency into widespread disillusion with the explanatory power of psychoanalysis in general, and with the effectiveness of psychoanalytically oriented approaches to the treatment of delinquent youth in particular.

By the early 1990s, competing theoretical models sought to explain the problems of delinquent youth:

1. Sociocultural models (see, e.g., Cloward & Ohlin, 1960; Wichstrom, Skogen, & Oia, 1996) identified the significance of socioeconomic class; ethnicity; family size; access to social, medical, and psychiatric services; child-rearing and socializing practices; and modes of exposure to alcohol and drugs.

2. Family interaction models (see, e.g., Patterson, 1982; Patterson, DeBaryshe, & Ramsey, 1989) emphasized the importance of parental violence, severe marital discord, and parental inadequacies in providing children with structure, supervision, and emotional involvement.

3. Neurobiological models stressed genetic influences (Brennan, Mednick, & Jacobsen, 1995; Christiansen, 1977), neuropsychiatric vulnerabilities (Lewis, 1983; Lewis, Shanok, & Balla, 1979), attentional deficits (Cantwell, 1981), and depression (Kovacs, Feinberg, Crouse-Novak, Paulauskas, & Finkelstein, 1984a; Kovacs et al., 1984b; Riggs, Baker, Mikulich, Young, & Crowley, 1995).

In a similar fashion, a number of alternative perspectives were proposed to explain the pathogenesis of personality disorders, particularly borderline personality.

A decade earlier, empirical studies had already helped to detach borderline personality disorder from schizophrenia, which, at least in the child arena, was a notion derived from Mahler's "mild or incipient psychosis" model. A shift in focus to the affective lability and dysphoria of borderline patients led to the concept of borderline as an affective disorder spectrum condition. Klein (1977), for example, proposed that a subgroup of borderline patients, whom he referred to as "hysteroid dysphorics," suffer from a problem in affective regulation that gives rise to emotional lability and heightened sensitivity to rejection. According to Klein, manipulative relationships and other maladaptive interpersonal tactics *result from* rather than cause the affective dysregulation. This view gained strength after studies by Stone (1979), Stone, Kahn, and Flye (1981), and Akiskal (1981) found a high prevalence of affective disorders in the relatives of borderline patients and identified features suggestive of borderline personality in the offspring of affectively ill patients.

As evidence mounted, however, that a linkage between affective disorder and borderline personality was neither uniform nor especially strong (Gunderson & Zanarini, 1989), a number of authors proposed instead that borderline personality could best be conceptualized as an impulse spectrum disorder—that is, as a disorder linked to attention-deficit/hyperactivity disorder, substance abuse, episodic dyscontrol, and cognitive processing difficulties, such as developmental reading disorder and other problems sharing a propensity for the immediate discharge of affect in action (e.g., Andrulonis, 1991).

Yet again, prospective studies pointed out that, just like most children with an affective disorder or the psychosocial "vulnerabilities" associated with delinquency (e.g., poverty, parental discord), many, if not most, impulsive children manage to survive childhood without developing severe personality disorder or manifesting serious delinquency problems.

The search for an alternative explanation brought the focus to maltreatment, particularly sexual abuse. A number of studies found a very high incidence of sexual abuse in the background of adolescents and adults with borderline personality (Famularo, Kinscherff, & Fenton, 1991; Goodwin, Cheeves, & Connell, 1990; Herman et al., 1989). Indeed, when clinicians focused on the possibility of sexual abuse, an astonishing number of borderline adolescents were found to be marred by abuse, their lives appearing to be not an empty house devoid of sufficient internalization of parental functions, but rather a haunted house (Zanarini, Gunderson, Marino, Schwartz, & Frankenburg, 1989) filled with the terrifying ghosts of caregiver brutality and boundary violations. In Terr's (1991) view, exposure to repeated traumatization—such as physical and sexual abuse—evokes defensive operations and experiential distortions that lead to severe personality disorders. Still, as a number of studies demonstrate (e.g., Paris & Zweig-Frank, 1992, 1997; Zanarini & Frankenburg, 1997), although sexual abuse seems to be an important factor in the etiology of borderline personality disorder, abuse alone is neither necessary nor sufficient to develop borderline or other severe personality disorders.

The time seems ripe to consider an integrative perspective (Cicchetti & Cohen, 1995), the point of view of developmental psychopathology. This framework considers how the full array of biopsychosocial factors interact with one another to generate both the *protective* and the *risk* factors that shape the direction of adaptive or maladaptive developmental trajectories. From this perspective, all behavior, including maladaptive behavior, is evaluated not simply from the standpoint of what a person does, but also in reference to how behaviors are organized in respect to one another and in reference to context. Likewise, development is not regarded as the *addition* of new capacities but as an unfolding *organization* of capacities. Finally, personality is conceptualized not as a collection of traits but as the organization and structuring of attitudes, values and goals, coping strategies, relationship patterns, modes of feeling and response, and ways of processing experience across contexts (Sroufe, 1989).

In particular, the point of view of developmental psychopathology allows us to investigate the protective mechanisms bestowed by the evolution of the human species to cope with biological vulnerability and environmental misfortune. Examining these children against the background of developmental psychopathology offers the promise of a framework that integrates psychoanalytic, cognitive, social–cultural, family systems, and neurobiological perspectives in a new paradigm that can serve as the basis of better understanding and more effective treatment.

2

Attachment and Reflective Function

In every nursery there are ghosts. There are the visitors from the unremembered past of the parents; the uninvited guests at the christening. . . . The intruders from the parental past may break through the magic circle in an unguarded moment, and a parent and his child may find themselves enacting a moment or a scene from another time with another set of characters.
—FRAIBERG, ADELSON, AND SHAPIRO (1975, p. 387)

GHOSTS IN THE NURSERY
AND ATTACHMENT PATTERNS

In their classic 1975 paper, "Ghosts in the Nursery," Fraiberg, Adelson, and Shapiro evocatively describe how some people's lives are haunted by the "ghosts" of brutality and insensitivity they encountered in their childhood. These ghosts intrude at "unguarded moments," after these children grow up and become parents themselves, compelling them to reenact abusive interactions, with their own children in the role of the victim.

Yet perhaps the most important question raised by Fraiberg and colleagues concerns resilience. How is it that some people exposed to similar abuse, or to other types of early misfortune or disadvantage, manage not only to contain the "ghosts" and protect themselves from severe maladjustment but also to protect their children from the transgenerational transmission of the misery that marred their own early life? This capacity has long baffled investigators seeking a clearer understanding of the development of the severe personality disorders.

Researchers have identified a host of factors that allow children to develop and adapt successfully in circumstances often associated with maladjustment and dysfunction (Fonagy, Steele, Steele, Higgitt, & Target, 1994; Rutter, 1987, 1999; Werner & Smith, 1982). These protective factors include not only individual qualities such as high intelligence (Masten & Garmezy, 1985; Masten et al., 1988; Rutter, 1987) and easy temperament (Rutter, 1985; Smith & Prior, 1995) but also features in the children's social environment and developmental context such as parental warmth (Smith & Prior, 1995), caregivers' emotional responsiveness and competence (Wyman et al., 1999), perceived social support in childhood (Anan & Barnett, 1999), positive educational experience (Rutter & Quinton, 1984), and family involvement in organized religious activity (Baldwin, Baldwin, & Cole, 1990; Comer, 1988; Ianni, 1989). Last, but certainly not least, researchers have identified factors that arise *in the interactions* of children and their caregiving environment, particularly attachment security (Booth, Rubin, & Rose-Kransnor, 1998; Elicker, Englund, & Sroufe, 1992) and maternal reflective function (Fonagy & Target, 1997).

Understanding these protective mechanisms is crucial because the mental health field is pushed by both socioeconomic pressures and scientific and clinical developments to embrace *prevention*. In particular, clinicians are asked to "do something" about those patterns of behavior that give rise to the greatest societal distress and consumption of resources (i.e., violence, self-destructiveness, drug abuse, illegitimate births, and child maltreatment) that are characteristic of problems faced by those with severe personality disorders.

These protective factors leading to resilience are unlikely to exist in isolation. As Stein, Fonagy, Ferguson, and Wisman (2000) suggest, resilience is best regarded as a dynamic interactive process that unfolds over time. Quoting Sroufe (1997), Stein argues that, from a developmental perspective, resilience is not something some children have in abundance while others have little. Instead, it is a capacity that evolves over time, within the total context of biological and environmental influences affecting children's development. As Sroufe points out, "The capacities for staying organized in the face of challenge, for active coping and for maintaining positive expectations during periods of stress are evolved by the person in interactions with the environment across successive periods of adaptation" (p. 256). This capacity for resilience does not remain static but is continuously influenced by changes in the context.

These contextual changes are not simply the result of adding protective factors and then subtracting the accumulation of adversities and risk factors. Instead, Stein and colleagues (2000) argue, it is individuals' capacity to construct their experience of themselves and their environment that directs them toward various developmental pathways and outcomes.

Fonagy (2000a) states these ideas more boldly: Evidence now indicates that individuals' capacity to appraise themselves and the environment is not only a *consequence* of genetic predisposition and environmental factors but also a central factor in shaping the environment and triggering gene expression. It is the significance of these mechanisms of appraisal, representation, and construction of meaning that explains the poor correlation between childhood experience and adult functioning (Kagan & Zentner, 1996). What matters most appears to be not what happens to children but how they can appraise and construct what happens to them (Elman et al., 1996). In the next two chapters, I discuss some of the evidence from human and primate research supporting this hypothesis.

But before venturing into the task of finding support for this premise, I should first present the key implication of this proposal: that the crucial protection humans have evolved against vulnerability and adversity is generated in the context of attachment bonds. This "protection" consists of the capacity, as articulated by Fonagy (2000a), to develop a mind that can interpret the world in human, meaningful terms. Through this capacity, children acquire the ability to represent themselves and other people in terms of understandable intentional attributes that permit social reciprocity. Severe personality disorders in children and adolescents result from distortions or dysfunction in these appraisal and representational capacities that render youngsters unable to preserve a psychologically grounded sense of self and others in the context of close human connections.

A starting point of this conceptualization of severe personality disorders is the concept of attachment and the primacy of social experience in triggering gene expression and developmental outcomes. Over the past three decades, a growing body of research (Bowlby, 1969, 1973, 1980; Bretherton, 1991; Carlson & Sroufe, 1995; Sroufe, 1990, 1996;

Stern, 1985, 1995) has indeed begun to document how the crucial protective mechanisms that humans have evolved against trauma and vulnerability develop in the context of the attachment system.

Infancy research amply validates Fairbairn's (1952/1954) seminal notion about the primacy of the human craving for sustaining connections. Both observation and research document a powerful tendency in the human species, from the beginning of life, to seek out and elicit engagement with others because of a built-in motivation for "social fittedness" (Emde, 1989). As Stern (1985) noted, neonates are preprogrammed to recognize people, to prefer human stimulation above all other, and to develop the behavioral repertoire of attachment. Disruption of an infant's attachment produces distress that escalates to overwhelming anxiety and organismic vulnerability (Bowlby, 1969, 1973; Spitz, 1945; Spitz & Wolf, 1946). Moreover, the very maturation and capacity of the brain to perform its basic modulating and regulatory functions are contingent on the *ongoing* presence of a human, interactive environment (Kandel, 1983, 1998). As Perry and Pollard (1998) noted, the evolutionary process has shaped and "designed" the human brain to be organized by social experience.

The specific ways that the human brain is organized by social experience are becoming increasingly clear. Obviously, at birth and throughout infancy, human beings are not capable of regulating their arousal and emotional reactions, of gratifying their psychological needs, of soothing and comforting themselves, or of maintaining psychophysiological homeostasis. A regulatory system develops only when caregivers grasp and respond to infants' signals of moment-to-moment changes in their subjective experience and psychophysiological state.

Early psychoanalytic thinking about development assumed that normal newborns existed in a state of perceptual and cognitive undifferentiation—unable to differentiate what is me and what is not me—and were generally uninvested in the environment from which they were thought to be shielded by an inborn "contact barrier" (Freud, 1950/1966) or an "autistic shell" (Mahler et al., 1975). This shell was seen as a quasi-physical barrier shielding the newborn from the outside world.

Contemporary infancy research paints a radically different picture. As Colombo, Mitchell, Coldren, and Atwater (1990) have pointed out, not only are there no empirical data to support the view of infants as uninvested and unresponsive to outside stimulation, but also there is actually a significant body of evidence to demonstrate that learning on the basis of external stimulation occurs from the beginning of life. Evidence points to a very strong innate bias in infants to seek out and recognize social stimulation and contingencies associated with such responses, that is, to grasp the cause-and-effect connection between their behavior and environmental–social events (Murray & Trevarthen, 1985; Neisser, 1991; Watson, 1972, 1979, 1985, 1994, 1995).

A growing body of research documents that 3-month-olds can differentiate between *perfect* contingencies—such as a live video image of themselves—and imperfect contingencies—such as a delayed video image (Bahrick & Watson, 1985; Rochat, 1995; Schmuckler, 1996).

Meltzoff and Moore (1977, 1983, 1989, 1994) provide evidence that, from the beginning of life, infants are aware of the match—or mismatch—between their behavior and that of others. Meltzoff (1990) has demonstrated that the greater the degree of match in the adult partners' actions, the more interested and attentive infants are in the interaction. This ability to differentiate between perfect and imperfect contingencies is acquired early and may be one of the mechanisms available to infants to distinguish self from others (Watson, 1994). Watson argues that the initial "target" of the infants' innate disposition toward contingency— which he calls the "contingency detection device"—is to seek out *perfect* response–stimulus contingencies in order to identify the range of self-generated stimuli. This "device," claims Watson, allows for the construction of the primary representation of the body self.

At about 3 months of age, however, a significant change is noted in the infant's search for contingencies. The preferential target of contingency seeking switches from *perfect* to *high but imperfect* response–stimulus contingencies. This change points to a crucial shift in infants' orientation as they now more easily recognize, prefer, and seek out social responses that *reflect* their own behavior closely but not perfectly. Not surprisingly, caregivers' responses associated with this shift are predominantly *modified* facial imitations, responsive vocalizations, and other actions that reflect back to infants the adults' grasp of infants' categorical affect, intensity, rhythm, tempo, and other aspects of the "architecture" of infants' internal state.

Caregivers' contingent responses to their infants are, of course, by necessity, imperfect. As Gergely and Watson (1999) point out, no matter how well attuned caregivers are to the baby's internal state, their facial and vocal responses will never match perfectly the temporal, spatial, and sensory parameters—the architecture—of the infant's state.

Caregivers "select" certain aspects of the infant's responses, such as the gestures and expressions they perceive as most vigorous (Trevarthen, 1979), and also show significant individual differences in the aspects of their infant's response to which they can respond with more or less vigor and accuracy. Some caregivers, for example, respond with great sensitivity to the infant's elated affect, while others show greater effectiveness in responding to subdued or distressed affect (Stern, Hofer, Haft, & Dore, 1985).

Gergely and Watson (1999) used this body of research to propose that contingency-detection mechanisms moderate key developmental acquisitions, such as self–other differentiation and the orientation toward the social environment. The innate dispositions to recognize, prefer, and seek out human stimulation and high but imperfect contingencies join hands to moderate the acquisition of additional, critical developmental achievements: the capacity for emotional self-regulation and the sense of the self as an active, causal, self-regulating agent; and the achievement of awareness of one's own internal states and understanding of one's self and others as intentional beings whose behavior is determined by psychological states.

This developmental sequence can be summarized as follows: Infants' emotions are initially a prewired, stimulus-driven, automatized process of psychophysiological activation embedded in procedures. Such automations are inflexible and operate outside of infants' conscious awareness.

Caregivers, however, repeatedly respond to infants' states, for example, states of distress and dysregulation, with reflective displays of attuned affect and behaviors designed to soothe, comfort, and restore infants' homeostasis. Such responses, in turn, reduce infants' distress and restore a state of regulation.

Infants can register the high degree of contingency between their emotional expression and the caregiver's affectively attuned reflective displays. These registrations arguably bring about a sense of causal efficacy in controlling and *producing* the caregiver's reflective behavior that in turn reduces distress. It thus can be hypothesized (Gergely & Watson, 1999) that repeated, successful, emotion-regulating, distress-reducing interactions involving infants' expressions of distress and caregivers' responses with affectively attuned, reflective, and regulating behavior will provide the experiential basis for the sense of self as a self-regulating agent. The previously inchoate, automatized process becomes to infants a signal capable of producing both a social response and a change in internal state.

Furthermore, the repeated presentation of an *external* reflection of the internal state—the caregiver's attuned affective response—serves to sensitize infants to the recognition of their own internal states. Gergely and Watson (1996, 1999) refer to this process as a form of social bio-feedback training. Caregivers who can "read" accurately their babies' internal states provide attuned responses that infants can correlate with their internal state. By being provided a less than perfect match of its internal state, the infant's perception of the caregivers becomes a secondary representation of the internal experience—the same, and yet not the same. This type of processing opens the path to the development of explicit symbolic processing that, as I discuss in Chapter 3, is flexible and accessible to conscious awareness and can be governed by higher-level cognitive functions to override automatisms.

Gergely (1995), Stern (1985), and Stern and colleagues (1985), among others, have investigated how caregivers direct the infant's attention to internal states rather than to overt behavior. Stern notes that caregivers typically reflect some aspects of the architecture of the infant's behavior using a different modality. For example, Stern and colleagues describe a baby reaching for a toy just beyond his reach. As the baby stretches his body in an obvious effort to reach the toy, the mother says, "Uuuuuh . . . uuuuuh!" with a crescendo of vocal effort, accelerated breathing, and a lift of the shoulders that matches the architecture of the infant's physical effort.

Gergely points out that caregivers *"mark"* their affect as reflective behaviors to make them distinguishable from the expression of their *own* internal state. This marking is typically achieved by producing an exaggerated version of the emotional expression, similar to the "as if" marking of affective displays in pretend play.

The effect of the partial matching and the "marking" on the part of caregivers may be to help infants decouple the automatic process of psychophysiological activation from a *mental representation* of such experience. Such decoupling will eventually permit youngsters to move away from automatic, procedural expression to a flexible, reflective–symbolic mode of functioning.

This developmental framework is obviously rooted in Bowlby's (1969, 1973, 1980) attachment theory. Bowlby's conceptual model postulates that the evolution of the human species has resulted in an inherent bias to generate, organize, and pattern psychological experience resulting from interactions in an interpersonal context. Bowlby (1973) designated as *internal working models* the psychological processes that infants utilize to encode and retrieve memories of experiences of interpersonal interaction, and the expectations generated by those same interactions.

Bowlby's (1969, 1973, 1980) attachment theory postulates a biological preparedness in the human infant to seek proximity, to signal distress, and to enter into reciprocal relationships with caregivers who are disposed to understand, give meaning to, and respond to the infant's signals by holding, caressing, comforting, smiling, feeding, and so forth. The outcome of these interactions, as described earlier, is that infants subjectively experience security, restored equilibrium, and satisfaction. These interactions create the memories that infants synthesize in internal working models.

Internal working models—and the expectations from them—can be observed in the "Strange Situation," an experimental procedure designed by Mary Ainsworth and her collaborators (Ainsworth, Bell, & Stayton, 1971; Ainsworth, Blehar, Waters, & Wall, 1978). In this situation, infants are briefly separated from, then reunited with, their caregivers while in an unfamiliar environment. The infants' responses to the Strange Situation can be classified by one of four attachment patterns: (1) secure, (2) anxious/avoidant, (3) anxious/resistant, or (4) disorganized/disoriented.

Infants classified as *secure* will readily explore the unfamiliar environment in the presence of the caregiver. During the caregiver's absence, however, they become distressed and anxious in the presence of the stranger. The return of the caregiver quickly reassures them, and they promptly resume active exploration.

Anxious/avoidant infants show little distress at being separated from their caregiver. But on reunion, they may avoid the caregiver's efforts to attract their attention or reestablish contact.

In contrast, *anxious/resistant* infants appear preoccupied with the caregiver's whereabouts even while the caregiver is present, which limits their exploratory activity. These infants are enormously distressed by separation and cannot settle down even after the caregiver returns, continuing instead to cling, cry, and fuss.

Finally, the *disorganized/disoriented* infants (Main & Solomon, 1986, 1990) appear difficult to classify because they show disorganization or disorientation in the very presence of the caregiver. Their behavior comprises a mix of approach, avoidance, and "trance-like" activity.

ATTACHMENT AND DEPRIVATION
IN HUMAN AND NONHUMAN PRIMATES

The Strange Situation offers a controlled environment where the infant's response to separation can be observed systematically. These observations substantiate the views of Spitz (1945) and Bowlby (1969) about the distress and dysregulation experienced by infants on being separated from their caregivers. Bowlby's (1951, 1969) pioneering studies demonstrated that, following such separation, human infants go through a period of agitation, increased arousal, and automatic activation—the stage of *protest*—that includes behaviors that serve to draw the caregivers to the children. This phase involves an activation of the hypothalamic–pituitary–adrenocortical axis, as evidenced by sharp increases in plasma cortisol and corticotropin (ACTH) levels, and by increased turnover of the noradrenergic system, as measured by decreased cerebrospinal fluid levels of norepinephrine (NE) and an elevated heart rate, pointing to sympathetic arousal.

This arousal stage is followed after several hours or days by a stage that Bowlby referred to as *despair*, during which motoric and emotional expression are restricted, rapid eye movement (REM) sleep is decreased, overall sleep is disrupted, and autonomic measures fall below normal baseline (Hollenbeck et al., 1980). But while the behavioral and physiological components of the protest–despair response sequence appear fairly consistently in normal infants, there are dramatic, constitutionally based individual differences in the intensity and duration of the resulting distress. Some children, particularly vulnerable to separations, experience extreme distress and much greater intensity of physiological responses than the average infant. Instead of being comforted by the reappearance of their caregivers, they continue to display profound autonomic and behavioral reactions even after reunion. These children tend to be inhibited; they fear change and avoid the unfamiliar. In well-controlled studies, they present much greater autonomic and hormonal reactivity to change, stress, or separation than do matched controls (Kagan, 1994).

But aside from such extremes, a proneness to become distressed on separation appears "prewired" into the normal human brain. Kandel (1983) has pointed out the likely innate neurobiological readiness to trigger or downplay a fight-or-flight sequence of hyperarousal, anxiety, and anger in response to the respective absence or reappearance of caregivers. Other humans, says Kandel, evoke a built-in, ready-to-be-activated signal of safety. A basic root of anxiety and a basic prototype of trauma thus appear to be the biologically "programmed" tendency to respond to separations with anxiety and to reunions with relief.

Human infants, of course, are not unique in experiencing distress on separation from their caregivers. Other, nonhuman primate infants exhibit similar distress and give a specific cry to evoke their caregiver's protection and proximity. This "cry of separation" in all primates powerfully summons parental involvement via a response that involves autonomic and limbic–hypothalamic activation (Panksepp, Meeker, & Bean, 1980).

Although the behavioral and physiological dysregulation of infants following separation from caregivers is well documented, research on nonhuman primates has allowed a more systematic examination of the long-term effects of deprivation of caregiving. Fifty years of research on nonhuman primates offers abundant and unequivocal evidence that early disruption of caregiving substantially reduces the long-term capacity to modulate psychophysiological arousal and cope with social stressors (Kraemer, 1985). Such effects correlate with abnormal neurochemical responses of catecholamines, cortisol, serotonin, and opioids to subsequent stress (van der Kolk & Fisler, 1994).

Beginning with the groundbreaking work of Harlow (1958), accumulated evidence has shown that nonhuman primates separated from their caregivers eventually exhibit grossly abnormal social and sexual behavior. As adults, they do not produce offspring and, if artificially inseminated, will mutilate or kill their babies; they become socially withdrawn and unpredictably aggressive; and they develop self-destructive and self-stimulating behavior such as self-clasping, self-sucking, and self-biting (Harlow & Harlow, 1971). In short, they exhibit behavior and adjustment strikingly reminiscent of humans with a severe personality disorder. Of particular interest from the standpoint of the development of reflective function (see below) is the finding that these deprived monkeys fail to discriminate social cues (Mirsky, 1968). Remnants of this deficit persist throughout their lives, in spite of later exposure to responsive caregivers.

Although separation evokes a nearly universal pattern of protest in monkeys, less uniformly followed by despair (apparent only in some species), the age at which protracted separation occurs is crucial in determining both the intensity of the short-term response and the severity of any long-term consequences. With some variations, deprivation of caregiving at the end of the first year—roughly equivalent to the third year of life in human infants—tends to have severe and permanent consequences (Suomi, 1984).

Yet these consequences are not entirely irreversible. Suomi and Harlow (1972) demonstrated that rearing deprived monkeys with peers could eliminate most of the grossly maladaptive behavior. After 3 or 4 years of living with peers, the initially deprived monkeys are nearly indistinguishable from normally reared monkeys (Suomi, Harlow, & Novak, 1974). However, their adaptation is vulnerable: Under stressful conditions requiring complex social discrimination, the deprived monkeys revert to socially inappropriate behavior, becoming either withdrawn or aggressive while engaging in self-injurious and stereotypical activities. Even under normal conditions, isolated monkeys persistently show clear-cut deficiencies in coping with novelty and social behavior, including an ongoing inability to tease out subtle social messages (Suomi, 1997).

But if deprivation of early nurturance handicaps monkeys' development, an unusually nurturing start can turn otherwise vulnerable infants into future leaders of their groups. In a fascinating series of studies, Suomi (1984, 1991, 1997) demonstrated that monkey infants with "behaviorally inhibited" or "physiologically reactive" temperaments (similar to those of the inhibited babies described by Kagan, 1994), if reared by "supermothers," that is, foster mothers that are both exceptionally nurturant and encourage independence, will develop secure attachments and grow up to become unusually adept at recruiting support and mediating conflict. These monkeys tend to rise to the leadership position in their groups. This developmental success contrasts the outcome of infants with similarly reactive temperaments raised by "normal" or less nurturant foster mothers. These monkeys develop insecure attachments, display extreme reactions to environmental change and stress throughout their lives, and usually end up at the bottom of their group's hierarchy. These studies suggest that the "physiologically reactive" temperament may be a marker of an exceptional innate capacity to read social cues—a capacity that ensures success as leaders—but that innate ability requires a specific quality of caregiving to become an adaptive advantage rather than a vulnerability. In Chapter 6, I discuss a possible correlate of such physiological reactivity in humans, arguably as an indicator of a constitutional proneness to unusual mind-reading abilities.

ORGANIZING THE BRAIN FOR DISSOCIATION

Research with nonhuman primates opens a window onto the significance of attachment in human development. Peering through that window raises several questions: What are the mechanisms by which a lack of caregiver response sets the stage for long-term maladjustment? What are the components of the caregiver response that mediate the short-term restoration of the infant's psychophysiological equilibrium and may account for long-term adaptive success, perhaps even for turning a vulnerability into an advantage?

The first question requires that we look again at the responses of infants to separation from caregivers. As previously discussed, following separation, human infants go through a period of agitation, increased arousal, and autonomic activation. This stage of *protest* (Bowlby, 1969) is terminated fairly rapidly—except in temperamentally vulnerable infants—by the presence and "appropriate" response of the caregivers. The protest response, with its increased arousal and autonomic activation, is an expression of the fight-or-flight alarm system that Kandel (1983) postulated as biologically programmed to be activated by the absence of people. Yet infants, obviously limited in their capacity to fight or flee, are thus restricted to a relatively small repertoire of responses to modulate their own agitation and hyperarousal: gaze aversion, self-sucking, and, particularly, dissociation.

Dissociation (i.e., the segregation of experience into poorly integrated or nonintegrated components) counters the brain's normal proclivity to integrate available information (see Chapter 3) and to seek contingencies, as previously discussed. This failure of integration, however, makes good adaptive sense under conditions of overwhelming threat. Dissociation permits individuals to "escape" otherwise inescapable horrors and optimizes their chances of fighting or fleeing, unencumbered by pain or distraction.

Several solid lines of research establish the association of a history of trauma with increased levels of dissociation (Putnam, 1985, 1996). Various studies (e.g., Coons, Bowman, & Milstein, 1988; Dell & Eisenhower, 1990; Loewenstein & Putnam, 1990) establish that 85–100% of adults with dissociative identity disorder report a history of severe childhood trauma.

A second set of studies (Branscomb, 1991; Briere & Runtz, 1988; Chu & Dill, 1990; Irwin, 1994) documents traumatized individuals' significantly higher levels of dissociation compared to nontraumatized controls. Within the traumatized group, variables such as duration, severity, and life-threatening nature of the trauma correlate significantly with the extent of dissociation (Kirby, Chu, & Dill, 1993; Putnam, 1985).

Considerable controversy still surrounds several aspects of dissociative phenomena, particularly questions of whether pathological dissociation differs only in extent from normal dissociation. Other questions include the following: Is there a particular type of dissociative individual who presents discontinuities of experience that rarely occur in normal people? What is the role of genetic factors in the proclivity to extreme and/or pathological forms of dissociation? What is not controversial is the fact that maltreated children have significantly higher levels of dissociation than age-matched, normal children. In comparison, few normal children (about 6–7%) develop high levels of dissociation in the absence of severe trauma or loss (Putnam, 1996).

The developmental trajectory leading to this dissociative proneness is becoming increasingly clear. As Perry (1997) suggests, the repeated failure of human response to the infant's signals of distress organizes the developing brain in the direction of a bias to activate the fight-or-flight mechanism, particularly the dissociative component more readily available to infants. Such brain organization can be compared to the neural pathways the developing brain produces during the first few months of life in response to exposure to a specific language environment. Edelman (1987, 1992) postulates that neural networks within the brain "compete" with one another, with the most functional network surviving. For example, infants' exposure to a particular language (e.g., its unique syntax, sounds, rhythms) "selects" certain neural pathways leading first to selective attention to the specific sounds and subsequently to the ability to understand and speak the language. It is plausible that a similar facilitation toward a dissociative response may occur, perhaps more easily, in children who are temperamentally vulnerable to separations and change, as well as in those who may be constitutionally predisposed to dissociation (Perry & Pollard, 1998; Schwartz & Perry, 1999).

In Chapters 4, 5, and 6, I examine the implications of this particular trajectory for children's adjustment. Of note now is that the early steps in this journey show the harbingers of future problems. The disorganized/disoriented pattern of attachment may represent the behavioral expression of this early proneness to dissociation brought about by a lack of response, perhaps interacting in varying degrees with a constitutional predisposition to intense reactivity. Disorganized/disoriented infants show gaze aversion, contradictory intentions toward caregivers (e.g., sometimes clingy, sometimes unresponsive), lack of orientation to the environment, and periods of sudden immobility or "freezing" associated with a dazed expression that has been referred to as a "trancelike" state. But more than neglect is necessary before infants develop a disorganized/disoriented attachment. Although about 15% of a normative sample of infants present disorganized/disoriented attachment, the prevalence among maltreated infants is as high as 80% (Main & Solomon, 1990). In Chapter 4, I discuss the role of trauma, genetic factors, and caregivers' own dissociative tendencies and the putative pathways leading from this aberrant attachment pattern to some severe personality disorders.

REFLECTIVE FUNCTION AND THE "PSYCHOLOGICAL BIRTH" OF THE HUMAN INFANT

The failure of human response arguably organizes the infant's brain toward a proneness for dissociation and is at least an element in the development of disorganized/disoriented attachment. We are left to ponder the particular components of the caregiver's response that promote the development of the infant's psychobiological organization.

The psychoanalytic perspective emphasized that psychological organization and self–other differentiation are achieved when infants slowly shift their investment and attention from internal to external stimuli (Mahler et al., 1975). In Mahler's influential description, during the first 10–12 months of life, children gradually put together in their mind fragments of their mother's and their own image. The vague feeling of being one with mother (Mahler's symbiotic phase) recedes as children develop an increasingly more sophisticated sense of what is inside and what is outside, what belongs to them and what belongs to mother.

Differentiation results as the innately designed maturation of cognitive, perceptual, and motoric abilities join forces with children's inner feelings and sensations, and with their experience with caregivers, to push them in the direction of a slow coalescence of fragmented self-image into a core sense of self. Thus, according to Mahler and colleagues (1975), children develop by the end of their first year a growing capacity to experience themselves as distinct and separate from their mothers. In other words, they develop mental self-representations that have boundaries and are differentiated from the representation of the mother. This, to Mahler, is the moment of "psychological birth" of human infants, the point when human beings can begin to conceive of themselves as separate individuals.

Developmental research, however, as pointed out, turns this formulation around. Rather than beginning in an undifferentiated state and gradually moving toward differentiation, contemporary research suggests that infants *first* acquire a sense of their distinct, separate self *before* they are able to conceive of ways of sharing their internal experience with others.

According to Stern, during the first 2 months of life, infants rapidly organize a core sense of self as "a separate, cohesive, bonded, physical unit" (1985, p. 10). The *reflection* of the infant's internal states embodied in the highly contingent, imperfectly matched, and specifically marked behavior of the caregivers will then provide the impetus for the development of a sense of ongoing affectivity and continuity over time. This development, as we will see later, leads to the capacity to *represent* memories of the self and others in a personal narrative that has coherence and permits the understanding of other people as psychological beings, with mental states not only similar to but also different from those of the self.

This developmental path thus begins with the capacity of the caregivers to provide a behavioral reflection of the infant's internal state. Attachment researchers have assumed that the development of psychological organization is an outgrowth of secure attachment that results from the infant's experience with sensitive, attuned, and responsive caregivers. Sensitivity, attunement, and responsiveness are thought to foster the expectation that needs will be met and that states of hyperarousal and dysregulation—states of activation of the fight-or-flight mechanism—will not become overwhelming but will lead instead to caregivers' responses that restore control and equilibrium. More generally, sensitivity, attunement, and responsiveness promote the infant's trust that it is safe to explore because the caregiver will offer a "secure base" (Bowlby, 1969, 1973, 1980) to which the infant can return for soothing and nurturance.

Yet evidence of a rather modest, *direct* link between security of attachment in infancy and the quality of subsequent relationships and personality functioning in childhood and adolescence (Elman et al., 1996; Rutter, 1985; Thompson, 1999) is shifting the focus of inquiry from the type of experience to the acquisition of specific mediating capacities and mechanisms that in turn affect psychosocial development and organization.

What then are the mechanisms that make it possible for caregivers to attune to their infants and respond in a highly but imperfectly contingent way that closely matches the infant's internal state? The study of the specific elements of the attuned responses has sought to answer this question.

Caregivers are generally effective in reading their infants' displays of emotion and tend to attune their own affective responses to modulate their infants' emotional states (Tronick, 1989). Stern (1985) demonstrated that attunement occurs regularly in normal mother–infant interactions. In his studies, about half of the mothers in his sample were rated as *highly* to *very highly* attuned. When these mothers interacted with their infants, their blood pressure and other physiological measures paralleled those of their infants. Stern went on to demonstrate how mothers naturally and effortlessly "read" the qualities of their infants' internal states as expressed in the architecture of the children's behavior: the intensity, tempo, rhythm, categorical affect, and other features of the experience. A high level of attunement is generally found in ordinary caregiver–infant interactions, notwithstanding the caregivers' individual patterns of response that reflect their personalities and current circumstances, their own relationship and emotional history, and their expectations regarding their infants (Stern, 1985).

As noted earlier, Stern emphasized that the caregivers are not simply imitators of the infant's outward behavior. They only partially match some of the features of the architecture of the infant's behavior and typically respond in a different modality (i.e., the infant's motor "stretch" to grasp a toy is converted by the caregiver in a visual and vocal response of shrugged shoulders and vocalizations).

But attunement is far from a unidirectional process. For example, while caregivers typically recognize their infant's optimal range of stimulation at a given moment, infants will avert their gaze to cut out stimulation that has risen above the optimal range and then reestablish gaze and positive affect when they seek to "prompt" the caregiver to provide a higher level of stimulation (Bigelow, 1998). This is only one instance of how infants appear disposed to "help" their caregivers recognize and respond to their internal states.

Evolution has guaranteed a finely tuned complementarity between caregiver and infant morphology and behavior. As Kaye (1982) points out, this complementarity is evident in the very anatomy of human nursing:

> The newborn comes equipped for sucking with a suitably shaped mouth; strong buccinator muscles; rooting, sucking and swallowing mechanisms; and the ability to coordinate these with breathing. None of these would be of value if human mothers did not come equipped with nipples of an appropriate size and shape for the newborn's oral cavity, suited to just the kind and amount of expression produced by the sucking movement, responsive to the range of sucking pressures infants happen to create. (p. 25)

Indeed, evolution seems to have designed caregivers to comprehend and respond to infants' physiology, behavior, *and* internal states.

Drawing from such ideas, Fonagy and his collaborators (Fonagy, Steele, & Steele, 1991; Fonagy, Steele, Steele, Moran, & Higgitt, 1991; Fonagy & Target, 1996) have built an impressive body of research and conceptualization that centers on understanding the development of psychological organization and personality and, in particular, the developmental pathogenesis of severe personality disorders, a remarkable human capacity: reflective function. Reflective function is also referred to by developmentalists as *theories of mind* (Baron-Cohen, 1994; Baron-Cohen, Tooby, & Cosmides, 1995), *mentalization* (Fonagy & Target, 1997), or *interpersonal interpretive mechanism* (Fonagy, 2000a). Reflective function is the biologically prepared and nearly universal capacity of humans, including very young humans, to interpret the behavior of all agents, themselves as well as others, in terms of internal mental states.

This capacity should not be confused with introspection, insight, or the ability to explain our own or other people's motives. It is instead the moment-to-moment "reading" of other people's minds. Without any particular conscious effort, such ability permits caregivers to "read" their infant's internal states (e.g., feelings, desires, intentions) and to "make sense" of them (e.g., a baby's crying and fussing may signal an internal state that calls for stroking, rocking, feeding, and verbalizations such as "Oh, honey, you are so hungry."). As Brazelton, Koslowski, and Main (1974) noted, in playful exchanges with their infants, mothers normally coordinate their level of arousal in a subtly organized way, based on their moment-to-moment reading of the infant's level of arousal, and thus avoid being out of phase or unattuned. Reflective function is therefore the capacity underlying the normal interpretation of interpersonal situations that allow for the relatively smooth reciprocity and mutual adjustment that is part and parcel of normal interactions.

It is hardly surprising that a species "designed" by evolution to be organized by social experience would come equipped with the capacity to read social cues and grasp the internal states that give direction to the behavior of other human beings. An innate biological disposition affords human beings the capacity for intersubjective engagement, and affective connectedness and differentiation from others (Hobson, 1993b).

The fundamental relationship between reflective function and human functioning and development is readily apparent in instances when reflective function does not operate properly, particularly in early childhood autism. As Baron-Cohen and colleagues (1995) and Hobson (1993b) suggest, perhaps the key deficit of autism is a brain-based limitation in reflective function.

Autistic infants and children appear impaired in both the capacity to convey their internal state to others in understandable ways and the ability to be sensitive to the inner states of others. As Hobson (1993a, 1993b) points out, the pathognomonic feature of autism is a severe disruption in intersubjective coordination. Hobson goes on to suggest that this disruption is the central factor in the failure of these children to develop creative symbolic imagination, to evolve awareness of self and others as separate centers of consciousness and intentions, and to acquire a full understanding of the forms and functions of language. Gergely, Magyar, and Balazs (1999) postulate that autistic children's defective contingency detection mechanism and "blindness" to less than perfect contingencies render them unable to grasp the less than perfect match of social responses.

The current dominant view in developmental research holds that caregivers and infants indeed form an affective communication system from the beginning of life (Beebe, Jaffee, & Lachman, 1992; Beebe & Lachman, 1988; Harris, 1994; Murray & Trevarthen, 1985; Papousek & Papousek, 1987, 1989; Sroufe, 1996; Stern, 1985; Tronick, 1989). But extensive use of microanalytic methods makes evident the bidirectionality of the attunement process (Beebe & Lachman, 1988; Beebe et al., 1992). Studies of face-to-face exchanges of affective signals between infants and their caregivers make apparent how ready normal infants are to grasp the affective states of others. Careful analysis of these transactions demonstrates that *both* caregivers and infants are sensitive to each others' state of mind and regulate their expression on the basis of the *anticipated* reaction of the other. Beebe and collaborators have shown that the facial expression of babies and mothers can be predicted by the facial expression of the other one-twelfth of a second before it occurs. Clearly, both interactive partners are able to predict and modify the other's behavior. A central contention of this book is that the capacity displayed by caregivers—and in an embryonic form, by the infants as well—of making sense, sharing experiences, and predicting the other is an expression of reflective function.

Reflective function is the developmental acquisition that permits people to respond not only to other people's overt behavior but also to their *conception* of their beliefs, intentions, feelings, and the like. By attributing mental states and intentions to themselves and others, human beings make people meaningful and predictable.

As Dennett (1987) pointed out, normal human beings seem inherently inclined to understand each other in terms of mental states and intentions in order to make sense and anticipate each other's actions. Dennett's theory is that explaining human behavior in terms of intentional states provides human beings with a shared and accessible basis to use in anticipating each other's behavior.

THE ACQUISITION OF REFLECTIVE FUNCTION

Baron-Cohen and Swettenham (1996, p. 158) raise a fundamental question: "How on Earth can young children master such abstract concepts as belief with such ease, and roughly at the same time the world over?" Arguably, the answer is that in infants biologically prepared to acquire reflective function, it is triggered by close proximity with caregivers who exercise their own reflective capacities in their interaction with the infants (Fonagy & Target, 1996; Gergely & Watson, 1999); that is, the development of the infant's reflective capacity depends on the presence of caregivers who not only understand the infant's internal state but also respond in ways that convey that external behavior is meaningful and intentional ("Oh, honey, you are so hungry.").

The infant's awareness of having a mind, and of other people also having minds, seems to require that the caregivers first represent in their own minds their infant's internal state and then respond in accordance with such representation. The developmentally correct formulation of the psychological birth of the human infant, according to Fonagy and Target (2000), requires a restatement of the Cartesian dictum from "I think therefore I am" to "He/She [the caregiver] *thinks that I think, therefore I am.*" Such an idea was expressed earlier by Winnicott (1967), when he stated that babies find *themselves* when they look at their mother's face.

In countless interactions, babies "find themselves" in the reflection of caregivers who grasp the full range of the babies' internal states—or fail to grasp and subsequently attempt to repair the failed communication. This discovery is not sterile information processing that utilizes biologically prepared tools. Rather, it is drawn out of the passions stirred up in the context of attachment: in interactions that regulate or fail to regulate, soothe or fail to soothe, restore equilibrium or fail to do so, bring about safety, pleasure, and satisfaction, or leave infants feeling overwhelmed and miserable.

Affect likely plays a crucial role in activating reflective function. Interactions that organize and regulate overwhelming and dysphoric affective states reinforce the attachment system and promote security of attachment. Inversely, as Fonagy's work has demonstrated, and as I elaborate in Chapter 3, secure attachment is a key correlate of reflective function (Steele, Steele, & Fonagy, 1996).

As the studies of Stern (1985), Gergely and Watson (1996), and others demonstrate, attuned, soothing responses from caregivers that rapidly signal a sharing of the infant's affective state are generally followed by a restoration of the infant's homeostasis. This attunement, as discussed earlier, is typically expressed through a *different* modality than the one used by the infant to express an internal state, yet the caregiver's behavior preserves the "amodal" qualities (e.g., tempo, rhythm, intensity) of the infant's affective state. In addition, the caregiver adds a "twist" of his or her own (a touch of humor, a shrug, and the like) that "marks" the response and perhaps also reflects a capacity to cope with the infant's inner state.

By using a different modality of expression to signal attunement, caregivers indeed shift the infant's focus of attention from the outward behavior to the inner state (Stern, 1985). Then, by adding a different "twist," the caregivers ensure that infants recognize their experiences as being analogous with, but not identical to, the infants' own.

Gergely and Watson (1999) argue that the special "marking" of a caregivers' affective–reflective display leads infants to set up mental representations of these responses that are uncoupled from their representation of the caregiver who is displaying them. In other words, the affect–reflection will be represented as "not being about" a particular caregiver's actual emotional states, but because of the high contingency control infants experience between their emotional state and their caregivers' attuned reflective responses, their representation of a response becomes a *referent* that points to their own internal state.

It appears likely that the association of affective–reflective displays with restored homeostasis acts as a catalyst in the evolution of the contingency detection mechanism. Children will then shift from a preference for perfect contingencies to high but imperfect ones and, in the process, yoke their development to the functions and mechanisms that are generated in interactions with responsive human beings.

In Gergely and Watson's (1999) terms, infants internalize their caregivers' attuned reflective responses as a secondary representation of the caregivers' interpretation of the infants' own internal state. If infants could verbalize their experience of observing a caregiver's expression, they would say: "So that is what I am feeling!" This experience is made possible by an interaction with another person who attunes to the infant's internal state and responds in a way that communicates back to the infant, "I get what you are feeling and I share your experience." Trevarthen and Hubley (1978) designate this emerging domain of relatedness as the domain of "intersubjectivity," a term that points to a developmental path eventually leading to the capacity of *both* interactive partners to represent in their minds each other's mental states.

This secondary representation process "pulls" the infant's primary affective experience of psychophysiological arousal and procedural expression toward a mentalized or reflective experience. The pull toward experiencing a mental state instead of raw affect is fostered by the sense of contingency control—"I can produce an effect"—and restored regulation, homeostasis, pleasure, and comfort in relation to the caregiver's attuned reflective response. At the same time, the secondary representation begins to separate psychological experience from procedural, motoric expression.

Children thus develop the precursors of the capacity to label and find their own psychological experiences meaningful in the process of observing another person's interpretation of their own internal state. The caregiver's "reflection" promotes infants' ability to represent their affect mentally, while it also conveys that internal states can be communicated, understood, and managed to a large degree by the process of sharing them, assigning them meaning, and representing them as mental constructs.

The representation of the caregiver's attuned reflective response promotes the sharing of internal states and also becomes a referent to the other person's internal states. By directing children's attention to the caregiver's internal state, the infant's representation of the caregiver's response sets the stage for the use of the caregiver as a "reference" point to guide the infant's affective assessment of novel experiences, a phenomenon described as "social referencing" in the developmental literature (Campos & Stenberg, 1981; Sorce, Emde, Campos, & Klinnert, 1985). A 1-year-old, for example, confronted with a "visual cliff" (i.e., an arrangement that simulates a cliff at the end of a table) will proceed across the "cliff" if the caregiver looks relaxed, but will freeze if the caregiver appears anxious. Hobson (1993b) emphasizes that the crucial issue in social referencing is the infant's dawning appreciation of the distinction between the concrete world-as-given and a world in which objects and events can have person-related meanings (e.g., a world in which the same situation can be either "dangerous" or "inviting"); that is, in any personal situation, the "meaning for me" is not necessarily the "meaning for her."

In Chapter 3, I review how reflective function promotes the emergence of symbolic thought and vice versa. At this point, however, I would like to mention that the mutual cueing just described is, from the infant's standpoint, prereflective. Infants do not yet represent in their minds the mental state (e.g., beliefs, intentions, desires), of their caregivers when they anticipate their caregivers' actions based on facial expressions or when using caregivers as a "reference" to inform their own internal state. A more fully reflective position involves a capacity to conceive of and represent the other's mental state, separate from one's own, and to take it into account.

This milestone, normally reached when children are between 3 and

4 years of age, is marked by the understanding of false beliefs. This capacity involves the awareness that others' behavior may be understandable even when based on mistaken and even irrational beliefs and assumptions. For example, a 3½-year-old shown a bag of candy and asked what it contains will respond: "Candy." If the bag is then opened and shown to contain a pencil, the child will be able to predict accurately that his friend waiting outside the room will reply "Candy" to the same question, demonstrating a reflective capacity to anticipate his friend's mistaken belief. Such development is nudged along by several mediational processes, most prominently by play and pretend, peer and sibling interactions, and talking.

Empirical evidence supports the link between pretend play and reflective function. Three-year-olds who engage more readily in joint pretend play demonstrate superior capacity to "read minds" and understand other people's emotions (Astington & Jenkins, 1995; Youngblade & Dunn, 1995). An independent body of longitudinal studies demonstrates that preschool children who were securely attached to a primary caregiver in infancy are significantly more capable of engaging in fantasy play than are children with anxious attachment patterns (Main, Kaplan, & Cassidy, 1985). This variance provides evidence that security of attachment not only directly promotes the development of reflective function, as discussed earlier, but also enhances the chances of reflective development by fostering processes, such as interactive fantasy play, that are, in turn, fertile ground for reflective growth.

Playing, from its modest beginnings in games such as peekaboo, requires exquisite synchronicity of mental states, affect, and tempo. As play progresses to the realm of pretend (e.g., when a 2-year-old takes a stick to stand for a gun), the child is assigning a self-selected meaning to the stick (his conception of a gun) alongside his recognition of the stick as an object. Then, as children become able to engage in *interactive* pretend play, they jointly transform reality by creating a shared representation that differs from actual reality but is shared by those participating in the pretend play. Children engaged in such play have to hold in mind both the shared pretend reality and the actual reality, while keeping an eye, moment-to-moment, on the minds of the others sharing in the pretense.

Beyond providing increased opportunities for pretend play, interactions with peers and siblings create a powerful impetus for reflective function. As noted earlier, primate research suggests that peers can partially overcome the maladaptive consequences of deprivation of caregiving.

W. Corsaro, quoted in an article by Gladwell (1998), illustrates how children take their cues from each other and thus come in contact with sources that stimulate their reflective function. Corsaro describes watching two 4-year-old girls, Jenny and Betty, playing house in a sandbox by putting sand in pots and teacups. Suddenly, a third girl, Debbie, approaches. Debbie watches Jenny and Betty for about 5 minutes, then circles the sandbox and watches again before moving closer and reaching for a teacup. Jenny takes the cup away from Debbie and says, "No." Debbie backs away and again watches Jenny and Betty. She then stands next to Betty and says: "We are friends, right, Betty?" Betty, not looking up at Debbie, continues to put sand in the cup and says, "Right." Debbie now moves next to Betty, takes a pot and spoon, begins putting sand in the pot and says, "I am making coffee." "I am making cupcakes," responds Betty. Betty now turns to Jenny and says, "We are mothers, right, Jenny?" "Right," answers Jenny. Such interactions help children acquire complex strategies of approaching, avoiding, sharing, and competing, while they also become able to grasp cues about the intersubjective meanings being created and exchanged.

Language undoubtedly plays a central role in such exchanges. More generally, language both promotes and is promoted by reflective function. Smith (1996) suggests that the availability of verbal–symbolic referents to name mental states is crucial for the acquisition of mind-reading ability. Harris (1996) makes the more general claim that the experience of engaging in conversations, irrespective of whether they make reference to mental states, alerts children to the fact that people are receivers and providers of information who *differ* in what they know, believe, and feel about a shared topic.

Yet to extract the actual meaning conveyed, children must learn to integrate verbal communication with the total context of cues. Bruner (1983, 1990) quips that any 5-year-old "knows" what even sophisticated language-recognition computers struggle with: that when Aunt Sally asks Billie if he would be "kind enough" to pass the salt, she is not making an inquiry into the limits of the boy's compassion but simply wants the boy to pass the salt shaker. This capacity of normal 5-year-olds to "get it" contrasts with that of a 20-year-old man with a mild-to-moderate pervasive developmental disorder who, desperate to "score" sexually with any girl, asked plaintively: "When a girl says something to you, it can mean 10 different things, so how do you know what she means?"

Yet for children with a normal biological preparedness, perhaps the critical factor needed to develop reflective function is the ongoing capacity of their caregivers to retain reflective function while negotiating the multiple tasks and challenges of day-to-day life and development. The ability to "read" the moment-to-moment changes in a child's mental states allows caregivers to treat the child's behavior *as if it is* meaningful and intentional. Such treatment is the foundation of secure attachment. Securely attached children, in turn, are optimally positioned to explore their caregiver's mind—and to find there a mental conception of their own behavior.

The acquisition of reflective function thus appears to be the outcome of intersubjective transactions between infants and their caregivers that is potentiated by subsequent transactions with other significant people, such as peers, siblings, and other adults. Caregivers activate their children's reflective function (and usher in their psychological birth) by pervasively and nonconsciously ascribing agency to their behavior and representing the children in their own minds as psychological beings. When caregivers respond to their children on the basis of their own reflective function, they open the door for their children to step into a world of complex possibilities that affect the most uniquely human aspects of development.

Psychological Organization and the World of Mental Representations

PATTERNING AND ORGANIZATION OF EXPERIENCE

The emergence of reflective function provides a catalyst for one of the human brain's key functions: to generate, organize, and structure psychological experience and to employ the resulting psychological structure(s) as the matrix for its regulating and modulating activities. Indeed, the brain is as prewired to create organization leading to self-regulation as the pancreas is designed to produce insulin in order to regulate glucose metabolism. As Emde (1989) remarks, the infant comes into the world "with biologically prepared active propensities and with organized capacities for self-regulation" (p. 38).

Along these lines, Stern (1985, 1995) notes that babies show an innate tendency to develop predictable patterns and to connect mentally ("to put together") what goes together in reality. Pairing what goes together in reality, however, is a daunting task. Stern (1985) delineates the multiplicity of processes and tendencies involved in creating organization: innate perceptual, cognitive, affective, and attentional biases—particularly the bias toward recognizing and engaging other humans; the predisposition to organize and transfer information from one modality to another; and the ability to grasp what is variant and what is invariant in order to create schemas. Evidence of an innate contingency detection module or mechanism (Gergely & Watson, 1996, 1999; Watson, 1994, 1995) speaks also of a built-in tendency toward control, self-agency, and organization.

These biologically prepared capacities, brought to life by the presence of reflective caregivers, lead to the active construction of mental schemas that represent the infant's grasp of the common or invariant features of specific types of transactions with specific significant others. From the standpoint of psychological development, a particularly relevant type of transaction occurs when the infant's dysregulation and hyperarousal are met by an attuned caregiver who conveys that he or she can grasp the infant's internal states, can handle them, and can ascribe intentionality to behavior, while responding to restore the infant's homeostasis. Such transactions are the likely basis of the internal working models (Bowlby, 1980) that underlie the secure attachment pattern.

A significant body of research demonstrates that, as early as 2–4 months of age, infants can construct schemas of reality and have expectations about interactions with others and the likely "fit" between different aspects of experience. Spelke (1979) and Spelke and Owsley (1979), for example, demonstrated that infants can respond to the congruity between auditory and visual stimuli. When 4-month-old infants were shown two cartoon films projected side by side, but only one had a sound track synchronic with the image, the infants preferred to look at the synchronized film. Other studies (e.g., Dodd, 1979) have demonstrated that infants can spot a discrepancy as small as 400 milliseconds between expected sight and sound (e.g., a slight delay in the sound track of a film of a person talking), and these infants then present a distressful response when the expected experiential congruity is violated. (For more information on this point in regard to trauma, see Chapter 4.) It is worth noting that the evolutionary function of early mental schemas—and the bias to seek out congruity—seems to be the anticipation of what is going to happen, particularly what other people will do or look like. This bias toward anticipation is shown in the previously mentioned preference that infants demonstrate for experiences that match their expectations, and in their aversion and distress when faced with experiences that fail to match those expectations.

STERN'S PROTO-NARRATIVE ENVELOPE
AND ATTACHMENT PATTERNS

Daniel Stern (1985, 1990, 1995) offers an extraordinary guide to the world of the infant's subjective experience. Drawing on a meticulous examination of empirical evidence and his own rigorous observations, Stern invites us to venture on a journey into the mind of infants, a journey that offers new vistas into how infants generate, construct, and organize their subjective experience.

Stern is particularly interested in better understanding how infants come to represent their experiences of being in relationship with others. As he points out, experiences of relationship differ from experiences with the inanimate world in several important respects, including their affective intensity and interactive nature. I would like to add that evolution has uniquely predisposed human infants to crave the company of other humans and to seek them out to mediate all the motivational systems built into human beings (e.g., attachment and security, physiological regulation and need satisfaction, sensual gratification and exploration, the bias to create patterns and organization; Emde, 1988; Lichtenberg, 1989). These motivational systems come into being around vital daily life activities such as eating, regulating affect, playing, sleeping, and exploring the environment.

Stern (1995) demonstrates that infants have both the capacity and the proclivity to schematize the basic elements of an experience, as well as a strong bias toward linking schemas together. In his review of infancy research, Stern shows that infants as young as 3–4 months of age, if not younger, can represent perceptual schemas (e.g., visual images, auditory stimulation); sensory–motor schemas (which coordinate motor acts with sensory experiences); event sequences (i.e., an invariant set of events represented as a single scenario); and affect schemas in the form of "temporal feeling shapes" (i.e., a representation of the quality and quantity of feeling that accompanies an experience). Such schemas include what Stern calls "vitality affects," which encompass the "shape" and temporal contour of the unfolding feeling states and their hedonic tone and arousal level. Finally, a superschema can represent the whole experience as a coherent happening. Stern also refers to conceptual schemas (e.g., symbols, words) that develop later (these are addressed in the section in this chapter on symbolic processing).

Stern (1995) emphasizes the notion of *emergent properties of mind* to describe the inherent tendency of the brain to create a mental organization that "renders coherent experiences made up of many simultaneously occurring, partially independent parts" (p. 89). Specialized areas and centers of the brain process simultaneously or in parallel each component of a given experience—the sense of the body in space, affect shifts, arousal levels, visual images, and so forth. From this complex mental activity, says Stern, an emergent property of the mind is created through coordination and integration of schemas; that is, the diverse aspects or schemas of processed experience are linked in a coherent, unified whole. Stern suggests that this whole assumes a meaning.

The "meaning" that Stern refers to is more likely a proto-meaning, based on the inherent capacity of infants to apprehend intuitively the intentional states of agents—that is, the biologically prepared substrate of reflective function. For Stern, the representational format that "holds" this integrated set of schemas in a coherent, meaningful, narrative-like mode is what he calls the *proto-narrative envelope*. This "envelope" contains organization the way the brain is designed to construct it: with the structure of a narrative. It is, however, a story without words or symbols, with a silent plot visible only through the perceptual, attentional, and motoric strategies to which it gives rise.

The notion of the proto-narrative envelope is intimately linked, as Stern (1995) explains, with the concept of goal-directed motivation underlying all human behavior. When the motive (e.g., safety, pleasure, exploration, regulation, mastery) is enacted in an interpersonal context, it "creates" or brings about a narrative-like structure: a "plot" with an expected sequence of events over time. Bruner (1990) points out that this narrative unit is the basic unit for comprehending human behavior, arguably reflecting the very way the brain grasps and organizes experience. Narrative-like structures may be the counterpart of intentionality, but they precede the capacity of the infant either to "comprehend" intentionality fully or to produce verbal–symbolic narrative structures.

Indeed, proto-narrative envelopes are presymbolic and do not involve a full grasp of intentionality on the infant's part beyond a basic, intuitive grasp of the goal directedness of human behavior. They are constructed and stored as implicit, nonconscious, procedural memories (Kihlstrom & Hoyt, 1995; Rochat, 1995; Schacter, 1992; Squire, 1987, 1992). This form of processing, in contrast to the symbolic processing and autobiographical memory systems that develop later (see next section), is nonvoluntary, nondeclarative, and nonreflective, and is dominated by emotional, impressionistic, motoric, and perceptual information—that is, the types of schemas described by Stern (1995).

Procedural memory, which is underpinned by its own relatively homogeneous neurological system, stores the "how to" of executing motor, affective, and perceptual strategies in response to specific cues. This knowledge is "in the body" or in "the guts" and is context bound; that is, any one of the concrete elements stored in any one of the schemas— a specific physical sensation, affective "shape," or visual cue—that are contained in a proto-narrative envelope can *"open" the envelope and make it accessible to enactment.* The proto-narrative envelope's proto-stories come to life only in *the performance* of specific perceptual–motoric–affective strategies. Within these strategies is embedded the knowledge that neuroanatomically depends on specific sensory and motor systems, as well as the cerebellum and the basal ganglia (Kandel, 1998). The "infantile amnesia" described in the psychoanalytic literature is thus more likely related to the predominance of implicit–procedural processing during the first years of life than to the effects of repression.

Procedural knowledge of the self in relationships has been referred to as *implicit relational knowing* (Stern, 1998; Stern et al., 1998). This kind of knowledge is about how to "be with someone." Stern (1998) and Stern and colleagues (1998) describe how infants come to know what form and intensity of approach, state of activation, affect, desire, and so forth will be welcomed or rejected by the caregiver at any given moment. This "implicit relational knowledge" continues through life as a nonsymbolic, nonconscious foundation of the symbolic and potentially conscious aspects of mental representations. For example, it is the "sense" we have of whether we can approach another person in a light-hearted, teasing fashion at a given moment and match the other person's mood and disposition. As Tronick (1989) has argued, relationships are based on the mutual regulation of states of affect, desire, activation, and so forth, that take place through microexchanges of implicit–procedural information.

The attachment patterns elicited by the Strange Situation tap into this implicit–procedural knowledge and memories. The "pattern" of attachment is evoked by a particular caregiver in a sequence of presence, absence, and reappearance. The pattern is thus a motoric, perceptual, and affective strategy acquired in, and activated by, a relation to a

particular caregiver in a specific interpersonal situation. It is worth remembering, as we strive to figure out ways to help people—particularly
those with a severe personality disorder—to alter relationship patterns
in which they find themselves trapped, that the basis of attachment patterns is the automatic, procedural, nonreflective strategies that spring to
life without reflection, triggered by specific internal and interpersonal
cues.

By the second half of the first year of life, these "working models"
of implicit–procedural memories underlying attachment patterns serve
not only to anticipate reality but also to *cope* with the expectations generalized from the aggregate of multiple interactions with a caregiver.
Children with an anxious/avoidant attachment, for example, develop a
coping strategy that involves an active shift of attention away from their
caregivers—and also away from these infants' own dependency and desire for response. This coping pattern appears to result from the expectation that any bid for access will be ignored. In contrast, the anxious/
resistant pattern is a coping strategy that *overemphasizes* the caregivers
and the infant's dependency on them at the expense of the infant's sense
of self-agency.

FROM IMPLICIT–PROCEDURAL TO EXPLICIT–REFLECTIVE: THE MIRACLE OF SYMBOLIZATION

Stern (1995) raises the question of how we go from the schemas contained in what he calls a proto-narrative envelope to fantasies and autobiographical narratives. Stern's question refers to the elucidation of the
path leading from a network of schemas, each representing categories of
invariant elements in specific aspects of lived experience (i.e., sensory–
motor or affective schemas generated in particular interpersonal interactions), to symbolic processes. In other words, "What is the process of
going from history to narration, from fixed serial order to arranged re-
orderings, from one pattern of emphasis and stress to a new pattern,
from objective events in reality to imaginary events in virtual time?"
(p. 94).

Symbolic processing contrasts with concrete processing in that instead of an "envelope" of schemas activated by elements stored in the
schemas, symbolic processing permits the active and flexible *selection* of
elements, moving attention freely between various schemas. Thus, at-

tention can be directed to two or more schemas at the same time, and the elements of various schemas can be combined, with one schema in the background while the other is in the foreground, and then vice versa. A child engaging in pretend play, for example, takes a stick to stand for a sword and sustains in his or her mind simultaneously the dual schema of a self-selected meaning conferred on the stick—the child's conception of "sword"—together with the recognition of an actual stick belonging to a "stick" category.

The possibilities of forming new schemas that are not limited to concrete, lived experiences become endless; that is, the elements of any one schema can be combined and recombined with those of others, creating new networks of schemas for purposes of defense, pleasure, sharing, or adaptation. The capacity to create fantasies is one of the outcomes of this symbolic transformation of the concrete schemas. As symbolic capacities grow richer and more sophisticated, fantasies can also become more elaborate, complex, and ever more fantastic. This view obviously contrasts with the notion that the earliest mental productions are also the most fantastic (Klein, 1952a, 1952b, 1957, 1958).

Even at its most rudimentary level, during the second and third years of life, symbolic processing, hand in hand with reflective function, allows young children to respond not only to the behavior of others but also to their own *conception* of others' beliefs, feelings, attitudes, desires, hopes, knowledge, imagination, pretense, deceit, plans, intentions, and other internal states. For example, children can begin to create stories, such as "Mommy does not respond to me *because* she is tired."

Yet the key outcome of the growth of symbolic capacities and reflective function during the second and third years of life may be the further development of the sense of agency (Crittenden, 1994; Fonagy & Target, 1997). Children can now *select* or *create* mental schemas to mediate their own behavior and can respond adaptively to particular demands that emanate from their reading of their own and others' mental states. Such active selection or creation of mental schemas or, more properly, of such *mental representations*, generates a subjective conviction of owning one's behavior that contrasts with the passive sense derived from procedural schemas activated by concrete, context-dependent cues. Children no longer feel as if their behavior "happens to them." Whims and urges, wishes and needs are transformed into more sustained and active experiences of decision and intentionality. As Ogden (1989) points out, the achievement of the capacities for subjectivity and symbol formation proper allows one to experience oneself as a person thinking one's thoughts and feeling one's feelings. In this way, thoughts and feelings are experienced to a large degree as personal creations that can be understood. Thus, for better or for worse, one develops a feeling of responsibility for one's psychological actions (thoughts, feelings, and behavior).

This development, as we see in subsequent sections of this chapter, paves the way for an integration of wishes, needs, motives, roles, and relationship patterns into a more coherent sense of self and others, with continuity over time. Arguably, this psychological construct underlies affect regulation, impulse control, self-monitoring, and the capacity for planning and setting goals, values, and ideals. Out of these elements, "the emergent property" creating coherence and organization now gives rise to *autobiographical narratives*, that is, more or less conscious and more or less cohesive models of ourselves, the world, and other people.

The narrative-like structures that children can now create enable them to integrate the older, nonverbal "proto-narrative envelopes" with the more recent, verbal–symbolic story lines. This occurs in a manner analogous to Freud's (1900/1953) "secondary revision"; that is, the inchoate images, sounds, and affects of dreams initially produced during sleep are transformed into the story-like dreams that can be made conscious, remembered, and described to others.

Thus, the explicit–symbolic mode does not *replace* the implicit–procedural mode but instead creates a new integrating thrust. Indeed, both modes of organizing experience are modes of integration and containment that shape and modify one another in a dialectical back and forth between immediacy and concreteness, and symbolization and multiple meanings. The integrating thrust of both modes contrasts with the discontinuity of experience and splitting of linkages that characterize the response to trauma (which I discuss in Chapter 4).

ATTACHMENT, REFLECTIVE FUNCTION, AND SYMBOLIC PROCESSING

Symbolic processing allows children to create increasingly complex stories about themselves or autobiographical narratives that rely on a different form of memory processing, the *explicit memory system* (Perner & Ruffman, 1995; Squire, 1987, 1992; Squire, Knowlton, & Musen,

1993). Explicit memory differs significantly from the implicit memory system that emerges earlier and forms the basis of concrete–procedural processing.

Like implicit memory, explicit memory is also based on a relatively homogeneous neurological and psychological system, one that involves the hippocampus and the medial temporal lobe. The explicit memory system, however, encodes information about *what* things are, compared to the implicit–procedural memory about *how* to do something. This memory of autobiographical events and factual knowledge *is accessible to conscious awareness* and is expressed through *verbal and symbolic referents*, instead of through "procedures," that is, perceptual–motoric strategies or affective discharges. Explicit memory opens a path for symbolic processing by permitting the separation and flexible combination and recombination of particular elements of objects and events from the schema in which such objects and events are grouped together.

Explicit memory stores details of specific events that build an individual's autobiography, which has the features of self and time. Once a particular bit of information becomes part of a person's autobiography, it tends no longer to be available as a separate, discrete entity, but instead tends to be actively transformed on the basis of associated and subsequent experiences. It is also transformed by frame of mind and context, including the meaning the individual ascribes to that context at the time of recall. Such autobiographical memory fits with Schachtel's (1947) definition of memory as a function of the personality that can be understood as the capacity for the organization and reconstruction of past experiences in the service of present needs, fears, and interests.

Explicit–autobiographical memories are the building blocks of the "narrativization" of experience (Siegel, 1999), that is, the creation of a sequential account that has the potential to be told verbally to others— and oneself—and that gives meaning and coherence to one's subjective experience. Siegel argues that creating an autobiographical narrative, a process that invariably is a coproduction involving intersubjective exchanges with attachment figures, is the way the brain's parallel processing of patterns of neuronal activation, which largely results in nonconscious processes, is transformed into a subjectively manageable and interpersonally useful process. As we see later, such autobiographical narrative is arguably a key not only to a sense of identity but also to affect regulation, the capacity to cope with trauma and vulnerability, and the ability to set goals, tolerate frustration, and accept limits.

A consideration of the nature of symbols is relevant to this discussion. Simply put, as Hobson (1993b) proposes, a symbol "refers to something or someone" (p. 171). But how do children come to create symbols that carry particular conception(s) of objects or events? For example, how does the word "juice" come to carry the conception of "juiciness" to refer to a category of liquids?

There is solid agreement that the "harmoniousness" of the mother–child relationship is a key contributor to the emergence of symbolic thought (Bretherton, Bates, Benigni, Camaioni, & Volterra, 1979), pointing to a link between attachment and symbolization. As noted earlier, Hobson (1993b) draws attention to the phenomenon of "social referencing" to illustrate how infants relate to another person's observable psychological reaction to visually shared objects and events.

The important point in social referencing is that the internal state of the infant in reference to an object or situation—such as a disconcerting "cliff"—is altered by the infant's "read" of the caregiver's internal state in reference to the cliff. The infant is thus relating not only to a perceptually specified world but also to another person's psychological relation to that same world. Infants can "triangulate" their own perception with their view of the other person's perception of the same object or event.

Bretherton (1991) has shown that between 6 and 18 months of age, children become increasingly able to "match" their caregiver's mental state in reference to an object, person, or situation. The crucial point in regard to the development of symbolic processing is that through such exchanges, infants acquire the recognition that given objects and events can have multiple, person-related meanings. Social referencing enables infants to see literally other people's orientation to the world. Out of such awareness, they begin to construct a sense of self in relation to others and of others in relation to the world. The door thus opens to the recognition of the distinction, as Hobson (1993b) points out,

> between the world-as-given, on the one hand, and the nature of persons who have potentially different psychological orientations, on the other. Here is the beginning distinction between "thought" (or at least "psychological attitude") and "thing." Before long, and perhaps as a result of recognizing this very distinction, the child comes to exercise his or her own powers as a "meaning-conferring" person, imparting new person-dependent meanings to objects in creative symbolic play. (p. 172)

Such creative, meaning-conferring capacities come to life in the domain of transitional objects and experiences, which Winnicott (1953) described as an intermediate area of experience between reality and fantasy, where reality can either be acknowledged or repudiated. The *process* by which children identify the impact of their caregiver's psychological orientation on their own internal state, particularly in relation to feeling soothed, comforted, and returned to a state of homeostasis, plays a key role in the acquisition of self-regulating capacities (Cicchetti & Tucker, 1994). Such identification is a prerequisite to the "assignment" of such psychological orientation—and its concomitant capacity to affect the children themselves—to objects and activities more under the children's control (e.g., a blanket or a teddy bear to which children can "assign" the caregiver's capacity to provide comfort at bedtime).

I concur with Fonagy, Steele, and Steele (1991), who hypothesized that secure attachment is a marker of the quality of the caregiver–infant relationship associated with the optimal opportunity for infants to "observe" their caregiver's mind, intentionality, and psychological orientation toward objects and events, as well as toward themselves.

The association between attachment security and reflective capacity was first suggested by Bowlby (1969), who recognized the significance of "the child's capacity both to conceive of his mother as having her own goals, and interests separate from his own, and to take them into account" (p. 368), a developmental step that he saw as emerging in the context of a secure attachment. In an investigation of Bowlby's assertion, Moss, Parent, and Gosselin (1995) reported that security of attachment with the mother was a good predictor of children's metacognitive capacity. Prospective studies by Fonagy and colleagues (1997) demonstrated the strong relationship between children's secure attachment to mother at 12 months and to father at 18 months, and their capacity to pass "theory of mind" tests at 5½ years. Of 92 children assessed at 12 months in relation to their mothers, 64% of those classified as secure passed a test of reflective function 4½ years later, whereas 67% of those classified as insecure failed the same test. Of the infants classified as secure with father at 18 months, 77% also passed the test. The possibility of an additive relationship between secure relationships was suggested by the fact that 83% of children with *two* secure relationships passed the test, while only 60% of those with *one* secure relationship successfully performed the reflective task. This and other studies (e.g., Meins, Fernyhough, Russell, & Clark-Carter, 1998) confirm that security of attachment is powerfully linked to symbolic capacities in general and to reflective function in particular.

What is the source of this association? Two synergistic processes appear to explain this developmental link. First, security of attachment serves as an indicator of an interpersonal context that is more likely to provide children with the social–developmental opportunities that indirectly promote symbolic functioning and reflective capacities. Second, security of attachment may be a marker of the quality of the caregiver–infant relationship that *directly* facilitates the development of reflective function (Jenkins & Astington, 1996). As noted earlier, securely attached children have easier access to experiences that foster symbolization and reflective function, namely, *play and pretense*, *peer interactions*, and *talking*—both talking specifically about mental states and using language in general.

One crucial contribution of secure attachment to the development of reflective function seems based on infants' confident expectation that they are effective in bringing about an appropriate response from the environment (e.g., that others will eventually be responsive). This expectation, of course, results from repeated experiences of regulation and positive affect that follow the infants' signaling of distress to their caregivers.

Sroufe's (1983, 1989, 1996) prospective developmental studies and observations suggest that the experience of competence in eliciting responses and reestablishing inner regulation leads to *other* social–developmental opportunities. As an illustration, Sroufe relates an incident at the Minnesota Preschool Project, where several children were dancing to recorded music. When other children arrived, one of them approached a dancing child and asked to join the dance. When the child said no, the child who had made the request withdrew to a corner to sulk. Another child then entered the room and also asked to join the dance; he was also turned down. This child, however, persisted until he located a child who agreed to let him in. The second child, who had a history of secure attachment, showed far less evidence of feeling rejected, but instead modeled a persistence presumably borne out of the conviction that he was worthy and that others would ultimately be responsive. A similar persistence and hopeful expectation were displayed by the girl who wished to join in playing house in the sandbox, as described in Chapter 2.

A wealth of research confirms this observation: Children who are securely attached in infancy carry forward an image of themselves as worthy and effective, and an image of others as available and valuable. These children are consistently found to be more enthusiastic, more confident in solving problems, and more open in their approach to the environment; they are also more curious, independent, self-possessed, and capable of skillfully using their teacher's help (Sroufe, 1989).

Several points can be made about these studies. First, it is clear that securely attached children are primed to take advantage of social and developmental opportunities that in turn foster the development of symbolic and reflective capacities. Second, as securely attached children's symbolic and reflective capacities develop, they begin to *generalize* expectations from one set of relationships to others. Thus, the person-specific responses characteristic of the attachment patterns at age 1 are replaced by more generalized patterns of relatedness with associated expectations and attitudes at age 3. Third, proto-narrative envelopes and internal working models serve the function initially of *anticipating* reality (at 2–4 months of age) and then of *coping* with reality during the second half of the first year of life. But by age 3, children demonstrate a tendency to *organize* reality to conform to their expectations.

Thus, as in Sroufe's preschool dance, securely attached children persist until they obtain an interpersonal response that matches their sense of worth and of other people's eventual positive response. In this fashion, earlier patterns of dyadic organization begin to forecast specific patterns of subsequent adaptation (e.g., the organization of coping strategies, expectations, behaviors, feelings, and relationships that *create* experience by evoking particular responses from the environment). But while these mediating experiences may be a critical catalyst in the development of reflective function, the foundation of this developmental acquisition is more likely to be built *directly* on the bedrock of the caregiver–infant relationship.

Fonagy, Steele, Steele, and colleagues (1991) have demonstrated that both mothers and fathers with a high reflective capacity, as assessed *before* their child's birth, were three to four times more likely to have securely attached infants than were parents with a low reflective capacity. The assessment of caregivers' reflective function predicts their children's security of attachment, independent of the parents' own early deprivation. In one follow-up study (Steele et al., 1996), mothers were divided according to the degree of their childhood deprivation. *All* the children of deprived mothers with high reflective capacity were securely attached to their mothers, while *almost none* of the children of deprived mothers with low reflective function ratings showed a pattern of secure attachment to their mothers.

This evidence suggests that the key to children's development of secure attachment *and* reflective function is the moment-to-moment capacity of the caregiver to nonconsciously conceive of the full range of the infant's internal states; that is, caregivers must strive to maintain a reflective stance in spite of stress or other changes in the infant's mental state or in the state of the caregiver–infant relationship. And when, inevitably, they fail, they must seek fairly rapidly to repair the breakdowns in reflective function that occur in the course of everyday life. Unfortunately, some caregivers consistently are unable to retain a reflective perspective under various circumstances, such as when their infants become distressed, seek proximity, or strive for autonomy or mastery.

Arguably, children's experience of being treated as an intentional being in multiple, diverse internal states and dyadic transactions (e.g., when feeling distressed and in need of self-regulation, when joyfully sharing a playful mood, when venturing to explore a new environment, when the caregiver is tired, happy, frustrated, or eager to respond) is the fundamental developmental trigger of their reflective capacity. This trigger operates through several interrelated mechanisms to link their children's safety, pleasure, and self-regulation with their experience of someone understanding their behavior on the basis of their underlying intentions, affects, and wishes. Caregivers' reflective function also serves to release children's reflective capacity by signaling that, by and large, internal states are safe for exploration and reflection. Moreover, caregivers trigger children's reflective function by providing a model of "mind reading" as a particularly effective way to transform distress into safety and regulation, to enhance pleasure and mastery, and to strengthen human connections.

The pervasive, nonconscious, moment-to-moment capacity of caregivers to conceive of infants' internal states thus permits children to conceive of *themselves* as intentional beings, in addition to opening the path to their capacity to read the minds of others. As Winnicott (1967) and others have pointed out, it is in the face (i.e., mind) of the mother that infants find an image of themselves as mindful, intentional beings.

DEVELOPMENT AND REFLECTIVE FUNCTION

Becoming Human: Empathy, Intersubjectivity, and Self-Agency

The mythical "test" that identifies an individual as an "undead" yet not alive vampire is the being's failure to produce a reflection in a mirror. The ability to see ourselves reflected in other people's eyes and our reciprocal capacity to reflect other people's internal states in our own mind creates a bond of shared feelings and empathy with others that requires no conscious reflection. Reflective function serves to integrate explicit–symbolic processing about the self in relationships with implicit–procedural relational knowledge. This integration allows people, on meeting others, to engage in active mutual regulation of their own and others' states, which forms the basis of smooth, back-and-forth communication and the creation of shared meanings.

Between 3 and 5 years of age, children develop reflective–symbolic capacities that enable them to advance to a qualitatively different level of psychological organization. This new level is based on the ability to conceptualize the implications of one's own feelings, thoughts, and intentions toward one person from the point of view of a third person. Likewise, children can now conceptualize for *themselves* the implications of the feelings, thoughts, and intentions that a person to whom they are attached has for a third person. This realization, as Britton (1989, 1992) pointed out, is not simply an enlargement of awareness and knowledge, but is instead a fundamental disruption of the child's psychological world. This qualitative change in reflective function effectively transforms the child's world from a dyadic to a triangular and then a multifaceted one.

For Britton and other modern Kleinian thinkers, such psychic reorganization is an outgrowth of the depressive position, that is, the acquisition of the capacity to recognize that multiple, contradictory affects such as love and hate can be directed at the same person. This occurs as children gain awareness that the other person has continuity of existence over time, space, and situation—continuity not influenced by changes in the children's own internal states.

Britton (1989, 1992) makes the crucial point that this integration of experience is essential to accepting disappointment and frustration and to recognizing the difference between aspiration and expectation. In turn, these distinctions permit children to appreciate the difference between the psychic and the material. In the absence of such a capacity, children experience frustration as a concrete, physical state that can be eliminated only through physical action. This situation is the same one that Segal (1981) described as the failure of symbolization that results in "symbolic equations," that is, in new objects and events being experienced as identical to the original objects and events.

The disruption of the children's existing psychic world, brought about by their unfolding reflective–symbolic capacities, enables them to enter into that cauldron of passions and complexity that the psychoanalytic literature describes as the Oedipus complex. Britton's (1989, 1992) formulation implicitly suggests that what is most important about the oedipal situation is *not* the specific content of children's mental states but rather their very capacity to conceive simultaneously of several psychic realities. Thus, oedipal children can both conceptualize and tolerate the conceptualization of a caregiver as not only someone they sometimes love and sometimes hate, but also as someone who is at times nurturing and gratifying and at times frustrating and punitive. Children can also see caregivers as people who have relationships with other people from which they are excluded.

From this vantage point, children are prepared to construct a more complex autobiographical narrative that can encompass the multiplicity of feelings and roles that they encounter in the broader social world outside the family. A crucial development in this respect is the evolution of defensive adaptations. Increasingly, children become able to shift attention away from the content of particular mental states. The prototype of this type of defensive adaptation is repression. These defense mechanisms are directed at experience that has been processed in a reflective–symbolic fashion. In contrast, earlier defensive adaptations are directed not at particular mental states but rather at the blotting out of a way of mental functioning, one that involves reflective function. This defensive adaptation, modeled on the dissociative response to trauma, described in Chapter 4, consists of the inhibition of reflective or symbolic functioning. Repression does not require an inhibition of the reflective–symbolic function but instead preserves the capacity to stay connected with others and to engage in intersubjective regulation.

The developmental literature documents the links between secure attachment, reflective function, and social competence afforded by an evolution of coping strategies that permit the preservation of a reflective stance. Sroufe's (1996, 1997) prospective studies show that both preschoolers and school-age children with a history of secure attachment are more engaged with their peers and more capable of responding to others' bids for interaction. These children develop deeper relationships and show a greater capacity to recognize others' feelings. They demonstrate concern for reciprocity and fairness, and they are considerate of other children; for example, they avoid taking advantage of them (Block & Block, 1980). Sroufe (1996, 1997) concludes that securely attached children have a history of empathic (reflective) responsiveness, from which they internalize the capacity and the disposition to be empathic themselves.

Arguably, reflective function serves the evolutionary "purpose" of permitting human beings to exist in communities and social groups with relative concern for one another's welfare. The pervasiveness of violence, brutality, and lack of concern that humans have exhibited throughout history in all cultures attests to the vulnerability of a reflective perspective. As I discuss in Chapter 4, reflective function is normally inhibited under conditions of intense arousal and the fight-or-flight response. For most people, however, the failure of reflective function and of the capacity to conceive of others as human beings is an intermittent phenomenon. In Chapters 4, 5, and 6, I discuss how reflective function is selectively and intermittently *inhibited* in children and adolescents in response to internal or external cues. It is worth mentioning at this point, however, that *anyone* can lose reflective functioning under the "right" circumstances, activating the fight-or-flight response. The truly horrifying message derived from documented human atrocities, from the Holocaust to the "killing fields" of Cambodia, to the "ethnic cleansing" of Bosnia and Kosovo, to the mutilation of children in Sierra Leone, is indeed, as Hannah Arendt (1994) pointed out, the banality of such evil. Ordinary human beings can turn into "monsters" unable to conceive of others' humanity—and thus able to treat others not as individual human beings but as "things," "enemies," "Jews," or "Muslims," who can be gassed, mutilated, raped, or "reeducated."

For most ordinary people, such a transformation occurs in a context that drowns reflective–symbolic processing under a cacophony of concrete procedural "noise" and triggers the fight-or-flight response. Under conditions of intense emotionality and a heightened sense of collective threat, coupled with a pressure to act and a shared vision of the other as belonging to a concrete category, reflective capacity is frequently inhibited, even in people who, up to that moment, were regularly empathic. The frightful implications of such transformations—that anyone can become an inhuman monster—might serve to evoke a measure of empathy for the plight of children with severe personality disorders. It should also stand as a warning sign to clinicians venturing into the treacherous terrain of their treatment: Buffeted by the implicit–procedural pressures that are the currency of relatedness of these children, even well-trained clinicians will find themselves compelled to shut off their ability to conceive of others' minds reflectively.

This loss or inhibition of reflective function carries with it a loss of the sense of ownership over one's own behavior, a feature common to persons participating in atrocities: Their behavior seems to have "happened" to them. In contrast, as we saw earlier, reflective capacity is key to developing and maintaining a sense of agency. Stern (1995) describes how infants' sense of agency begins with their recognition that they are the authors of their intended actions. "Instrumental crying" at 3 months is an example of such goal-oriented behavior. Yet, as Ainsworth and Bell (1974) and Sander (1975) point out, given infants' physical and cognitive limitations, their ability to carry out their intentionality and thus acquire the beginnings of ownership over their behavior depends on the presence of alert, "mind-reading," responsive caregivers.

The recognition of internal states of intentionality by caregivers appears critical in making infants' intentions "real" for them. The self-as-agent is built on the foundation of transactions with reflective others that promote the inner sense that our behavior results from our own decisions, wishes, thoughts, feelings, and intentions. Such an inner sense gives us the capacity to "contemplate" these mental states relatively unburdened by threat or anxiety. On the other hand, when reflective function breaks down, we find ourselves deprived of a capacity to experience our actions as truly belonging to us; thus, we are cut off from the bond of shared humanity that allows us to recognize ourselves in others and others in ourselves.

Self-Regulation: Limit-Setting and Direction-Giving Systems and Self-Esteem

Self-agency, reflective function, and symbolic capacities weave together the fabric of an increasingly richer matrix of autobiographical narratives during the third and fourth years of life. Among other things, this matrix mediates the translation of needs, impulses, wishes, and whims into

action. Normally, the experience of intention grows from the capacity first to inhibit the expression of impulses into action. The impulse, need, or wish—whichever motivational state initiates behavior—commands or fails to command attention, then gains or loses significance as it is balanced against and integrated into more enduring aims, values, motivational constellations, and representations of the self and the self in relation with others (i.e., the evolving autobiographical narrative). It is as if the person were to "ask" him- or herself, "How does this wish of the moment fit with what is going on in my life; with my goals, ideals, and relationships; with who I think I am; and with what I wish to become in the future?"

Such processing, often conducted outside conscious awareness, allows the momentary urge to act to be suppressed, delayed in its expression, turned away from awareness, or modified so that it can become a more acceptable or better fit. Alternatively, the impulse can be given access to action and woven smoothly into the experience of "what belongs to the self." This very processing boosts the sense of agency and decision, and contributes to the ongoing evolution of the person's autobiographical story.

The autobiographical narrative builds on the concrete–procedural schemas that dominate mental life during the first year of life. With increasingly complex symbolic representation, this narrative provides children with what Erikson (1959) calls a sense of "me-ness," which is subjectively experienced by school age, if not before, as cohesive and continuous over time. Children have a sense of "I am me, the same that I was yesterday and am likely to be tomorrow," which is relatively independent of their feelings of the moment, the state of their relationships with others, or their awareness of their own developmental changes.

In contrast, as we will see later, children with severe personality disorders typically experience a pervasive sense of a lack of genuineness, continuity, or coherence. In Chapter 5, I discuss the development of, and the maladaptive consequences for, children with severe personality disorders of the "false self" (Winnicott, 1965), the feeling of hidden defectiveness, incompleteness, and phoniness. Some consequences can be gleaned by examining the role of a coherent sense of self—a relatively well-integrated autobiographical narrative—in the development of self-regulating functions.

The emerging coherence of the self, pointed out earlier, serves as a matrix into which to incorporate new capacities. This incorporation occurs as children "triangulate" their conception of their caregivers' *conceiving of them* as capable of executing the homeostatic, regulating functions performed by the caregivers and their own mental model of themselves actually executing those self-regulating functions.

The reflective stance of caregivers enables them to envision capacities in their infants that are not yet present but are likely to emerge soon. Caregivers in tune with their infants' emerging capacities align themselves with what Vygotsky (1962) calls "the infant's proximal zone of development." Irwin Rosen (personal communication, March 27, 1990) characterizes caregivers operating in this zone as a sort of "Panasonic mother," a reference to that corporation's advertising promise to be "just slightly ahead of its time." Most likely, caregivers' interpretation and treatment of their infants, as if they had already become what they are only *about* to become, promotes the organizational changes occurring within the infants.

Kierkegaard (1938) beautifully described this capacity of caregivers to encourage their children to take that developmental step forward for which they are almost ready:

> The loving mother teaches her child to walk alone. She is far enough from him so that she cannot actually support him, but she holds out her arms to him. She anticipates his movements, and if he totters, she swiftly bends as if to seize him, so that the child might believe that he is not walking alone . . . and yet she does more. Her face beckons like a reward, an encouragement. Thus, the child walks alone with his eyes fixed on his mother's face, *not* on the difficulties in his way. He supports himself by the arms that do *not* hold him and constantly strives toward the refuge in his mother's embrace, little suspecting that in the very same moment that he is emphasizing his need of her, he is proving that he can do without her, because he is walking alone. (cited in Mahler et al., 1975, p. 72)

I would argue that the child's eyes, "fixed on his [or her] mother's face," allow the child to grasp the caregiver's belief and acceptance of his or her capacity for independent locomotion. Caregivers' attunement with children's emerging capacities—and the pride and acceptance children evoke in their caregivers when they demonstrate increasing mastery and autonomy (which normally coalesce with the maturational burst in cognition, language, and independent locomotion during the second and third years of life)—prominently includes the blossoming of reflective and symbolic functioning. Such convergence provides children with an extraordinary new tool for achieving mastery, self-regulation, and experiential coherence, and for creating far richer representational models of themselves in relationship with others.

The growing development of reflective–symbolic functioning allows children increasingly to replace their need to observe directly the caregiver's conception of them as capable (i.e., the eyes fixed on the parent's face) with *symbolic models* that they can "triangulate" with their own conception of their abilities as they seek to master and respond to adaptive challenges. Using a mental model of how to perform self-regulating functions as a road map, children can compare and seek to match the representation of their *actual* self with the model. Joffe and Sandler (1967) refer to these models as the "ideal self." Accordingly, the ideal self is the "shape" of a self-representation associated with or encompassing a sense of safety, competence, satisfaction, and optimal connection with others. The ideal self thus conjures up experiences of mastery, experiential integration, and ability to meet adaptive demands. Such an ideal self transacts pleasurably with available and reflective others. The effort to match the ideal self is arguably an elaboration of the contingency-seeking mechanism described earlier as instrumental in achieving self-agency and an orientation toward the social world. Both of these aspects of development serve as the underpinnings of this process of anticipation and preparation for further growth and mastery.

What are the building blocks of the ideal self? According to Joffe and Sandler (1967), the ideal self is a composite of (1) memories of actual experiences of pleasure, mastery, and satisfaction (with particular emphasis on memories of successfully evoking caregiver responses that led to restored regulation and well-being); (2) fantasies about such experiences (which become increasingly more elaborate as reflective–symbolic capacities grow and allow for more elaborate reconfiguration of experience, thus serving adaptive and defensive purposes); and (3) the models provided by other people who are loved, feared, or admired (models derived not only from these persons' outward behavior but also from the children's own "reading" of other people's mental states). Children's reflective capacities allow them to build a mental representation of their own characteristics, the actual self, a representation significantly built as the basis of inner sensations and perceptions of the self, and the myriad verbal and nonverbal messages given to children, consciously and unconsciously, that convey other people's conception of them. The actual self serves as a matrix to seek "self-like" objects

(Tyson, 1982) as models to construct the ideal self. An example of this representational composite is found in the following vignette.

> A 2½-year-old boy protests loudly when his parents, both busy profession-als, leave on certain evenings to attend "meetings." The parents, attempt-ing to comfort their child, and driven as much by guilt as by empathy, tell him, "We have to go to a meeting, dear, but when you wake up, we will be back." A few weeks later, the boy is happily riding up and down the drive-way on his brand-new tricycle. "I'm going to a meeting," he proudly an-nounces to his father. Rather sheepishly, the father replies, "Great, Johnny, have fun." The father's endorsement, however, only elicits the child's scorn. "No, no, Daddy," the child chides his father with exasperation, "cry!" When the chastised father finally "gets it" and "weeps" in distress, the child trium-phantly says, "It's OK, Daddy, when you wake up, I'll be back."

This vignette illustrates how a model derived from the child's re-flective capacity to put himself in his parents' shoes serves as a blueprint to guide children's efforts to reverse states of helplessness and passivity, and to reestablish self-regulation, safety, mastery, pleasure, and a sense of connectedness. (See Chapter 4 for a review of the significance of these processes.) In this vignette, the child is no longer the one being left but is instead the one leaving. Rather than being the recipient of the comforting, he is the one attempting to soothe. The mental representa-tion of the ideal self provides an internal model that children can at-tempt to match or approximate. In the process, they gain new adaptive capacities and tools to relate more effectively with others.

According to Joffe and Sandler (1967), a particular form of vulnera-bility, *narcissistic* vulnerability, results from the "mismatch" or incon-gruence between the ideal self and the actual self. The actual self is roughly equivalent to the person's autobiographical narrative, that is, the conscious and unconscious sense that individuals have of their characteristics, history, relationships, capacities, and ability to respond to adaptive demands. The tendency toward experiential coherence and contingency seeking we have observed as a constant theme of mental functioning now encompasses both external and internal reality (i.e., the match between the model of what the world is expected to be and what the world turns out to be), as well as the match between the actual and the ideal self.

From a subjective standpoint, narcissistic vulnerability thus refers to a painful state of self-appraisal, whose affective correlate is the feeling of shame. Narcissistic vulnerability, as we see later, is a crucial component in the maladjustment of children and adolescents with a severe personality disorder. Shame, as the prototypical affect of narcissistic vulnerability, reflects the sense of deflation accompanying the inability to measure up to an ideal.

On the other hand, narcissistic well-being or *self-esteem* results from the successful shaping of the actual self to approximate the ideal self. The "incentives" to match the ideal are fueled by interpersonal validation and greater proximity with caregivers. Their pride and pleasure in children's approximation to their own ideals, which normally also reflect the caregivers' ideals because they are based on how children think their parents view them, promote children's identificatory efforts while also bringing children and caregivers closer together. Again, self-regulation and attachment, or in psychoanalytic terminology, narcissistic regulation and object relations, potentiate each other in a developmental process in which intrapsychic models and interpersonal context are constantly shaping, modifying, and reinforcing one another.

In order for this identificatory process to promote growth and adaptation, two conditions must be met:

1. The model provided by the ideal self must be "reachable" by the child, using actual and potential capabilities and real attributes. The ideal self in effect *partially replaces* the "checking" with the caregiver (i.e., social referencing) and the reliance on the caregiver's attunement to the child's emerging capacities as the "proximal area of development"; that is, the ideal becomes a preview of the person the child is about to become.
2. Successful matching or approximation of the ideal self results in better self-esteem *and* interpersonal validation. A parent, for example, will serve as an effective model only when that model proves "reachable" and the child experiences it as regarded by others as worthy and competent. Parental pride and pleasure in children's identificatory efforts greatly reinforce the positive affective coloring and the narcissistic value associated with the self becoming more like the ideal (see Figure 3.1).

Every step in development, which inevitably includes maturational changes and new psychosocial demands, opens anew the "gap" of narcissistic vulnerability. Self-esteem regulation is not a developmental task "settled" at any particular stage in life. The ideal self (when reflective–symbolic functioning is available) is constantly reshaped on the basis of

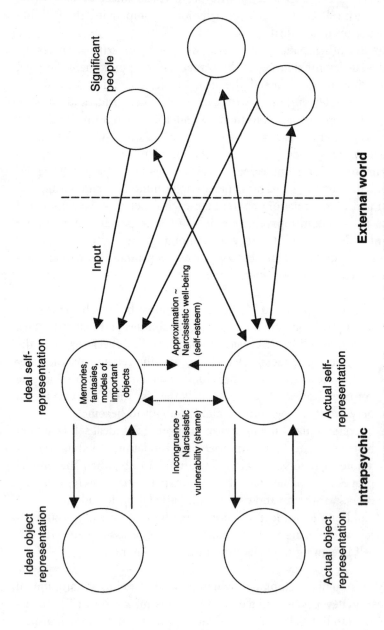

FIGURE 3.1. Regulation of narcissistic well-being/self-esteem.

newly created and *shared* meanings, and the reconfiguration of the models of the past. Using the ideal self as a map in life's journey permits us to reshape the self-representation (i.e., the autobiographical narrative) in order to find new solutions to life's dilemmas, to explore different ways of being in the world and relating to others, and to attempt behaviors and attitudes that promise greater mastery, better connection with others, more effective coping, and increased pleasure and adaptation.

Play serves as a prominent way to anticipate the future. While play can serve multiple developmental and defensive purposes, one important aspect of play is as an experiment in which "anticipatory" identifications (Alvarez, 1992) are tried. As Vygotsky (1978, p. 102) pointed out, "In play, a child always behaves beyond his average age, above his daily behavior; in play it is as though he were a head taller than himself. As in the focus of a magnifying glass, play contours all developmental tendencies in a contoured form and is a major service of development." Play and the efforts to match an ideal self become the children's proximal zone of development, performing internally the facilitating function caregivers had performed in the past. In this process, children seem to internalize the capacity of the caregivers to conceive of them as taking the developmental step for which they are almost ready.

Kernberg (1976) described the progressive abstraction that takes place in the ideal self in healthy development as it becomes not only an effective direction-giving system but also a limit-setting psychological system. Although this system remains open to interpersonal influences, it becomes somewhat depersonified and relatively autonomous from external validation and reinforcement.

The following exchange illustrates the principles involved in internalizing the limit-setting and direction-giving functions of caregivers:

> Three-year-old Billy has been told repeatedly that his favorite snack is available only after dinner. One day he experiences an acute longing for the special succor that only the favorite morsel can bring. As a result, he attempts—unsuccessfully—to seduce his mother into breaking the family rule. When mother is unmoved by his charm, he himself ends the exchange by loudly declaring, "Billy, you cannot have fruit bars before dinnertime!"

Effective limits that are based not only on stopping the children from misbehaving but also on a reflective view of the underlying internal state promote children's use of mental models to acquire a self-limiting capacity. As we will see later, a failure to "internalize" limits often stems from caregivers who react procedurally and automatically to their children's behavior, with *no* reflective connection to the mental state behind it. Such "coercive cycles" (Patterson, 1982), aimed at squelching behavior, only further alienate children from the internal sources of their own behavior and thus from the psychological mechanisms that produce self-regulation.

On the other hand, "reflective" limit setting promotes children's capacity to understand what goes on in the caregiver's mind when setting limits. Children can then use this conception of the caregiver's mind as a model to establish their own limit-setting capacity. Eventually, no loud declaration will have to reach the children's ears—even from the children themselves—because a silent psychological process will replace it. By the end of adolescence, more abstract principles, rules, and values (e.g., self-restraint, healthy habits) will replace the internal representation of a parent admonishing the child to wait until after dinnertime to indulge his or her cravings.

In summary, from the bedrock of concrete, procedural "working" models, reflective–symbolic processing guides the development of representational models of the self in relation to others (i.e., autobiographical narratives with both conscious and unconscious aspects). As children acquire the capacity to "read" their own—as well as other people's—behavior in terms of underlying mental states, they become able to flexibly activate or combine in a new configuration the self–other representation(s) best suited to respond adaptively to particular demands. These self–other representations derive from the multiple sets of such representations contained in a child's autobiographical narrative, that is, built and constantly reshaped by reflective–symbolic functioning, and underlie the capacities for affect regulation, impulse control, self-monitoring, and the experience of self-agency (the building blocks of self-regulation). Thus, by the time children are 4 or 5, they possess the psychological organization of coping, experiencing, and relating patterns of a developing personality.

From Dyadic to Triangular Relationships and Beyond

The oedipal situation, as described earlier, is based on the psychological revolution introduced by the capacity to conceive simultaneously of several interacting psychic realities. For both boys and girls, longing for the love and attention of the same-sex parent coexists with competitive feelings toward that parent. Boys with overbearing mothers and/or distant or devalued fathers will have difficulty seeing their father as a role model. Boys also can retreat to an identification with the mother that is spurred by fear of being hurt in competition with a harsh father, by guilty feelings of damaging a weak and ineffectual father, and/or by concern about losing control in the face of an overly seductive mother. Girls, on the other hand, may find themselves struggling with their feminine identification, particularly if the feminine model is associated with early frustration, misattunement, or a sense of inadequacy related to being a woman.

Normally, however, boys compete with the father yet long for his company, enjoy his love and attention, and admire his skills and competence. Girls' competitiveness with their mothers coexists with a persistent dependence on mother, wishes for her love and companionship, and admiration of her as a role model. Children's investment in preserving and deepening their identification with the same-sex parent is reinforced by their fears of retaliation for their erotic and hostile wishes, and their desire for exclusive possession of the other-sex parent, as well as their feelings of guilt and shame associated with those wishes and their feelings of narcissistic mortification. Both boys and girls find it painful and frustrating that guilt, fear of retaliation, and their own limitations conspire against the possibility of actualizing oedipal fantasies. Thus, children are thrust into relinquishing their desire to possess exclusively the other-sex parent and instead begin to seek alternatives to their oedipal strivings that seem more attainable—and that may close the gap of narcissistic vulnerability, allowing for the preservation of attachments to both caregivers and assuaging feelings of guilt, shame, vulnerability, and fear.

The change from a dyadic reflective perspective to a triangular one is crucial in this evolution. The capacity of both boys and girls to set up the same-sex parent as a model of identification is predicated not only on the relationship of children to the same-sex parent but also on parents' comfort with their femininity or masculinity, with the relationship of each parent to the other, and with the value each parent places on the child's relationship with the other-sex parent.

Obviously, identification with the other-sex parent and a strong attachment to the same-sex parent play a major part in building the ideal self. These identifications, however, are often strongly defined during school age and early adolescence, particularly by boys, whose peer culture punishes with narcissistic mortification and ostracism any hint of effeminacy. Such identification surfaces, however, in the struggles and conflicts of adolescents with closeness, intimacy, and sexuality. It also makes possible the development of mature relationships. As Tyson (1982) points out, men eventually accept and encourage the femininity of their lovers, wives, and daughters. Women can similarly learn to conceive reflectively and to nurture the masculinity of their mates, husbands, and sons.

The development of reflective–symbolic capacity helps children find a solution to their oedipal dilemma. The acquisition of gender stability (Kohlberg, 1966), that is, the knowledge that boys become men and girls become women, is grounded not only in cognitive maturation but also in an ability to grasp the subjective world of caregivers and their representation of how to navigate the transformation from childhood to adulthood. Such knowledge builds the inner conviction of a possible future, when boys (in identification with their fathers) can become fathers themselves and have a woman like their mother, and girls (in identification with their mothers) can become mothers and have a man like their father.

Children's growing reflective–symbolic capacity affords them the ability to put emotional and cognitive distance from their awareness of experiences that are emotionally painful, conflictive, or anxiety producing; that is, the children become capable of repression. Repression contrasts with earlier modes of defensive adaptation, which are, as we review in the next chapter, based on the prototype of the fight-or-flight response (i.e., the psychobiologically prepared response) to trauma or threat. This response comprises hyperarousal, numbness, and a tendency to dissociate, as well as a "shutting off" of reflective–symbolic functioning. Repression, on the other hand, while creating a cognitive–affective distance, allows for the preservation of reflective–symbolic functioning and the consideration of multiple, person-related meanings.

Repression paves the way for higher-level defensive adaptations (A. Freud, 1936/1966; Kernberg, 1976), such as reaction formation, sublimation, or displacement, that serve to "dispose" of unacceptable or threatening mental content without suspending symbolic and reflective processing. Such adaptive capacities, in turn, coalesce with children's greater cognitive abilities and the motivational thrust—based, in part, on defensive needs—to expand their social horizons beyond the family. By school age, peers and other adults become attachment figures and alternative sources of support and identification. The adaptive tasks of the wider world of school and peers evolve into increasingly important regulators of narcissistic well-being and form a crucial context in which to define identity.

The growing use of repression and, more generally, of symbolic processing allows children, as noted earlier, increasingly to abstract the direction-giving and limit-setting functions contained within the ideal self. As a result, a process of depersonification (Kernberg, 1976) and symbolic integration takes place. Under optimal conditions, by mid- to late school age, rules and prohibitions become more flexible, functional, and abstract.

Adolescence, Narcissistic Vulnerability, and Pathological Narcissistic Regulation

The vicissitudes of narcissistic vulnerability and normal and pathological narcissistic regulation come into sharp focus during the passage through adolescence. The confusion and contradictions that pervade the psychological world of the adolescent are perhaps surpassed only by the formulations created to explain them. Psychoanalytic writers (e.g., Blos, 1967; A. Freud, 1958) state that psychic turmoil and regression are not only normative but also essential for healthy development. Such emphasis led Adelson and Doehrman (1980) to quip that, in the psychoanalytic literature, the adolescent is depicted as "miraculously holding on to his sanity, but doing so only by undertaking prodigies of defense" (p. 105). From this vantage point, it may be difficult to differentiate the normative—and necessary—crises of adolescence from the symptomatic manifestations of disturbed youth.

On the other hand, the psychological literature waxes eloquent on adolescents' relentless expansion of cognitive, normal, social, and adaptive capacities. The view from this perspective reveals young people mostly committed to a quest for truth, intolerant of adult hypocrisy, and feeling passionately and intensely about relationships and ideals.

The paradoxes of adolescent development can be better appreciated through the window of narcissistic regulation and narcissistic vulnerability. Perhaps like no other phase of life, the passage through adolescence bears the telltale signs of narcissistic vulnerability: a proneness to embarrassment and shame, acute self-consciousness and shyness, and painful questions about self-esteem and self-worth. How is this vulnerability different from pathological narcissism?

The sources of the heightened narcissistic vulnerability of adolescence are not hard to discern. Biological, cognitive, emotional, sexual, and psychosocial changes impose a complex array of adaptive demands that adolescents feel ill equipped to master and integrate. The very core of the self requires reorganization, because the youngster has to integrate dramatic neurohormonal and physical changes, heightened sexuality and newly acquired reproductive capacities, and profoundly transformed affective experience and cognitive capabilities.

Reflective function and the associated capacities of sense of self and others, and of sense of agency and self-regulating capacities, are compromised by the transformation of adolescence, which complicates the integration of aspects of the self-experience and challenges the capacity to grasp other people's states of mind. The adolescent's ability to grasp the internal states of others, particularly those of other adults and most especially those of caregivers, is eroded by a growing need to disengage from the parent, as both a real and an internal presence.

This need for disengagement is fueled by progressive pressures to emancipate and gain greater autonomy and self-reliance, which stem, in turn, from psychosocial demands and expectations, and from the adolescent's own forward thrust. Disengagement from one's parents is also grounded in a defensive need to distance from the real as well as the internalized image of the parents that is associated with regressive longings for dependency, threats to personal boundaries and autonomy, and reactivated conflicts from all stages of development.

The regressive pulls of adolescence are not generated by the adolescent's internal changes alone (Bleiberg, 1988). The caregivers are also changing. They are often aroused by, and envious of, the energy and attractiveness of these youngsters, who are freshly facing the excitement of intimate relationships, erotic passion, and life's possibilities. The caregivers, on the other hand, must contend with the decline of their strength and vigor, and come to terms (however painfully) with life's limitations that mark middle age. At no other point in life, except adolescence, is the gap between the actual self and the ideal self as painfully wide as in middle age.

Regressive and defensive pulls in the caregivers will potentiate adolescents' regressive and defensive tendencies, and vice versa. As Adelson and Doehrman (1980) have pointed out: "The child's nubility may awaken conflicted, unconscious emotions of rivalry and desire, along with a sense of time's passing and the waning of one's own power and beauty. One will often discern, even in households characterized by self-control, a certain amount of semiconscious, semierotic 'gesturing' between parents and their adolescent children" (p. 105).

The adolescent's moves to distance from the parents and their internal representations thus come from both progressive pressures and defensive pursuits. In time, such distancing diminishes the effectiveness and authority of the parents as models incorporated into the adolescent's ideal self. The power of these models is also under attack from the adolescent's recently acquired critical capacities. Using only thoughts and words, adolescents can project themselves mentally into the future (the realm of the possible), and, in so doing, can explore the full range of possibilities inherent in a problem. As Anthony (1982) has explained, new categorizing and argumentative language emerges, with adolescents subjecting their own and other people's beliefs to systematic scrutiny and criticism. Such scrutiny regularly exposes the inconsistencies and contradictions of parental values, ideals, and behavior.

Thus, adolescents are uncertain about who they are. They feel torn between progressive and regressive trends, and are bereft of a clear road map to guide their transition into adulthood. Although many adolescents welcome a moratorium on this journey (Erikson, 1959, 1968), they are also aware of the relentless psychosocial and developmental demands on them to separate from their family, to find an independent niche in the world, and to engage in sexual and emotional intimacy.

Clearly, one of the central developmental tasks of adolescence is the creation of a new direction-giving, self-esteem-regulating system (Wolf, Gedo, & Terman, 1972). This task is not beyond the reach of normal adolescents. For them, the self-regulating functions and capacities that were internalized during childhood have achieved a significant degree of depersonalization. Self-soothing, limit-setting, direction-giving functions are far less bound to the internal presence of a parent. Thus, normal adolescents can contemplate disengagement from their internalized parents without concomitantly finding themselves bereft of their self-regulating capacity.

Furthermore, in spite of squabbles and conflicts with parents, and the reorganization of internal relationships, normal adolescence does not require a total cutoff from parental figures. In healthy development, youngsters typically manage to construct mental representations of their parents that are imbued with love and respect. Parents, in general, provide their children with reasonably competent models for their efforts to negotiate reality and so are experienced as generally supportive of their children's growth and autonomy. Thus, normal adolescents maintain basically good relationships with both their real and their intrapsychic parents.

Normal adolescents build an ideal self by selectively using their own memories, fantasies, parental models, and new extrafamilial objects of their expanding world. They construct an internal ideal that matches their real talents and characteristics, and the realities of their physical and social world. In other words, adolescents are normally not subjected to extreme narcissistic vulnerability. They can build a reflective–symbolic mental model of an achievable future, and they can take steps to approximate their own ideals, resulting in greater competence, self-esteem, and adaptation.

In contrast, as I discuss in Chapters 5 and 6, youngsters whose previous solutions to narcissistic vulnerability are grounded in the illusion of omnipotence, the replacement of reflective function with coercive, nonreflective models, and the dissociation of vulnerability find the pressures of adolescence difficult to bear. Their need to feel omnipotent jeopardizes their ability to take advantage of the developmental opportunities of adolescence, thus exacerbating their predicament. Unable to achieve real competence and effectiveness, they only intensify their claim to omnipotence and coerciveness, and so are thrust into an even more extreme grandiosity—hidden or overt—and a variety of desperate defensive maneuvers directed at protecting a precarious self-esteem and an illusory sense of control.

Needing to devalue, idealize, or manipulate others, fearing closeness, and burdened by needs for perfection and a driving concern to protect themselves from vulnerability and humiliation, adolescents with severe personality disorders fail to construct an ideal self that approximates their talents and opportunities. They feel like persistent failures, lacking a realistic road map to adulthood, while they strive to achieve impossible goals. They denigrate their parents for their inability to live up to ideal standards, yet they cannot truly separate from them because they are convinced that their family will collapse if they do. They enviously watch their peers move on, propelled by a passion and a search for love and intimacy. But closeness only brings anxiety, leaving these adolescents feeling worn out and jaded, longing to get away, or choked by dependency. In the end, the crowning achievement of adolescence, the capacity for love and intimacy, eludes their grasp.

4

Trauma, Vulnerability, and the Development of Severe Personality Disorders

TRAUMA, ORGANIZATION OF EXPERIENCE, AND SYMBOLIC PROCESSING

A growing body of research demonstrates that maltreatment impairs the development of reflective function, thus undermining children's capacity to experience themselves as mindful, self-regulating agents who can relate to other persons who have minds of their own. Schneider-Rosen and Cicchetti (1991) report that abused toddlers show less capacity to recognize themselves in a mirror—and less positive affect on recognizing their own reflection. Beeghly and Cicchetti (1994) document the deficit of maltreated children in using words to describe internal states—and the concrete, context-dependent nature of their language. Studies of maltreated children (e.g., Cicchetti & Toth, 1995) identify deficits in reflective functioning in maltreated youngsters, particularly those with a history of sexual abuse or a combination of physical and sexual abuse.

But to fully appreciate the impact of maltreatment on reflective function, it is useful to consider first how traumatic experiences affect the capacity to symbolize and maintain a reflective stance. The awareness of such impact can be traced back to the pioneer work of Pierre Janet (van der Kolk & van der Hart, 1989), as well as to Freud's original concept of trauma. In his first conceptualization of hysteria, Freud (1896/1962) claimed that the key mechanism underlying hysteria was the dissociation of traumatic memories. In *Studies in Hysteria*, Breuer and Freud (1893–1895/1955) stated that an event becomes pathogenic when it is incongruous with the "dominant mass of ideas" (p. 116), which they defined as the organization of a person's values, attitudes, and concepts—a conceptualization that served as a precursor of "representational models," "autobiographical narrative," and "ideal self." Because of this incongruity, the event in question cannot be integrated and processed through the normal psychological mechanisms. The memory of the event persisted, instead, according to Freud and Breuer, "unmetabolized," seeking expression through somatic or symptomatic channels.

Hysterics, claimed Breuer and Freud, "suffer mainly from reminiscences" (1893–1895/1955, p. 7). But these reminiscences are not readily available to the patient. "In the great majority of cases, it is not possible to establish the point of origin by a simple interrogation of the patient . . . principally because he is genuinely unable to recollect it and often has no suspicion of the causal connection between the precipitating event and the pathological phenomenon" (p. 3).

In his subsequent conceptualization, Freud (1926/1959) defined "trauma" as the experience of being overwhelmed by an adaptive demand that renders the ego passive, helpless, and unable to anticipate and cope. According to Freud, the "essence and meaning" of the traumatic situation consists of the subject's "admission of helplessness" (p. 166). As an important corollary, Freud also described a self-righting tendency of the ego, that is, a universal tendency to turn around such passivity and helplessness, and eventually regain activity and control.

Freud (1914/1958) believed that the ways and adaptive consequences of this turning around depend largely on whether the person *remembers* the trauma. In cases in which the trauma is *not* remembered, the affected person "reproduces it *not as a memory but as an action*; he repeats it, without, of course, knowing that he is repeating it . . . and in the end we understand that this is his way of remembering" (p. 150, emphasis added).

Contemporary research and clinical observation have lent substantial support to Freud's views on trauma, even though Freud shifted his theoretical focus and interest from *traumatic events* to *intrapsychic conflict*, and from *dissociation* and *fragmentation of experience* to defensively motivated *repression*. In contemporary terms, Freud's formulation of trauma defines it as an event that overwhelms the capacity to organize and store experience at an explicit–reflective–symbolic level. Instead, trauma is organized, at least initially, as sensory fragments and intense emotional states that have no linguistic components (van der Kolk, Burbridge, & Suzuki, 1997; van der Kolk & Fisler, 1995); that is, the normal integration of implicit–procedural and explicit–symbolic processing is disrupted and replaced by a fragmentation or discontinuity of experience, more specifically a dissociation of implicit–procedural and explicit–symbolic processing (Siegel, 1999). Dissociation indeed appears to be an intrinsic component of traumatic experience. The unintegrated sensory fragments and emotional states associated with the traumatic event continue to intrude as flashbacks or nightmares, activated by concrete reminders of the trauma—a particular smell, physical sensation, or sound. In these altered states of consciousness, the shock, helplessness, hyperarousal, and loneliness of the trauma are relived, unintegrated with an overall sense of self that can be felt to have continuity, affectivity, and a sense of agency.

In van der Kolk and Fisler's research (1995), *all* the childhood trauma subjects, and 78% of those traumatized as adults, reported that they initially had no narrative memory of the event. According to van der Kolk and Fisler, their subjects could not tell a story about what had happened to them "regardless of whether they always knew that the trauma had happened or whether they retrieved memories of the trauma at a later date. All these subjects, regardless of the age at which the trauma occurred, claimed that they initially remembered the trauma in the form of somatosensory flashback experiences, as visual, olfactory, affective, auditory, or kinestetic imprints" (van der Kolk et al., 1997, p. 103).

But as van der Kolk's subjects gained clearer conscious awareness of the traumatic events in their past, they evolved a capacity to *tell* what actually had happened. Multiple prospective and retrospective studies support the contention that memories of terrifying events remain in prolonged, unintegrated, implicit–procedural storage. As traumatic reminders elicit sensory, affective, and/or motoric procedural responses, traumatized individuals fail to use their own "procedural" reactions as cues to attend to incoming information and to select or create a mental representation of the situation—that is, they fail to achieve the normal integration of procedural and reflective–symbolic processing. Instead, their flashbacks, or their own arousal, trigger fight-or-flight reactions that take them, as van der Kolk and Fisler (1994) suggest, "from stimulus to response without being able to assess the meaning of what is going on" (p. 154). In other words, the fight-or-flight response triggered by traumatic reminders can obliterate individuals' capacity to maintain a reflective stance.

As it has become clearer that an overwhelming threat and extreme emotional arousal lead to a failure of the central nervous system to integrate the elements of the traumatic experience, growing attention has been directed to the neurobiology of traumatic memory (van der Kolk et al., 1997). Particular attention has been focused on the parts of the central nervous system that process and interpret the meaning of incoming information, and on the impact of the neurophysiological and neurochemical responses to stress and trauma on the activity of these structures.

Of specific interest are the structures involved in integrating ongoing experience, namely, the parietal lobes, which integrate information between different cortical areas (Damasio, 1989); the hippocampus, which is essential for encoding and retrieving explicit memory, and is believed to generate a "cognitive map" that allows for the categorization of experience and its subsequent integration into an evolving autobiographical narrative (Bremner et al., 1997; McEwen & Magarinos, 1997; Sapolsky, 2000); the medial temporal lobe, which is essential for processing explicit memory (Squire & Zola-Morgan, 1991; Squire et al., 1993); the amygdala, which is involved in the interpretation of the emotional valence of incoming information (Davis, 1992; LeDoux, 1996); the corpus callosum, which serves to transfer information between the two hemispheres and thus facilitates integration of cognitive and emotional aspects of experience (Joseph, 1988); the cyngulate gyrus, which is believed to amplify and filter incoming information, and is involved in the integration of experience (Devinsky, Morrell, & Vogt, 1995); and the prefrontal cortex and ventromedial frontal cortex, which are thought to oversee the integration of experience (Gershberg & Shimamura, 1995; Shimamura, 1995) and may be key structures involved in self-knowledge and reflective function (Damasio, 1998; Goel, Grafman, Sadato, & Hallett, 1991).

Among the most significant findings in the research on the neurobiology of trauma and posttraumatic disorders are the following:

1. Alterations in the hypothalamic–pituitary–adrenocortical (HPA) axis in individuals with posttraumatic stress disorder (PTSD) that are the opposite of those found in acute stress and major depression

(Yehuda, 1998), while classic descriptions of stress and major depression have demonstrated increased levels of cortisol (Kathol, Jaeckle, Lopez, & Meller, 1989; Sachar et al., 1973), decreased concentration and responsiveness of glucocorticoid receptors (Gormley et al., 1985), and a decreased sensitivity and progressive desensitization of the HPA axis to negative feedback—that is, the hypothalamus progressively becomes less able to stop producing stimulating hormones in response to increased levels of cortisol (Holsboer, von Bardeleben, Gerken, Stalla, & Muller, 1984; Stokes & Sikes, 1987). In patients with PTSD, on the other hand, there are *decreased* levels of circulating cortisol, *increased* concentration and responsiveness of glucocorticoid receptors, and *increased* sensitivity and progressive sensitization of the HPA axis to negative feedback (Mason, Giller, Kosten, Ostroff, & Podd, 1986; Yehuda, 1997, 1998; Yehuda, & McFarlane, 1995).

2. Release of endogenous opiates under a variety of stressful conditions that presumably produce analgesia and modulate response to fear (Glover, 1992). Investigators (Glover, 1992; Roth, Ostroff, & Hoffman, 1996) hypothesized that the chronic overproduction of endogenous opiates underlies the emotional numbing in patients with PTSD and severe personality disorders. The associated craving for such endogenous stimulation may play a role in the reinforcement of behavior, since self-cutting and other self-injurious behaviors trigger a release of endogenous opiates that momentarily abate the craving and relieve the feelings of numbness.

3. Increased autonomic arousal in response to threat and a proclivity to heightened intensity of autonomic activation in response to traumatic reminders in previously traumatized individuals, and oversensitivity of neural pathways controlling the fear response—particularly the amygdala—to potentially threatening cues—analogous to the kindling mechanism involved in seizures—in patients with PTSD (Post, Weiss, Smith, Li, & McCann, 1997), supporting the hypothesis that trauma exposure in general, and unresolved trauma in particular, quickens the response and heightens the amygdala's intensity of responsivity to threat signals (Whalen et al., 1998).

4. Reduced hippocampal function in trauma-exposed individuals with or without PTSD, with concomitant reduction in the encoding and retrieval of explicit memory, as well as evidence of reduced hippocampal volume in patients with PTSD (Bremner & Naranyan, 1998; Gurvits et al., 1996; Sapolsky, 2000; Stein, Yehuda, Koverola, & Hanna, 1997).

5. Alteration of Broca's area and other frontal cortex areas, with concomitant decline of language and symbolic processing in trauma-related arousal (Stein, Hanna, Koverola, Torchia, & McClarty, 1997), as well as hemispheric lateralization in response to personal trauma scripts (van der Kolk et al., 1997).

In summary, threat signals and traumatic experiences trigger a fight-or-flight psychobiological response characterized by increased arousal and activation of the sympathetic system and the HPA axis, leading to increased levels of circulating cortisol, activation of the amygdala and release of endogenous opiates, and a concomitant deactivation of the hippocampus and the cortical areas involved in explicit–reflective–symbolic encoding and processing. Thus, it appears that at a basic neurobiological level, the fight-or-flight system creates both hyperarousal that prepares the organism to fight or to flee and a disconnection between explicit–symbolic and implicit–procedural modes of processing and functioning. The fight-or-flight response seems "designed" by evolution to be a largely automatic, unreflective, procedural response to a signal of danger.

Normally, this state of activation is terminated by a series of negative feedback loops, including the inhibition of hypothalmic stimulation by increased circulating cortisol that, in turn, by negative feedback loop process, brings down the levels of cortisol. It appears, however, that the termination of the fight-or-flight activation may require the mediation of a *social* response that, in turn, appears essential to the resumption of explicit–symbolic processing and the capacity to generate symbolic information and narrative structures that use verbal–symbolic referents (Siegel, 1999).

Developmentally, children's experience of distress normally acts as a signal that evokes proximity, protection, and attuned reflective responses from their caregivers. As seen earlier, these responses not only generate soothing, comfort, and restored homeostasis but also promote a sense of self-agency in the children. Distress thus becomes an internal cue that prompts the activation of the prewired motivation to seek human connections and contingent, attuned reflective responses from others. To put it more plainly, the attachment system is reinforced by the pairing of distress with restored homeostasis, mediated by attuned responses from caregivers.

Caregivers' attuned responsiveness to their children's distress is thus the interactive context in which secure attachment develops. Secure attachment, in turn, marks the conditions under which reflective function can optimally develop and operate. As Fonagy, Steele, Steele, and colleagues (1991) put it, a secure attachment offers the most congenial conditions under which children can learn about minds by exploring those of their caregivers. Exploring the mental state of sensitive and responsive caregivers enables children to find in the caregivers' minds an image of themselves as human beings, motivated by beliefs, feelings, and intentions (Fonagy & Target, 1997).

Thus, the pattern of response described as "secure attachment" may be a marker of the development of self-agency and reflective functioning, a thesis supported by conclusive evidence from longitudinal research linking security of attachment with robust and/or precocious development of a wide range of capacities based on meaning—conferring or symbolic abilities, such as frustration tolerance, ego control, self-recognition, play, exploration, social cognition, and emotion regulation (Fonagy, Steele, Steele, et al., 1991; Fonagy et al., 1994; Laible & Thompson, 1998; Meins et al., 1998; Sroufe, 1996).

As attachment becomes more securely organized, the high reactivity of the HPA axis, present at birth, becomes better modulated (Gunnar, 1992). A circadian rhythm is established by 8 weeks (Santiago, Jorge, & Moreira, 1996) and cortisol reactivity decreases steadily between 2 and 15 months. More specifically, the presence of the caregiver reduces cortisol elevation in response to specific stressors (Nichols, Gergely, & Fonagy, 2000).

What happens when an attuned reflective response is not forthcoming? Observation of infants of depressed or otherwise unresponsive caregivers (Field et al., 1988; Lyons-Ruth & Jacobvitz, 1999; Main & Hesse, 1990; Murray, 1992; Murray, Fiori-Cowley, Hooper, & Cooper, 1996) documents the efforts of even very young infants to cope initially with a lack of response by engaging in distinctive strategies. It seems likely that the anxious/avoidant and anxious/resistant patterns of attachment represent the prototypes of these early coping strategies.

In anxious/avoidant attachment patterns, children shift their attention away from the caregivers and their own distress, and focus instead on aspects of the environment they can manipulate and control. This pattern appears to involve a response to stress with significant dissociation or shifting of attention away from some aspects of the internal environment and the internal experience, with relatively little or no arousal.

In contrast, children in the anxious/resistant pattern overfocus on the caregiver's presence or absence and experience profound distress and hyperarousal when they fail to conjure up the presence of the caregiver.

The degree to which infants respond to stress with an anxious/ avoidant or an anxious/resistant pattern varies from child to child and also across events for any given child. Most children respond to stress with various combinations of dissociation and hyperarousal, although a developmental shift appears to occur, from a relative predominance of dissociation in early childhood to a predominance of hyperarousal in late childhood, adolescence, and adulthood (Perry, Pollard, Blakely, Baker, & Vigilante, 1995).

Some children, however, show a distinctive tendency toward dissociative responses with significant hyperarousal—that is, to anxious/ resistant patterns of overfocus on the caregiver's presence and responses—while others become predisposed to dissociation with little arousal—that is, to anxious/avoidant patterns of shifting attention away from the attachment figures and the internal experience of distress and vulnerability. It seems likely that an interaction of constitutional predisposition and the specific caregiving environment determines the relative predominance of one coping strategy over the other. The greatest significance of these coping strategies, however, is that they serve as blueprints for the type of response available to children when their coping and organizational efforts collapse.

The developmental prototype of the collapse of coping strategies is disorganized attachment (Main & Hesse, 1990, 1999). Such collapse, according to Main and Hesse, occurs when children not only fail to produce contingent responses from their caregivers—that is, evoke attuned reflective responses that relieve their distress—but also find the caregivers themselves terrifying.

Children are terrified when they recognize hatred and a desire to destroy or get rid of them in their caregivers' behavior. As children find themselves cut off from a sense of self-agency and unable to modify their caregivers' responses, fight-or-flight responses gain the upper hand, with increased dissociation and/or arousal. Fight-or-flight activation, in turn, dissociates information processed symbolically and reflectively from information processed implicitly and procedurally (Siegel, 1999). Explicit–reflective–symbolic processing appears indeed blocked under conditions of extreme fight-or-flight activation and, as a result, traumatic experiences are stored primarily as sensory, somatic, motoric, and affective states (Bower & Sievers, 1998).

The disruption of reflective processing brings about a greatly diminished ability to understand mental states and human intention. This impairment in interpretive abilities is reflected in a loss of the preference for the close-but-imperfect contingencies characteristic of human interactions and a regression to a preference for *perfect* contingencies.

Fonagy and Koss's studies (see Fonagy, 2000a) show that securely attached 1-year-olds clearly prefer to look at the face of their mother rather than look at themselves reflected in a mirror. These children test actively their self-image only when their mothers are instructed to become unresponsive (the still face protocol). In contrast, children who present a disorganized attachment are drawn to their own perfectly contingent image even when given the choice of looking at a responsive caregiver. This preference for perfect contingencies in disorganized attachment anticipates the coercive patterns of relationships of youngsters with severe personality disorders. As we will see later, these children tyrannize others, compelling others to match perfectly a script of their own creation.

Main and Hesse (1999) and Fonagy and Target (1997) hypothesize that children presenting disorganized attachment recoil from apprehending the mental state of the caregivers because they are confronted with attitudes toward them that are unbearable. These caregivers are likely to engage in severe neglect and abuse. Defensively, these children learn to inhibit reflective functions actively, under conditions that engender terrifying behavior in their caregivers.

However, a poor ability to grasp mental states—both of the self and of others—heightens distress and thus amplifies the need for closeness and attachment. Fonagy argues that "the need for proximity persists and perhaps even increases as a consequence of the distress caused by the abuse. Mental proximity becomes unbearably painful, and the need for closeness is expressed at a physical level. Thus, they may paradoxically be drawn physically closer to the abuser" (Fonagy, Target, & Gergely, 2000, p. 111).

This paradoxical convergence of a need for physical proximity and mental distance is reinforced by the caregivers' usual alternation of abuse and neglect with caring behavior. Thus, inhibition of reflective function occurs only in the context of specific internal and interpersonal cues, with a resulting "fractionation" (Fischer, Kenny, & Pipp,

1990) of functioning: normal reflective function in some contexts and inhibited reflective function in others. In addition, when abuse alternates with caring, it leads to impairments in children's capacity to create a coherent representation of their caregiver. As Allen (2001) points out, children can "resolve" their inability to create coherence by resorting to splitting. Creating different representations of themselves and the caregiver interacting in either benevolent or terrifying ways generates coherence and predictability in specific relational contexts. The developmental price is a lack of sense of self and others—a personality torn apart (Freyd, 1996).

Chronic exposure to maltreatment exacerbates the vicious cycles just described, because children are often trapped in conditions of protracted, if not inescapable victimization. Such entrapment precludes the children's efforts to restore coherence, mastery, and self-agency to their lives.

Furthermore, children's fears of retribution, loyalty conflicts, and concerns about shattering the family (or prompting the intervention of outside authorities) all militate against disclosing and sharing with others the experience of maltreatment and also exacerbate children's sense of isolation and their difficulty in making sense of the abuse. Compounding their dilemma are feelings of pleasure, secret power, and specialness that mix in a confusing fashion with their pain, rage, shame, and helplessness.

But in their effort to preserve a sense of agency and attachment, maltreated children must create for themselves a conviction of a sense of badness and responsibility for their abuse. As Herman (1992b) points out, an internalized sense of badness preserves an attachment with the caregivers and, by taking responsibility for the misfortune that befell them, children can produce at least an illusionary sense of control and agency.

Not surprisingly, an abundance of research (Chu & Dill, 1990; Pynoos, Steinberg, & Wraith, 1995; Terr, 1991) demonstrates that chronic exposure to maltreatment creates enduring distortions in relationship patterns, subjective experiences, sense of self, and coping strategies.

VULNERABILITY AND EARLY EXPERIENCE

Although trauma—particularly the protracted traumatization often associated with physical and/or sexual abuse—places children at a significant risk for severe and persistent maladjustment, clearly, not every abused child grows up to suffer serious psychopathology and/or to become an abuser. Oliver's (1993) review of the literature shows that only one-third of parents who were abused as children abuse their own children. Likewise, Paris and Zweig-Frank (1992, 1997) show that, while physical and sexual abuse are clearly overrepresented in the background of individuals with borderline and antisocial personality, a large percentage, perhaps even the majority of survivors of childhood abuse, do *not* grow up to develop a severe personality disorder.

Such data beg the question raised by Fraiberg and colleagues (1975): How is it that some children protect themselves from severe maladjustment in spite of deprivation and maltreatment when others cannot? Efforts to answer this question have focused on genetic predisposition and the psychobiological alterations that *precede* children's traumatic experiences.

Yehuda's research strongly suggests that PTSD occurs only in individuals whose biological response to trauma is neither typical nor normative. Those who develop PTSD, as indicated earlier, show *lower than normal* levels of cortisol (Mason et al., 1986; Yehuda, 1998). Several studies cited by Yehuda (1998) show that only those individuals who responded to an acute trauma with *low* levels of cortisol were likely to develop PTSD. In her excellent review of the research literature, Yehuda shows that individuals who develop PTSD also present a larger than normal number of basal glucocorticoid receptors, which are the receptor sites for cortisol in its target cells throughout the body, including the pituitary gland and the hippocampus, which is rich in cortisol receptors and may be the structure that gives the signal to the hypothalamus to shut down the HPA axis during the fight-or-flight response. She then hypothesizes that an increase in glucocorticoid receptor numbers and activity is a primary deficit in individuals predisposed to PTSD. According to this hypothesis, increased cortisol receptor activity produces a negative feedback that leads to lower cortisol levels.

Yehuda cites evidence in support of her hypothesis, including increased suppression of cortisol after administration of dexamethasone—a finding replicated independently in children exposed to natural disasters, combat veterans, Holocaust survivors, and victims of childhood sexual abuse (Goenjian et al., 1996; Golier & Yehuda, 1999; Stein, Yehuda, et al., 1997; Yehuda et al., 1995).

Using neuroendocrine challenges, as well as data from other independent studies, Yehuda (1998) offers evidence that individuals with PTSD present chronic increases in the release of hypothalamic CRF (corticotropin-releasing factor), the hormone that stimulates the pituitary to produce adrenocorticotropic hormone (ACTH), which stimulates the adrenal glands to produce cortisol. Chronically increased hypothalamic stimulation of the pituitary leads to pituitary hyporesponsiveness, which explains the increased dexamethasone suppression and the finding of blunted production of ACTH.

Thus, according to Yehuda (1998), individuals predisposed to PTSD present an *enhanced negative feedback inhibition* of the HPA axis. They are prone to respond *abnormally* to stress, with both an inability to terminate effectively the brain's fight-or-flight response to a traumatic event (due to low levels of cortisol) and a subsequent hyperresponse to environmental challenges (e.g., subsequent stress or traumatic reminders) due to hypersensitive cortisol receptors. She believes that this cortisol receptor hyperresponsiveness, rather than direct cortisol toxicity, is the pathogenic mechanism behind one of the most dramatic findings in individuals with chronic PTSD, namely, hippocampal atrophy.

Yehuda (1998) thus proposes a chronic sensitization process of the HPA axis that renders people vulnerable to react to stress with an abnormal and maladaptive response. Similarly, identified predisposing abnormalities of other neuromodulatory systems (McFarlane, Weber, & Clark, 1993; Murburg, 1994; Shalev, Orr, Peri, Schreiber, & Pitman, 1992) point out that patients with PTSD often experience exaggerated psychobiological responses to neuroendocrine challenges, other stressors, and traumatic reminders. This disposition contrasts with the *decreased* negative feedback system of depressed individuals, characterized by increased cortisol and dexamethasone nonsuppression that are compatible with reduced sensitivity to environmental stimuli.

The origins of the biological alterations predisposing to PTSD are not clear. Evidence that the presence of caregivers modulates children's cortisol levels (Larson, White, Cochran, Donzella, & Gunnar, 1998) supports the hypothesis that early disruptions of attachments, particularly lack of caregiver emotional availability and reflective response, generate an unmodulated stress response in infants. The hypercortisolemia associated with this heightened stress may, in turn, initiate a cascade of dysregulation that eventually leads to the alterations Yehuda demonstrates in adults at risk for PTSD.

A growing interest in genetic risk factors has focused, in particular, on the role of the D_2 dopamine receptor gene, which may interact with early stressors. Since the early 1990s, evidence has accumulated that the D_2 dopamine receptor gene plays a role in addictive disorders (Noble, 1996, 1998). A particular allele of this gene, the D_2A_1, appears to be associated with a decrease in D_2 dopamine receptors. The hypothesis, originally conceptualized as the "reward deficiency syndrome" (Blum et al., 1996), postulates that individuals deprived of dopamine D_2 receptors, particularly in mesolimbic and mesocorticolimbic pathways (important in reinforcement and reward), seek to compensate for the deficit by utilizing substances that increase dopamine levels, such as nicotine, alcohol, or cocaine. Addicted individuals are indeed more likely to possess the D_2A_1 allele. The larger the number of addictive behaviors in an individual, the greater the chance that the D_2A_1 allele will be present (Blum et al., 1996).

More recently, the D_2A_1 allele has been studied in relation to its association with maladaptive responses to stress. Comings, Muhleman, and Gysin (1996) report that 60% of combat veterans with PTSD carry the D_2A_1 allele, compared with 5% of veterans without PTSD. Berman and Noble (1997) report that boys with the D_2A_1 allele are significantly more likely than boys with the D_2A_1 allele to respond to family stress with a decrease in cognitive performance. The Schneier and colleagues (2000) finding of low D_2 receptors in the striatum in individuals with social phobia adds to the evidence that D_2 receptor function plays a key role in modulating social behavior. These findings in humans parallel animal studies that demonstrate lower striatal D_2 binding in socially subordinate monkeys (Grant et al., 1998).

Thus, there is good evidence to conclude that the D_2A_1 allele serves as a marker for vulnerability to interpersonal stress and trauma. But in the absence of trauma, this marker does *not* appear to be associated with significant dysfunction or maladjustment. It can be argued that trauma is either the necessary trigger for the expression of the gene or that the gene signals a predisposition to inadequately process traumatic experience.

This point can be expanded further to suggest that early experience, particularly early attachment, interacts in critical ways to determine gene expression. As discussed in Chapter 2, temperamentally hyperreactive monkeys show poor adjustment, exhibit excessive aggression and poor social competence, and low cerebrospinal fluid concentrations of 5-hydroxyindoleacetic acid (Heinz, Higley, et al.,

1998; Heinz, Ragan, et al., 1998; Higley, Hasert, Suomi, & Linnoila, 1991; Higley, King, et al., 1996; Higley, Suomi, & Linnoila, 1996)—a neurochemical finding associated with proclivity to consume large quantities of alcohol and amphetamines that is manifested only when subjects are reared in a maternally deprived environment. On the other hand, if reared by exceptionally attuned and responsive mothers, equally inhibited and hyperreactive monkeys grow to display exceptional social skills and adjustment. A genetic disposition may thus be a marker of either vulnerability or strength, depending on the presence or absence of environmental conditions that promote the development of capacities necessary to process experience and respond to the environment.

There is a clear parallel between the inhibited hyperreactive monkeys described by Suomi and the inhibited children in studies by Kagan (1994). The inhibited children described by Kagan (1994) likely inherit a highly reactive amygdala and are at risk to develop separation anxiety disorder and social phobia (Biederman et al., 1990; Schwartz, Snidman, & Kagan, 1999). These children present a constitutionally lower threshold for limbic–hypothalamic hyperresponse to environmental changes or threats and are thus highly vulnerable to respond with great distress and dysregulation to separations or other disruptions of attachment. This hypersensitivity may be a marker of a heightened sensitivity to social cues and to the cues that signal people's internal states (discussed in Chapter 6). Their hypersensitivity makes them both more dependent on caregivers for psychophysiological regulation—because of greater proneness to dysregulation—and more keenly aware of their caregivers' misattunement, hostility, or rejection—because of heightened ability to "read minds." Research is needed to explore the link between these hypersensitive children with a putative heightened ability for "mind reading" and the previously discussed deficits in D_2 receptors.

Children with attention-deficit/hyperactivity disorder (ADHD) present constitutional vulnerabilities modulating arousal—perhaps linked to the dysregulation of the HPA axis hypothesized by Yehuda, in which low cortisol levels create an ongoing difficulty with *terminating* states of hyperarousal. These children also present problems of sustaining attention, which may be linked to dopamine deficits similar to those related to the D_2A_1 allele.

Children with ADHD are thus prone to develop what David Shapiro (1965) described as an "impulsive style." Several neurobiological models have been proposed to account for the deficits in attention and inhibitory control that children with ADHD present. Heilman, Voeller, and Nadeau (1991) propose that reduced dopaminergic tone in prefrontal–striatal circuits produces the inattention, impulsivity, and hyperactivity of ADHD by disrupting the executive and "gating" functions of the prefrontal cortex—arguably including reflective function.

An alternative model proposed by Pliszka, McCracken, and Maas (1996) implicates multiple neurotransmitter systems. According to this model, attentional functions are distributed into two distinct systems: a posterior attention system that orients to and engages novel stimuli, and is localized in the superior parietal cortex, the superior colliculus, and the pulvinar nucleus; and an anterior executive system in the prefrontal cortex and the anterior cingulate gyrus.

The posterior system receives sense noradrenergic input from the locus coeruleus, which links the system to stress and threat perception. The anterior executive system is modulated primarily by ascending dopaminergic fibers. Pliszka and colleagues (1996) propose that dopamine D_1 (DAD_1) receptors are particularly important in selectively gating input to the anterior executive system, thus reducing irrelevant neuronal activity. This capacity is likely a crucial underpinning of the selective and flexible reflective processing.

Impulsive children—and adults—translate their wishes, needs, and impulses into action directly and with minimal mediation. Because they short-circuit the integration of momentary internal states with a more enduring autobiographical sense, their own wishes cannot evolve into sustained intentions, anchored by a sense of stability and self-continuity. Instead, their impulsivity produces a vicious cycle of disruption of their capacity to develop a cohesive and continuous sense of self and others. Their low tolerance for frustration stems from an inability to connect or integrate momentary wishes with general goals and interests, or to form more enduring representations of the self and others.

Impulsive youngsters view their actions as happening to them instead of resulting from their choice—conscious or not. Thus, they experience little guilt or sense of responsibility. The world appears to them as a disconnected series of temptations and frustrations, possibilities for immediate gain and satisfaction, or obstacles to gratification. They experience other people and relationships in equally fragmentary and shallow ways, which results in a barren and undifferentiated inner life. As Marohn (1991) noted, such a youngster has "little awareness of an inner psychological world, cannot name affects or differentiate one affect from another, and often confuses thought, feeling, and deed" (p. 150). Their concrete, egocentric, unreflective mode of experience interferes with planning, symbolization, and generalization, and also forms the basis for their well-known difficulty in learning from experience.

In a similar fashion, the proneness to irritability, mood lability, and anger in children with mood disorders lends an ever-changing, kaleidoscopic quality to their sense of self and others. Biological vulnerabilities seem to increase the odds that children may respond catastrophically— and with potentially long-term maladaptive consequences—to stress and trauma. Arguably, these various vulnerabilities increase the odds of long-term maladjustment after exposure to stress and trauma by increasing children's tendency to fragment experience and to cut themselves off from meaningful relationships; that is, these vulnerabilities contribute to children's tendency toward dissociation or other forms of discontinuity of experience that tip the balance against the integration of experience and the protection afforded by reflective function and supportive connections. A tendency toward discontinuity of experience in the face of unmodulated stress in turn shapes the structuring of coping mechanisms and relationship patterns in particularly maladaptive ways, which I discuss in the next section. One clinical example serves to illustrate the plight of these children.

Travis's birth was haunted by the suicides of his father, a paternal uncle, and a paternal grandfather, all of whom suffered from bipolar disorder. Travis's father, after whom the boy was named, had pleaded with his wife to have an abortion. When she refused, he hanged himself 3 months before Travis was born. Travis was later told by his mother that his father had gotten so excited when he found out that Travis was coming, his blood pressure "went sky high" and he died of a heart attack. Not surprisingly, the boy became convinced that he had killed his father.

Mood lability was Travis's most striking feature when he was brought for consultation at age 7. One moment he bubbled with enthusiasm, swept up by an elated mood, while his thoughts raced ebulliently. Yet minor mistakes or frustrations triggered fits of rage or plunged him into abject self-loathing. Constant vigilance was needed to prevent him from hurting himself in an "accident."

Mood stabilizers significantly decreased the boy's affective storms. Yet his developmental problems—his fragile sense of self and others, his vulnerability to "lose" reflective functioning—remained glaringly apparent. Whenever Travis felt threatened, he valiantly tried to hold on to an image of himself as the heroic savior and protector of his beautiful mother. But if the image of the "protector" was challenged, he "switched" to a rageful foe of a mother that he perceived as guilt-inducing, self-absorbed, and depriving.

Travis's vignette points to the bidirectional process between biological vulnerabilities and the psychosocial determinants of reflective function. Obviously, constitutional factors play a crucial role in shaping children's experience of themselves and others, of their competence and of other people's reliability, of the safety or lack of safety of their emotional responses. These factors also reflect their ability to monitor emotional signals from themselves and from others, to cue others about their internal states, and to create reciprocal interactions. Last, but certainly not least, biological vulnerabilities provoke interpersonal conflicts and caregivers' frustration—in caregivers who often share similar constitutional vulnerabilities.

Thus, biological factors can limit the development of reflective function by generating environments in which maltreatment is more likely and parental reflective function is compromised. Children with biological vulnerabilities may fuel the chaos that often prevails in their families, exhaust their caregivers, and impose an added burden of frustration and distress while they wreak havoc on the minimal structure and boundaries their families can offer. Thus, they exacerbate the maladaptive consequences of their biological vulnerabilities by depriving themselves of the social supports and natural protection of reflective function.

In the following section, I propose a model of the way constitutional vulnerabilities and environmental forces generate severe personality disorders. It is worth pausing, however, to note that even against seemingly impossible odds, some people manage to retain an integration of the memories and the affects that were part of their experiences—including their experiences of maltreatment (Fraiberg et al., 1975). By retaining reflective function, even when presented with traumatic reminders, they are also able to retain adaptive connections with others and to experience enough empathy to protect their own children from the pain of parental misattunement.

The factors that enable some people to develop such resilient reflective capacity are not entirely clear. They may include a constitutional sturdiness, perhaps in the form of an exceptional innate capacity for reflective function (the opposite end of the spectrum from autism), and a greater than average capacity to modulate alarm responses.

But the crucial factor in explaining resilience may be the presence of people who respond reflectively to children at critical points in their development. Interaction with peers who promote reflective function—as opposed to reinforcing unreflective, impulsive behavior—is emerging as a critical factor in explaining differences in outcome (Stein et al., 2000).

Harris's (1998) observation that, in both normal and pathological development, peers fundamentally matter more than parents—aside from direct genetic influence—in shaping character and personality calls for critical examination. Given the realities of human development, which include a prolonged period of maturation and growth contingent on the presence of caregivers—and the substantial body of research supporting this very point, it is far more plausible that caregivers are essential to *activating* the crucial capacities on which subsequent development depends, including the capacity for reflective function.

Increasingly, after age 3 or 4, children become less and less interested in becoming like their parents, and more and more interested in seeking self-like models in siblings and peers (Tyson, 1982) to guide their search for competence, mastery, safety, connections, and satisfaction. In other words, peers gain an increasingly privileged position in children's evolving "ideal self." By seeking to approximate the model provided by peers, and through actual interactions with other children, even vulnerable children can grasp the intersubjective meanings created and exchanged in interpersonal relationships and can thus find alternative sources to develop reflective functioning.

Through access to peers, their own caregivers, and other adults—when they are able to function in a reflective fashion, vulnerable maltreated children can "tip the balance" between dissociating and fragmenting tendencies on the one hand, and the integration and adjustment promoted by reflective function on the other. Thus, even in the face of traumatic reminders—as the Adult Attachment Interview (AAI; George, Kaplan, & Main, 1995) research demonstrates—many people preserve the ability to create "stories" about themselves and their past that are populated by real human beings, people whose behavior remains meaningful and understandable. They are, therefore, in a position to remain attuned to their own children and to other people, and to experience them as real, intentional beings rather than as frightening or hated ghosts that evoke only a compelling need to escape or destroy.

THE PATH TO SEVERE PERSONALITY DISORDERS

A crucial determinant of children's resilience to genetic vulnerability and/or trauma appears to be the caregivers' capacity to retain reflective functioning in their interactions with their children—in spite of their own experiences of vulnerability or maltreatment. Empirical evidence strongly supports Oliver's (1993) conclusion that abused parents who are able to "face the reality of past and present personal relationships" (p. 132) are far less likely to perpetuate the cycle of abuse into the next generation. Van der Kolk and Fisler's (1994) subjects substantiate the fact that symptomatic improvement after a traumatic experience is associated with a growing capacity to create a narrative that "explains" what happened to them in a way that allows them to integrate the trauma into the fabric of their autobiography and the world of experience they share with others. The "turning around" of passivity and helplessness described by Freud seems to be, in light of contemporary understanding, essentially the very process of creating coherence and organization by weaving a narrative at a reflective–symbolic level that integrates the disparate procedural, sensory, and affective elements of the traumatic experience. Healing after a traumatic experience may have less to do with retrieving a factual memory than with restoring the capacity to process and integrate experience, and retain a reflective stance even in the face of traumatic reminders. This conclusion is consistent with the evidence emerging from the use of the AAI (George, Kaplan, & Main, 1985), which has proven to be a remarkable instrument for probing the links between attachment experience and adult functioning.

The AAI is a structured interview that asks subjects first to produce and then to reflect on their memories of early attachment experiences and their effect on subsequent functioning. Its scoring system (Main & Goldwyn, 1984, 1998) classifies individuals as *secure/autonomous*, *insecure/dismissing*, *insecure/preoccupied*, or *disorganized* with respect to attachment, loss, or trauma based on the structural qualities—coherence, relevance, completeness, clarity, and so on—of the subject's narrative of early experiences.

Secure/autonomous individuals parallel securely attached infants, valuing and presenting attachment relationships in internally consistent narratives. Their responses are clear, relevant, and succinct. Reflective function—or "metacognitive monitoring" in Main's (1991) terminology—is evident in subjects' responses indicating, for example, that their memories might be in error, that the person discussed might have a different point of view, or that their present beliefs may later undergo change. Such classification is unrelated to whether childhood experiences were largely positive or difficult and even traumatic.

Insecure/dismissive individuals minimize the importance of attachment but their narratives are filled with internal contradictions. Insecure/preoccupied subjects, on the other hand, exhibit a confused, angry, or passive preoccupation with attachment figures. Their responses are grammatically entangled, as if the subject were unable to remain focused on the interviewer's questions once memories were aroused. The disorganized category applies to individuals who present cognitive disorganization and disorientation specifically during discussions of potentially traumatic events, such as loss or maltreatment.

A body of research utilizing the AAI is providing additional empirical support to van der Kolk and Fisler's (1994) conclusion: Successful adaptation after adverse (or even overwhelming) life events requires—or at least is greatly aided by—the creation of a coherent narrative of one's experience based on the capacity to exercise reflective function. This narrative gives meaning to the past and restores the reflective processes that provide access to sustaining connections with others. The stories we create about our lives are woven into the fabric of the meanings extracted from interpersonal exchanges and the resulting flexible reconfiguration of mental representations. The exercise of reflective function enables us mutually to regulate interpersonal relationships. In turn, that capacity allows us to grasp the meaning of past and present events in a process that limits the automatic activation of patterns of experience and response.

This conclusion is validated by Fonagy's research. As previously noted, children of deprived mothers with high reflective capacity were securely attached to their mothers, whereas almost none of the children of deprived mothers with low reflective function show a similar security of attachment (Fonagy et al., 1994).

For some caregivers, however, their infants' distress becomes a traumatic reminder that triggers in them the fight-or-flight response, attachment disorganization, and the loss of reflective capacity. These care-givers are either compelled to escape their children's distress or driven to destroy the apparent source of their anguish: their own children.

One such mother, for example, reported that her 5-month-old baby's crying provoked uncontrollable panic and an overwhelming need to get away from and/or silence the disturbing noise. She found that she could best protect both herself and her baby by locking herself in the bathroom and turning on the shower to muffle the inconsolable—and unattended—cries of her baby. Weston (1968) confirms the paradigm suggested by this report with the finding that in 80% of instances of abuse cases, mothers harmed their infants in reaction to their crying. Eventually, however, caregivers "snap" out of the fight-or-flight mode and reengage their infants, albeit in a driven, desperate, overstimulating fashion, as the reflective and integrating tendencies present in most people begin to reassert themselves.

Some of these children cope by actively retreating from reflective functioning *whenever* they become distressed. In effect, these children prompt themselves to dissociate in response to their own hyperarousal—an active coping stance likely facilitated both by a constitutional pro-clivity for dissociation (Braun & Sacks, 1985; Kluft, 1984) and/or by a brain "trained" to dissociate by repeated experiences of neglect, as described in Chapter 2.

The active inhibition of reflective function—replacing the integrat-ing tendencies of reflective processing with the "tuning out" and frag-mentation of experience—evolves out of children's awareness that *some* of their own internal states can trigger terrifying internal states in their caregivers (e.g., a desire to destroy or abandon them). As Fonagy and collaborators postulate, "The infant may deliberately turn away from the mentalizing (reflective) object because the contemplation of the ob-ject's mind is overwhelming, as it harbors frankly hostile or dangerously indifferent intentions toward the self. This may lead to widespread dis-avowal of mental states by the child that further reduces the chances of identifying and establishing links with an understanding object" (Fon-agy et al., 1995, pp. 257–258).

The chaotic and contradictory features of approach and avoidance of the disorganized/disoriented attachment pattern characteristic of abused children appear to represent the early behavioral correlates of these coping strategies: an effort to inhibit their awareness of their care-giver's terrifying internal states, coupled with the anxious expectations of a blissful reengagement. Over time, these disorganized/disoriented children learn to "fractionate" (Fischer et al., 1990) or split (Kernberg, 1967) their access to reflective function across domains of interpersonal interaction, as their tendency to create discontinuities of experience evolves into what Ogden (1989) describes as a schizoid–paranoid mode of organization of experience.

In the Kleinian tradition, Ogden emphasizes that the schizoid–paranoid mode is born out of the anxiety generated by the realization that the object of love is also the object of hatred, a problem handled by "separating loving and hating facets of oneself from loving and hating facets of the object" (p. 24). I propose, instead, that the schizoid–paranoid mode is generated more generally as the built-in response to threats that overwhelm the person's capacity to integrate experience and call for the protective intervention of attachment figures. The content of these responses is likely modeled after the proto-narrative envelopes acquired in the process of adopting anxious/avoidant or anxious/resistant patterns of coping and relating.

In a schizoid–paranoid mode, there is no experience of historical continuity or integration of the immediate experience of the self and others with other aspects of the self and others in the past or in the present. When the person experiences hurt, fear, or anger, that is all he or she can see—with absolute clarity and unmitigated power. There is not, as Ogden describes, a shared experience of the history of the relationship to balance the anxiety and anger associated with a sense of endangered survival.

While words can be used, there is "virtually no space between symbol and symbolized" (Ogden, 1989, p. 25). This mode of quasi-symbolization creates a "two-dimensional form of experience in which everything is what it is. There is almost no interpreting subject mediating between the percept (whether external or internal) and one's thoughts and feelings about which one is perceiving" (Ogden, 1989, p. 25). Thus, mental states are not experienced as personal creations but instead as facts, as Ogden (1989) points out, as "things-in-themselves, that simply exist" (p. 25).

As a biologically prepared form of coping with an overwhelming threat, this mode of organizing experience is largely based on the principle of separating the endangering experience from the rest of one's experience. It is a mode of processing experience that, in contrast to the normal tendency toward coherence and integration, appears designed instead to create a *discontinuity* of experience, to isolate, so to speak, the traumatic event, in order to deal with it swiftly and without encumbrance. As Kluft (1992) explains about dissociation, it is a "defense in which an overwhelmed individual cannot escape [what] assails him or her by taking meaningful action or successful flight, and escapes instead by altering his or her mental organization, i.e., by inward flight" (p. 143). This disposition will subsequently be elaborated in the form of psychological defense mechanisms, such as splitting and projective identification, and in the active inhibition of reflective function that shapes the person's experience and relationships.

Discontinuity of experience and dissociation, however, are not unitary responses but are instead a spectrum of coping efforts that range from "turning away" from paying attention to some aspects of external reality to dissociative detachment that entails clouding of consciousness, to numbing of pain and other dysphoric internal states, to discontinuities of experience associated with amnesia, and, in more extreme forms, to a complete retreat from outer reality or a profound fragmentation of inner experience. It is not clear at this point how much the "choice" of the type of response is linked to a particular constitutional disposition, to the nature of the threat, to previous patterns of coping, to the presence or absence of protective factors, particularly reflective caregivers, to ongoing reinforcers of dissociation, or to a combination of all of the above.

In Chapter 5, I discuss how the dominant types of discontinuity of experience and varying degrees of hyper- or hypoarousal evolve into different model types of maladjustment within the cluster of severe personality disorders. At this point, however, I review how the coping efforts of infants and young children—who retreat from reflective function in response to specific internal and external cues—evolve into self-reinforcing patterns of maladjustment, that is, into a tendency to function at a reflective level in some contexts and domains of interpersonal interaction and internal experience but not in others.

Reflective function most likely develops as a skill within a specific context—in interactions with reflective caregivers. Given a favorable balance of environmental support, biological readiness is subsequently generalized to other domains. As these children actively switch to dissociated states or states of inhibited reflective function in specific interpersonal and internal contexts, they also keep reflective function absent from particular social and developmental domains. Over time, they organize subsets of mental representations of themselves in relationship with others that reflect this fractionation. Some of these mental representations are encoded with the normal integration of procedural and symbolic modes achieved by means of reflective function—and are thus part of the children's evolving autobiographical narrative. Other mental representations, however, appear concrete, impoverished of reflective function, and associated with procedural responses; in short, they are organized in a schizoid–paranoid mode. These later subsets of self- and other-schemas are acquired in the states into which these children retreat when faced with danger signals.

Relatedness in these disconnected states occurs predominantly in the form of projective and introjective identification (Kernberg, 1987; Klein, 1952a, 1952b; Ogden, 1979, 1982; Spillius, 1994), as interpersonal processes match the mode of schizoid–paranoid organization and coping. This form of coping, as I discussed earlier, is modeled after the quasi-automatic response of dissociation in the face of threat that infants evidence, for example, when they "space out" at times of unheeded—and thus overwhelming—distress. Such dissociation is based on the effort to separate the endangering or endangered aspects of the self and control them by disowning or "getting rid" of them.

In projective identification, there is a nonconscious effort to rid oneself of threatening internal states by evoking in others the very same disowned feelings and perceptual and procedural strategies. Projective identification becomes not only a coping mechanism but also a paradigm for a mode of relationship. The recipient of projective identification has a subjective sense of the coercive nature of the interaction. As Bion (1959, 1962) put it, the other person feels that he or she is playing a part in someone else's internal drama. It is as if other people are compelled to provide the perfectly contingent match that young infants and children with disorganized attachments seek.

This experience of the caregivers points to an additional complication in children's effort to rid themselves of intolerable internal states via projective identification. Typically, these children are engaged in relationships with caregivers who likewise respond to their distress, often precipitated by the children's own distress or their bids for attachment, with projective identification efforts to dispose of their threatening internal states.

Thus, the mental representations that children activate as they retreat from reflective–symbolic processing contain both repudiated in-

ternal states and states evoked by the caregivers' projective identification, that is, those responses that largely reflect the caregivers' own predicament. The results are mental states that confuse the children's own
feelings, intentions, and arousal level—including those feelings they
wish to get rid of—and the feelings, intentions, and arousal level that
others are coercing them to take on.

From ages 3 and 4, a variety of coping and defensive mechanisms
begins to evolve to maintain the discontinuity of experience created by
a retreat from reflective function. Splitting, for example, creates subsets
of self- and other-representations organized around a specific affective
quality (Kernberg, 1967), while denial affords the opportunity to obliterate from awareness a distressing reality.

The evolving mental representations, however, are cut off from the
integration of implicit–procedural and explicit–symbolic representations that, under the guide of reflective function, create an evolving
autobiographical narrative. Instead, these disconnected representations
of the self, confused about what belongs to oneself and what others are
attempting to impose on the self, grow as a sort of threatening internal
presence or "alien self" (Fonagy & Target, 1995). This sense of an alien
presence further creates a feeling of dyscontrol and pressures children
to seek to coerce others into behaving in ways that fit with their need to
dispose of their alien and threatening internal states.

Parent interviews (Solomon & George, 1996) suggest that, indeed,
the caregivers of children who are arguably on the path to consolidating
a severe personality disorder experience their children as increasingly
taking control over the relationship. Not infrequently, by the time these
children reach school age, a role reversal has occurred and they increasingly assume a caregiving role with their caregivers. The "caregiving,"
however, often takes the form of the children's maladaptive behavior,
which is reinforced by its ability to secretly comfort, distract, or protect
the caregivers.

The fateful step toward control of the environment becomes increasingly apparent between ages 3 and 6. As described in Chapter 3,
children begin to organize reality to conform with their expectations by
evoking in others the responses that support and reinforce their unreflective and dissociated mental representations. This observation suggests that, contrary to the view of personality disorders as based on
developmental "arrests" or "regression," these children have embarked
on a distinct—albeit maladaptive—developmental trajectory, with

self-perpetuating—and increasingly more complex—coping and organizing mechanisms.

By "creating" their environment, these children can achieve a semblance of self-righting to counter their helplessness, passivity, and lack
of experiential coherence: They do not wait *passively* for trauma to
overwhelm their reflective function, but instead retreat *actively* from
grasping mental states; they do not helplessly suffer the transformation
of other people into "monsters" incapable of perceiving them as real
human beings, but instead evoke unreflective, procedural responses
from others. In effect, they actively produce in others the very fight-or-
flight reaction that they so anxiously expect will lead to their being
harmed or abandoned. In so doing, of course, they vastly reinforce the
fractionation or splitting of their representational world and their ongoing need to retreat from reflective function and organize a portion of
their life around concrete, unreflective, coercive interpersonal exchanges. But as much as these coping and organizing strategies afford
children a measure of self-righting—an illusion, so to speak, of control
and integration—activating nonreflective interactions and their corresponding mental representation while withdrawing from a reflective
stance leaves children temporarily bereft of the adaptive capacities provided by reflective function. Thus, they struggle (1) to maintain a stable
and coherent sense of self; (2) to experience ownership and a sense of
agency over their behavior; (3) to self-soothe and otherwise contain and
regulate their affective experience; (4) to create a sense of direction and
an ability to set self-limits and tolerate frustration; (5) to experience
others as intentional, understandable human beings and thus feel connected to others through the sharing of meanings and mutually regulating mental states.

As these children reach school age and move into adolescence, the
developmental liabilities associated with a proneness to withdraw intermittently from reflective function turn into a more pronounced handi-
cap. In particular, the advent of the psychosocial and psychobiological
demands of adolescence challenge these youngsters with extraordinary
intensity. As they struggle with the requirement for more refined social
discrimination, an enhanced need to integrate multiple—and more
complex—sets of mental representations, and a greater frequency of
emotionally intense interactions, their coping, organizing, and relationship patterns become increasingly more rigid and self-perpetuating. The
psychosocial and developmental imperatives to separate from their fam-

ily, to find an independent niche in the world, and to engage in sexual and emotional intimacy only fuel their sense of subjective dyscontrol and emotional disconnection, thus exacerbating their need to organize their subjective experience even more rigidly and to evoke interpersonal responses that confirm, validate, and reinforce a set of internal convictions and representational models. Desperately, they hold on to an illusion of control and a precarious sense of relatedness to others.

By intermittently withdrawing from reflective function into a world of schizoid–paranoid discontinuity and procedural responses, some youngsters come to shape and reinforce the environment that shaped and reinforced their particular pattern of coping, experiencing, and relating. This shaping of the environment extends beyond their family to the school and the neighborhood, and, frequently, to protective services, the mental health system, and/or the juvenile justice authorities. Relentlessly, they become entangled in a tight web of interpersonal and social responses that narrows the scope of their functioning and precludes their taking advantage of developmental opportunities.

In Chapters 5 and 6, I discuss how this scenario leads to more specific patterns of disturbance within the cluster of the dramatic or severe personality disorders.

5

Antisocial and Narcissistic Children and Adolescents

Although children and adolescents who develop severe personality disorders share common features in their paths to maladjustment and clinical attention, they also display striking diversity of symptoms and levels of functioning. DSM-IV (American Psychiatric Association, 1994) identifies several types within the cluster of the dramatic personality disorders, reflecting various combinations of constitutional strengths and vulnerabilities that interact with developmental and environmental factors (see Figure 5.1). In this chapter, I describe the antisocial (ruthless), narcissistic configuration. This group comprises children seemingly unencumbered by guilt and capable of producing a great deal of pain in others, in contrast to narcissistic–histrionic youngsters, who crave attention from others (described in Chapter 6).

RUTHLESS–NARCISSISTIC CHILDREN

Ruthless–narcissistic youngsters—predominantly boys—respond to experiences normally associated with an increased need for attachment (e.g., experiences of vulnerability, hurt, or helplessness) with rather desperate attempts to create an *illusion* of control, largely based on turning others into helpless victims (Bleiberg, 1984, 1988). They carefully scan the environment for potential threats to their illusory control and are perennially haunted by the expectation of being attacked or blamed,

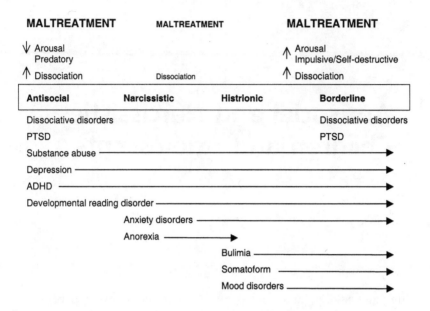

FIGURE 5.1. Cluster B (dramatic) personality disorders.

anticipating painful humiliation and vicious assault on any revelation of their shortcomings or failure to maintain control. They expect the same ruthlessness and lack of compassion from others that mark their own behavior. To them, dependency on others or efforts to secure protection or comfort from caregivers seem to lead only to more pain. Survival, on the other hand, appears predicated on the manipulation of other people, "toughness," self-reliance, and denial of vulnerability and dependency. That survival, however, comes at great cost. Although their apparent precocity gives them the appearance of miniature adults, they rarely experience real adults as protectors, soothers, limit setters, or effective interpreters of reality. Rather than being a matter for grief or regret, this perception forms the rationale for their efforts to hold on to an illusion of self-sufficiency.

The conviction that their survival requires vigilance and a readiness to lash out creates a deep reservoir of rage. They are callous and disrespectful of their victims and indifferent to human warmth. Noshpitz (1984) describes those who, when apprehended for wrongdoing, are "arrogant rather than repentant, angry, not crestfallen, haughty and demanding, instead of apologetic and guilt stricken" (p. 17).

Understandably, there is considerable reluctance in the field to label children and adolescents as "antisocial personalities." DSM-IV diagnostic criteria specifically require that the individual be *at least* 18 years of age *and* show evidence of a conduct disorder, with onset before age 15. Thus, ruthless youngsters are typically diagnosed as having a "conduct disorder" instead.

However, DSM-IV diagnostic criteria for conduct disorder scrupulously avoid any reference to developing personality features, such as relationship patterns, coping mechanisms, or organization of subjective experience. Instead, DSM-IV focuses on "a repetitive and persistent pattern of behavior in which the basic rights of others or major age-appropriate societal rules are violated" (American Psychiatric Association, 1994, p. 90). At this time, DSM-IV allows only for subtyping along the lines of age of onset. This allowance is based on studies that show childhood-onset antisocial and aggressive behavior to be predictive of adult antisocial personality (Farrington, 1983; Farrington, Loeber, & van Kammen, 1990; Robins, 1981).

Unfortunately, some dimensions of personality development, such as the capacity to form affectionate bonds and to experience concern for others (the basis of the distinction between *socialized* and *undersocialized* conduct disorder in DSM-III-R (American Psychiatric Association, 1987) have been eliminated because of inadequate empirical data. The designation "conduct disorder" shifts the focus away from internal states or developing psychological organization, in effect paralleling the very social responses that, as we see later, serve to reinforce and exacerbate these children's alienation from their own reflective capacities.

Yet a growing consensus in the study of juvenile offenders is that the conduct disorder category, as it now stands in DSM-IV, offers little assistance in identifying pathogenic factors or conceptualizing preventive or therapeutic interventions (Lewis, Yeager, Lovely, Stein, & Cobham-Portorreal, 1994; Steiner, Cauffman, & Duxbury, 1999). As Rutter and Giller (1983), Rutter and colleagues (1998), and Steiner and colleagues (1999) point out, focusing on degrees or types of personality disturbance offers the potential for more properly tailored forms of treatment and prevention. As Steiner and colleagues suggest, such a focus contradicts the current climate and its emphasis on *retribution* rather than *rehabilitation* in the treatment of juvenile offenders.

The need for finer discrimination is obvious: Consider that while one-third to one-half of all children and adolescent clinic referrals are for aggressive and antisocial behaviors (Robins, 1981), less than one-half of antisocial youth go on to become antisocial adults (Farrington, 1983). More significantly, as Wolfgang, Figlio, and Sellin (1972) demonstrated, antisocial behavior in children and adolescents is ubiquitous, yet only 6% of a total cohort of adolescents are responsible for 52% of all the offenses perpetrated in a community. I propose that these chronic offenders are predominantly children with the severe personality disorders discussed in this book, a portion of whom are ruthless youngsters in the process of organizing an antisocial–narcissistic personality disorder.

THE PATH TO RUTHLESSNESS

Several steps underlie the developmental pathogenesis of these youngsters' maladjustment. First, they turn away from the internal states that normally trigger attachment: distress, pain, vulnerability, and desire for closeness, soothing, and comfort. They actively inhibit reflective function because they come to experience these internal states and their own plea for attachment as leading to increased rather than lessened vulnerability: Their pleas are regularly ignored, and their efforts to secure closeness are ridiculed, precipitate abandonment or abuse, and often generate destructive, unreflective mental states in their caregivers. Some of these children will first develop *avoidant* attachment patterns, seemingly shifting their attention from internal states of vulnerability toward manipulation and control of the environment. When their coping efforts collapse, they develop *disorganized* attachment patterns.

The active inhibition of reflective function in response to their own attachment needs paves the way for these children to respond in a particular way to subsequent physical and/or psychological abuse: numbness. Lenore Terr (1991) captures how one boy obliterated self-aspects associated with pain, helplessness, sadness, and vulnerability. This chronically maltreated young boy was eventually removed from his mother and stepfather's home and placed with an aunt. Terr poignantly describes the situation:

> Frederick was 7 years old when he was sent to live with his aunt because his mother found out, through a tape recording set up to catch her husband at infidelity, that Frederick's stepfather had been throwing him against walls while she worked the evening shift. Frederick did not tell

anyone his yearlong story, despite two visits to the emergency room and one neighbor-instigated protective service investigation.

While in his aunt's custody, Frederick glanced down at the playground pavement one day and saw blood. After several seconds of searching for a wounded companion, Frederick realized that it was *he* who was bleeding. The boy realized he could feel no pain.

In a psychotherapy session I asked Frederick how he could make this sort of thing happen. "It jus' happens now," he said. "I used to pretend I was at a picnic with my head in Mommy's lap. The first time my stepdaddy hit me, it hurt a lot. But then I found out that I could make myself go on Mommy's lap (in imagination), and Winston couldn't hurt me that way. I kept goin' on Mommy's lap—I didn't have to cry or scream or anything. I could be someplace else and not get hurt. I don't know how many times Winston punched me out. I wasn't always payin' attention. Like I told you, first I'd be at a picnic on Mom's lap. Now if somethin' makes me bleed, I don't think of no lap at all. I jus' don't feel no pain." (p. 17)

Maltreated children such as Frederick discover that they can actively induce a self-hypnotic state to escape from pain, terror, and helplessness. This discovery leads them to take a crucial turn in the path to long-standing maladjustment, as this spontaneous dissociation sets the stage not only for anesthesia to bodily pain but also extreme emotional distancing.

It may be that an innate facility for dissociation and/or the early shaping of the brain in the direction of dissociation (as described earlier) plays a significant role in the development of these self-hypnotic states. Vigorous research seeks to elucidate both the neurobiological predisposition and the biological alterations brought about by the repeated traumatization that underlies this somatopsychic numbness (van der Kolk et al., 1997).

Frederick's description, however, points to the protection afforded by reflective function, as illustrated by the boy's capacity to conjure up the image of a reflective caregiver to comfort him and help him escape. Arguably, this boy may have a better prognosis than those incapable of such a feat because of his ongoing capacity to reflect on his own mental activities and to convey his internal state verbally and meaningfully—a capacity that is the likely outcome of constitutional strength and of having had a caregiver who treated him, at some point, as an intentional being.

As we will see here and in Chapter 6, however, this capacity to numb pain—physical as well as psychological—can lead to two distinct yet overlapping outcomes. In the pattern exemplified by Frederick, numbness to pain and self-hypnosis are triggered by concrete reminders of vulnerability or helplessness and are associated with self-anesthesia, little overt distress, and emotional distance. Persons so affected demonstrate a relative lack of psychobiological reactivity, as measured by galvanic skin response, heart rate, or blood pressure (Steiner et al., 1999). The second pattern is one characteristic of the borderline individual, in which numbness and self-hypnosis are associated with subjective dyscontrol, impulsivity, hyperarousal, and intense overt emotionality and distress—including distress about the sense of feeling "dead inside," brought about by psychic numbing and anesthesia.

This distinction is consistent with a model of delinquency and aggressive behavior that is gaining support in recent research based on animal models and studies of predelinquent aggression. This model differentiates between *predatory* and *affectively driven* violence (Dodge, 1991; Vitiello & Stoff, 1997; Wasman & Flynn, 1962). Affective aggression is characterized by increased autonomic arousal, threatening or defensive postures, and vocalization. It is typically reactive, situational, and not always goal directed. Predatory aggression, on the other hand, involves limited or no autonomic activation and is associated with stalking behavior, little posturing and vocalizations, and clear goal directness.

This differentiation fits with Meloy's (1988) categorization of Type I or Type II violent acts. Type I aggression, which is by far more common, consists of impulsive attacks carried out in a state of uncontrollable rage, with minimal provocation. Type II aggression, however, involves careful planning of the attack.

The predominance of boys in most samples of antisocial behavior—particularly of the predatory type—has raised questions about some inherent neurobiological disposition that places boys at greater risk for violence in general and for antisocial development in particular. Some differences in violence may be explained by biological variations between men and women, including differences in testosterone levels. However, the sharp increase in criminal activity and violence—including predatory aggression—among adolescent females over the past decade challenges this notion and suggests instead that the difference in violence rates may, at least in part, be mediated by differential patterns of child rearing and cultural reinforcement of different ways of expressing aggression. Women with backgrounds similar to those of antisocial boys are often diagnosed as borderline and are far more likely to attempt suicide, to deliberately harm themselves, and to choose partners who victimize them.

The work of Steiner and colleagues (1999) offers validation of the predatory–impulsive dichotomy. In their research with a sample of juvenile offenders, Steiner and colleagues have assessed two dimensions, distress and restraint, on the basis of which four subgroups can be distinguished. The low distress/low restraint subgroup, which Steiner and colleagues designate as the "nonreactive" subgroup, includes youngsters most likely to be rearrested after release. The low distress/high restraint subgroup, or the "repressor" subgroup, includes youngsters whose behavior is reminiscent of the controlled aggression found in "predatory" animal models. These youngsters commit fewer but more brutal crimes than do those in the other subgroups. A developmental antecedent of these "nonreactive" children can conceivably be found in their disorganized pattern of attachment, with a mix of avoidant features. Studies of these early attachment patterns (Sroufe, 1989) attempt to document the links between avoidant attachment and subsequent traits, such as minimal recognition of others' feelings, hostility, exploitiveness, and efforts to subjugate others physically and verbally.

Yet the biologically prepared disposition for attachment and for finding one's intentionality reflected in another person's mind refuses to disappear altogether. Like the Cheshire cat, the urge to seek attachment and to engage in reflective intersubjectivity leaves behind the disembodied grin of silent longings for responsiveness. If anything, attachment strivings are *intensified* by threat or unresponsiveness. Thus, a vicious cycle is set in motion: Abuse and neglect evoke the very longings for attachment that trigger the active disowning of vulnerability, pain, and attachment.

Abusive interactions such as those described by Frederick are processed and stored in the disconnected state brought about by inhibition of reflective function; that is, wishes for closeness and dependency, and the pain and vulnerability experienced in the context of abusive relationships are processed as concrete, nonreflective schemas, split off from integrated reflective–symbolic representations of the self and others. These nonreflective schemas contain affective, perceptual, and motor information, and an event sequence (Stern, 1995) of the abusive exchange. The scenario thus represented carries forward the malevolent presence of an *other* devoid of human feelings and unmoved by empathy with the child's plight, bent on destroying the child's terrified and helpless self.

In the grip of these schemas, children are unable to conceive of other people as amenable to being influenced by the communication of one's mental state. This is a prementalistic or prereflective world, where behavior is unencumbered and unmodified by reflection or meaning, leaving no room for more than one version of reality. Considering various points of view, changing one's mind, or constructing a shared understanding of a situation are unattainable and inconceivable. Under these conditions, the flexible, mutual regulation of interpersonal situations offered by reflective function is replaced by coercive efforts to impose rigid and unreflective patterns of interaction. Patterson and colleagues have built an impressive body of evidence documenting how an escalating cycle of coercive parent–child interaction leads to conduct disorders and violence (Patterson, 1982; Patterson et al., 1989).

The transactional nature of such coercive cycles is evident in the lack of consistent parenting behavior across time or across different children in the same family (Holden & Miller, 1999). Coercive cycles indeed appear to be aspects of a specific parent–child relationship rather than features present in the parents or the children alone. Parents' coerciveness is, in part, a response to their experience that their child is physically and emotionally punishing (Webster-Stratton & Herbert, 1994), and that the child's misbehavior is malevolent and deliberately intended to hurt them. The parents thus harbor negative expectations about the child and the family, and they feel that they have lost control in their role as parents (Baden & Howe, 1992; Johnson, 1996; Sanders & Dadds, 1992).

Parents thus appear disposed to respond to the particular cues of a specific child with an inhibition of their own reflective function. The ensuing coercive cycles provide a model of relationships that reinforces the deployment of aggression and coercive patterns of interaction in response to internal or interpersonal cues signaling heightened vulnerability.

Unreflective schemas of self and other become the nucleus around which these children organize the pained, dependent, vulnerable aspects of the self, while craving attachment and interacting with rejecting, dismissive, threatening, coercive, unpredictably abusive, humiliating caregivers. These schemas are split off from the evolving autobiographical representations that utilize reflective function to integrate implicit–procedural and explicit–symbolic processing. A sector of life, experience, and relationships is thus lived in a state of psychological void, creating a discontinuity in the sense of self that is experienced as an alien body, a ghost threatening to erupt, to "take over" and trap children in states of terror that are unbearable because they cannot be reflected on or processed. Fonagy and Target (1995, 2000), as discussed in Chapter 4, refer to these aspects of experience as the "alien self."

The only "escape" from this internal tormentor resides in children's ability to create procedurally unreflective and coercive strategies to externalize these schemas, that is, in their active enactment in the interpersonal world. Children are prone to this tendency because of the activation of the coercive patterns previously described. The externalization of the disowned and dissociated aspects of the self is the next step in the path toward a severe personality disorder.

From a remarkably young age, children headed toward developing a narcissistic–antisocial personality make excessive demands for control that can never be fulfilled (Egan & Kernberg, 1984). Unable to feel gratitude, even when their demands are met, they grow used to giving orders and setting the tone of the household. As Noshpitz (1984) points out, they insist on having their own way—and their parents are unable to manage them. These children struggle with all their might to be the center of everyone's attention and, when frustrated, they fly into a towering rage.

When such children enter school, their inability to expose their vulnerability interferes with schoolwork. Unable to acknowledge their limitations and to accept help from their teachers, they adopt the stance of refusing to work rather than admitting their shortcomings. Teachers are doubly frustrated: The verbal facility and charm of these children prompt expectations of academic achievement. But their verbal cleverness often expresses basically empty intellectualizations and word play. Tall tales and lies cover a limited capacity for sustained attention and difficulty in solving problems in reality. Language becomes a tool for exhibitionism and manipulation, a defense against shame, envy, and vulnerability, and a weapon to control, intimidate, and keep people at a distance.

Such children's attained illusion of control is supported by their capacity to elicit in others the helplessness and vulnerability they cannot tolerate in themselves. By imposing their dreaded and disowned self-experiences on others, they "rid" themselves of them and achieve the illusion that their vulnerability can be controlled and conquered rather than passively suffered. Control and intimidation over others thus confirm their power and invulnerability.

Aggression and coercive behavior, however, only demonstrate how these children are incapable of responding adaptively to distressing affect, which normally involves the activation of the attachment system. In their case, as we have seen, distress evokes a *retreat* from attachment and reflective function, leaving these children incapable of regulating intense negative affect except by the use of narrow and rigid strategies. This behavior, however, greatly increases the likelihood of peer rejection, which further impairs the children's capacity to find alternative attachments and to undo the negative impact of early disruptions in relationships. These children soon find themselves recreating coercive cycles not only with their peers but also with their teachers and other adults in the school system. Often, they become bullies (Farrington, 1993) and are shunned, which increases their drift toward deviant peer groups. Their association with deviant peers leads to a significant escalation of antisocial behavior and opens the path to substance abuse and delinquency (Dishion, Andrews, & Crosby, 1995).

Joe's case serves as an illustration. Thirteen years old when he began treatment, he was the only living child of parents divorced when he was 8 years old. A brother, born when Joe was 4 years old, had died at age 10 months from complications of congenital cardiac malformation.

Joe was brought for residential treatment after several years of outpatient treatment had failed to prevent the escalation of his antisocial behavior. His rather extensive history of drug abuse included the use of marijuana, cocaine, and alcohol. He had engaged in shoplifting and other forms of petty theft. In school, he was a bully and an exhibitionistic clown who demanded attention and refused to follow directions. When drugs were unavailable, he ate voraciously, at one point running up a $100 bill for hamburgers at his grandparents' country club.

Joe's parents' marriage had been a stormy affair, punctuated by the father's heavy drinking and brutal abuse of both Joe and his mother. As a young child, Joe witnessed fights almost daily between his parents. He sometimes attempted to divert his father's attention to prevent him from beating his mother. When he succeeded, his father would vent his anger on Joe, then pass out in an alcoholic stupor. More than once, Joe removed cigarettes from his father's hand after he had passed out or watched worriedly as his father nodded drunkenly at the wheel of the car. Joe's father also introduced Joe to drugs and alcohol. Joe's mother, heavily invested in pursuing her theatrical career and emotionally drained by her husband's abuse, provided Joe with little support or protection.

Joe, a handsome, appealing boy, appeared several years older than his age. His sharp wit and verbal cleverness rarely failed to charm and elicited reactions that only hinted at his enormous sensitivity to interpersonal nuances and his shrewd awareness of how to obtain the desired responses from others.

The beginning of treatment was marked by Joe's dismissiveness and mocking inquiries about whether I was a "faggot" and how much he despised my petulance and pathetic attempts to read his mind—his reply to the mildest efforts to clarify what he was trying to tell me. Almost in spite of himself, however, he began to feel more comfortable with me, even to look forward to the sessions, particularly since I was able to help him "save face" in school, where he had fallen hopelessly behind. Yet the desire for closeness was unbearable to him. Thus, he began carefully to look for "mistakes" (e.g., my interrupting him or "invading his space"), which triggered hateful barrages. He then let me know of his plans to run away from the residential treatment center and find my house ("I have good sources, you know"), so that he could set it on fire and burn it to the ground, but only after raping my wife and murdering my children with slow, intravenous injections of cocaine. He would spare my life, but only to ensure that I would suffer the loss of everything I held dear.

Joe's tirade spoke volumes about what the possibility of closeness evoked in him: a sense of his house/body being invaded and destroyed; a penetration that triggered burning, devastating feelings that would lead to total devastation; envy of my possessions and other relationships, with the associated rage at his own deprivation; and the overwrought striving to eliminate all possible rivals for my love and attention, and at the same time leave me as lonely, needy, and deprived as he was.

In the treatment section, I discuss a model of intervention that considers how to help children—and therapists—survive the exacerbation of dysfunction that almost inevitably follows when these youngsters begin to consider the possibility of trusting others. For now, however, I make only the obvious point that outbursts such as Joe's evoke intense responses in their treaters—as intense, in fact, as the responses they evoke in everyone else. Buffeted by the unreflective barrages to which these children subject therapists, caregivers, peers, teachers, and others respond in kind: with unreflective, fight-or-flight responses of their own, "fitting" in an unmodulated fashion the models that these youngsters attempt to impose on the world. Therapists, teachers, probation officers, and others typically experience dread of meeting with them, concern about being fooled or humiliated, and wishes to subjugate or outright hurt them. These experiences correspond with the children's efforts to intimidate, humiliate, and subjugate.

Alternatively, other persons may identify with the internal states these children seek to evoke and find themselves experiencing, at a visceral level, feelings of worthlessness, helplessness, and defeat. Perhaps more pernicious are the subtle ways in which these youngsters' manipulation and denial of vulnerability evoke a nonconscious envy of their ability to "get away" with breaking rules, which leads to covert collusion with antisocial behavior. These responses are examples of the mechanism of projective identification (Klein, 1952a), or what Spillius (1992) has called "evocative projective identification," the mechanism that Gabbard (1995) precisely describes as the emerging contemporary view of projective identification in the psychoanalytic literature. As summarized by Gabbard, projective identification involves disavowing an aspect of the self by "placing" that aspect in someone else and then applying interpersonal pressure to coerce the other person to identify with what has been projected.

In Chapter 9, I discuss the treatment implications of the patient's projective efforts. At this point, I want to draw attention to the nature of the responses these children evoke in others. Therapists' countertransference offers a glimpse of how these children shape the environment that will in turn shape and reinforce their maladjustment. These youngsters consistently evoke punitive, submissive, rageful, or collusive responses from others. The common element of these various responses, however, is that they tend to be unreflective, concrete, procedural responses to the youngsters' own unreflective behavior. Moreover, these responses disavow any consideration of the mental states underlying such behavior. The tit for tat of unreflective exchanges only reinforces and exacerbates these children's alienation from reflective functioning.

Joe's case also provides a good springboard to examining how much these children's apparent callousness and disregard for others' feelings reflect their own lack of awareness of those feelings. This idea is in line with Gabbard's (1989) notion of an *oblivious* type of narcissist, whose arrogance, aggressiveness, and self-absorption betray a gross insensitivity to others.

Observing children such as Joe makes plain, however, that they carefully scan the environment in search of clues of impending danger and are *exquisitely* aware of other people's motives and weaknesses. Often, as Tooley (1975) remarked, they are "self-possessed, convincing and attractive [and] demonstrate a capacity for cool reality testing and shrewd assessment of interpersonal situations" (p. 307). They do not hesitate to utilize their awareness of the "right buttons to push" to manipulate the environment. It would appear that, while generally *hypersensitive* and hypervigilant of other people's internal states in the context of *potential* closeness with others (i.e., in situations that may elicit a wish for dependency or intimacy), these children appear to inhibit their reflective capacity defensively. They not only numb themselves to feelings of vulnerability but also obliterate their awareness of the other person's mental states. This fractionation or splitting of reflective function explains the coexistence of striking sensitivity to interpersonal cues and the capacity to treat others as things rather than people.

Inhibition of reflective function in response to cues that signal vulnerability and/or a heightened need for attachment, coupled with hypervigilance to anticipate the possible emergence of such threats, explains the deficits in social–cognitive skills repeatedly demonstrated in this group of children (Coie & Dodge, 1998; Matthys, Cuperus, & Van Engeland, 1999). Their difficulties in processing social information include (1) encoding deficits, that is, a failure to pay attention to some social cues while being hypervigilant to others; (2) attributional bias, which consists of frequently assigning hostile intention to others' behavior; (3) misinterpretation of social cues, particularly misjudging other people's affect; and (4) social problem-solving deficits, that is, a limited capacity to generate effective and adaptive solutions to interpersonal conflict, and a preference for aggressive solutions.

Levinson and Fonagy (1999), in their study of imprisoned men, support this notion. Attachment interview narratives of violent men show a marked refusal, either spontaneously or in response to the interviewer's questions, to comment on mental states in the context of attachment relationships—either their own or those of their caregivers.

Fonagy (1999b) cites one such man, imprisoned for brutally assaulting his girlfriend. He described in clinical detail how his alcoholic father regularly emptied his bladder on him and his sister. When asked why he thought his father behaved as he did, he answered: "You tell me, you're the fucking psychologist." Throughout the rest of the interview, this man, like the other offenders, barely mentioned mental states—and then only to describe or explain how wardens, policemen, or other prisoners felt or thought. When discussing his girlfriend, his children, or his parents, he could address only their concrete circumstances, their physical environment, or their behavior. At no time could he give evidence that, in the context of attachment, he could comprehend the mental states that make human behavior understandable.

It should not be inferred from such descriptions that attachment relationships do not matter to such individuals. On the contrary, as Joe's story suggests, the response of the *attachment partner* to the intimidation or violence is a crucial component of these ruthless individuals' internal scripts. Perceiving the terror in the eyes of the victim is reassuring to them. The victim's struggling, pleading, and suffering are vital components of the interaction. Observing such interactions makes it readily apparent that provoking such responses in another person is one of the basic aims of the entire exchange.

At the very heart of the relationships these children establish is the necessity of feeling in control of the other person. The trigger for intimidating, bullying, or exhibiting frankly violent behavior is often some evidence that, in the context of a relationship that has grown close, the other person has a mind of his or her own. Some of these children can verbalize the rage they experience when the other person "escapes their control" and triggers in them a need to bring the other to heel and "teach him or her a lesson." The aim of "the lesson" is to keep the partner captive and available. Anything that reminds these youngsters that the other person has a separate intentionality is unbearable, because it threatens to reactivate their silent helplessness and vulnerability in the face of a malignant other who wishes to destroy or abandon them. A reflective stance in an attachment relationship is thus a disaster they must avoid at all costs.

On the other hand, when these children succeed in enacting the rigid script of their nonreflective schemas, they feel reassured and more real, coherent, and connected than at any other time. Like Joe, they check carefully and keep adjusting their actions until they produce the "right" response: that a disavowed personal aspect has come to life in the other person. Paradoxically, when they recognize in the other person a facsimile of their own internal state, they come close to experiencing the merger of subjectivities that is normally achieved only through the exercise of reflective function.

Thus, the seemingly unprovoked outbursts of violence and intimidation serve multiple functions in these children's homeostasis: They gain a measure of control by expelling and then controlling the unbearable helplessness and loneliness in the outside world; they provoke punishment and retaliation, which actively creates the trauma and abuse they otherwise expect will befall them passively; and last, but certainly not least, they turn violence and intimidation into the currency of intimacy and connection.

This developing personality organization, however, evolves into a range of levels of disturbance, from moderate severity and relative treatability to extreme lethality and untreatability. Stone (2000) proposes a schema of gradations of antisociality to evaluate the treatability and dangerousness of adults who exhibit antisocial behavior.

At the mildest end of Stone's spectrum are individuals who engage in some antisocial behavior that may be relatively infrequent and occurs in the context of another personality disorder. In the middle of the spectrum, Stone places antisocial personality without violence, while in the most severe—and intractable—end of the spectrum are psychopathy with violent sadism and murder, and even prolonged torture and murder. Stone's gradations resonate with Kernberg's (1992) notion of "malignant narcissism" to designate individuals with a narcissistic personality disorder admixed with antisocial and paranoid features. Kernberg's concept draws attention to the importance of narcissistic disturbances in the development and organization of antisocial personality and psychopathy. This connection was recognized in Cleckley's (1941) classic study of psychopathy, in which he used this term to describe individuals characterized by self-centeredness, flamboyance, superficial charm, lack of remorse, and contempt for social convention and rules.

As Stone (2000) points out, there are significant differences between the concept of antisocial personality, which is defined by DSM-IV largely on the basis of behavioral characteristics, and the concept of psychopathy, which is narrower and refers to a description of personality. Hare and colleagues (Hare, 1996; Hart, Hare, & Forth, 1994) have sought to clarify this distinction by developing a Psychopathy Checklist—Revised (PCL-R) that rates true descriptions of personality and includes those aspects of narcissistic disturbance that impinge on other people's rights.

Anchoring antisocial personality in constructs based on personality functioning makes possible (1) consideration of the links between antisocial and other personality disorders, particularly within Cluster B dramatic personality disorder; and (2) evaluation of antisocial personality using a dimensional and developmental approach that differentiates between the larger group of conduct disorders and children developing an antisocial personality.

Stone (2000) remarks that viewing psychopathic personality in dimensional terms makes clear that the mildest forms (exhibiting a few of the PCL-R items, such as charm, deceitfulness, and grandiosity) blend into the general population. Such traits can be associated, in fact, with very successful adaptation and may be essential components of the personality of entrepreneurs, politicians, and other leaders and innovators. Clearly, not all antisocial persons lack the capacities for successful adaptation and formation of meaningful attachments or the experiences of remorse, concern, and compassion. The presence of these capacities, in at least embryonic form, is a precondition for treatability (Stone, 2000). In its extreme forms, malignant or predatory narcissism, with its deceitfulness and pathological lying, cunning and manipulativeness, lack of remorse, callousness and lack of compassion, contempt and disregard for other people's feelings, and devaluation of others, including the treater, augurs poorly for treatability. Meloy (1988) offers a similar set of guidelines as contraindications to therapy for violent patients: (1) a history of sadistic behavior with injury, (2) a complete absence of remorse, (3) an IQ indicating either superior intellect or intelligence in the retarded range, (4) a lack of capacity for attachment, and (5) an intense countertransference fear in the therapist of the patient's predatory behavior.

Treatability thus appears to be contingent upon the degree to which a malignant narcissistic adaptation has obliterated the most basic human capacity to form attachments.

PATHOLOGICAL NARCISSISTIC REGULATION AND NARCISSISTIC DISORDERS

Defining the ruthlessness of some children as an extreme form of narcissistic pathology requires clarification of the elusive concepts of "narcissism," "narcissistic regulation," and "narcissistic pathology"—the core elements in the severe personality disorders.

Narcissus's fatal plunge in pursuit of his beautiful image turned him into a ready symbol of the perils of self-absorption. Delving into the literature on narcissism in search of clarity, however, while perhaps less perilous, is still a daunting and confusing challenge. The confusion arises, at least in part, from the diversity of meanings assigned to narcissism since Freud's (1914/1963) seminal paper "On Narcissism: An Introduction." Freud fueled the conceptual murkiness by using narcissism in various ways and in different contexts.

Pulver (1970) extrapolates four meanings of narcissism from Freud's writings: clinical, developmental, economic, and object relations. *Clinically*, narcissism was viewed as a sexual perversion, characterized by the preferential choice of one's body as a sexual object. *Developmentally*, it was the earliest stage of normal development, when infants were presumed to be unable to differentiate self and nonself, and thus could only invest their libido in themselves. Freud postulated that in this stage of primary narcissism, infants experience an "oceanic feeling" of boundless omnipotence, self-love, and overestimation of the power of their wishes. *Economically*, narcissism was the investment of libidinal energy in the ego, equivalent to self-love. In terms of *object relations*, it involved a type of object choice: the withdrawal of libido and identification with a lost object.

The *narcissistic object choice* includes people who love what they themselves are, were, or would like to be. Their aim is to be loved and gratified, while they regard the other person as only a means to satisfy their own needs. In the normal, affectionate relationship of parents to their children, Freud (1914/1963) found a "revival and reproduction of their own narcissism" (p. 91). Children, Freud claimed, are made the depositories of the wishful dreams of the parents: a narcissistic mode of relating to the environment that is characterized, in cases of illness, by the *withdrawal of libido* from the external world into the ego. Persons affected by pain, for example, may give up their interest and focus on the external world. In a regressive response to object loss, *identification* with the lost object (a narcissistic cathexis) replaces the love for the object. In relation to *treatment indications*, individuals manifesting the narcissistic neuroses were characterized by such self-absorption that they were unable to develop a transference and were thus not appropriate indications for psychoanalysis. These conditions included what nowadays would be described as schizophrenia, major depression, or hypochondriasis.

Over the past three decades, the trend in the psychological and psychoanalytic literature has been to look at narcissism less from the standpoint of drives and the hypothetical distribution of psychic energies, or the now largely discredited notion of a normal state of development characterized by lack of investment in others, and more in terms of the self. The self has proven to be a fruitful construct that draws together notions about the development (normal and pathological) of the person's conscious and unconscious mental self-representations; the mental processes underpinning such self-representations; the integration, continuity, and coherence of such mental representations; the individual's capacity for autonomous functioning and regulation; and the capacity for self-regard or self-esteem. From this perspective, Stolorow (1975) defined mental activity as narcissistic "to the degree that its function is to maintain the structural cohesion, temporal stability and positive affect coloring of the self-representation" (p. 179).

As previously noted, infants are biologically prepared to seek self-regulation and to create organization, and are traumatized when rendered unable to generate a sense of anticipation, coherence, and activity. Needless to say, such self-regulating tendencies are inextricably tied to the built-in disposition for attachment and congruity in a mutually reinforcing fashion. Sander (1975) and Ainsworth and Bell (1974) make the point that the infant's competence and self-regulation are contingent on the presence of alert and responsive caregivers. Not surprisingly, disturbances of narcissistic regulation invariably involve concerns about being ignored or not receiving attention, often coupled with doubt about one's ability to have an impact on or evoke a response from others.

Reflective function becomes the bridge between the complementary, innate urges to strive for self-regulation, contingency, mastery, and coherence on the one hand, and to seek attachments on the other. As noted previously, the growth of symbolic capacities and reflective function between the second and fourth years of life provides children with an extraordinary tool to guide their efforts to achieve both sets of aims: the creation of the "ideal self" (described in Chapter 3) as a blueprint to guide their efforts to achieve self-regulation and human connectedness more effectively.

Following Jacobson's (1964) concept, subsequently expanded by Joffe and Sandler (1967), I view the central feature of narcissistic disorders as a state of pain, overt or latent, caused by "a substantial discrepancy between the mental representation of the self and an ideal shape of the self" (p. 65). This discrepancy mobilizes a number of coping and defensive maneuvers that can assume maladaptive proportions. Needless to say, narcissistic injuries are an inevitable aspect of both normal and

pathological development. All children encounter them as they establish their personal identity, boundaries, and autonomy. Narcissistic vulnerabilities span the entire spectrum of psychopathology and are central
to a wide variety of clinical and developmental problems.

In what he describes as two poles on a continuum of narcissistic
personality disorders, Gabbard (1989) distinguishes between the *oblivious narcissist* and the *hypervigilant narcissist,* a distinction based on the
person's predominant style of interacting. The oblivious type *appears* to
have no awareness of the reactions of others. These individuals are arrogant, aggressive, and self-absorbed, constantly seek to be the center of
attention, and are seemingly impervious to having their feelings hurt.
The hypervigilant type is enormously sensitive to other people's reactions, inhibited and shy (sometimes to the point of self-effacement),
and prone to shun being the center of attention. Persons with this type
of narcissistic disorder carefully check the environment for evidence of
slights or criticisms that can hurt their feelings and cause them to feel
ashamed and humiliated. Gabbard's typology relates closely to Bateman's (1998) distinction between "thick-skinned" and "thin-skinned"
narcissism. It also overlaps to some extent with the differentiation between "predatory" and "affectively driven" destructiveness.

Beyond differences in overt style of relatedness among narcissistic
individuals, a lively controversy has surrounded the efforts to elucidate
the underlying developmental and dynamic features of narcissistic disorders. The major figures in this controversy have been Otto Kernberg
(1970, 1975) and Heinz Kohut (1971, 1972, 1977). Gabbard (1994) offers a crisp, point-by-point comparison of Kernberg's and Kohut's ideas.

Kohut anchored his conceptual framework on a supraordinate theory of the self, which he defined as the psychological center of activity,
initiative, and autonomy. According to Kohut, the primordial self of infancy is weak and unsteady, and lacks enduring structure, cohesiveness,
and continuity. Only parental intervention prevents the fragmentation
of the proto-self. Kohut coined the term "selfobject" to designate the
caregiver's support of the infant's self. This term highlights the infant's
view of the caregiver as only the supplier of regulating functions that
the infant is unable to perform.

The key to the attainment of self-cohesiveness and autonomy,
according to Kohut, is parental empathy. In particular, he stressed the
capacity of parents to respond with acceptance and pride (mirroring) to
their children's display of unique traits, talents, and evolving capabili-

ties, as well as the ability to convey their capacity to care for their children and prevent them from experiencing fragmentation.

Kohut claimed that parental empathy weaves the thread that binds the self into a cohesive whole capable of self-regulation. By gradually and emphatically reducing their regulatory role as caregivers, parents allow their infants to internalize bit by bit the conviction of their own reality, vitality, identity, and self-worth, as well as to develop an internal sense of competence, goals, and self-direction.

In this model, narcissistic disorders are placed between the neurotic disorders and the borderline and psychotic conditions. On the one hand, Kohut defined the neuroses as a group of disorders in which symptoms are manifestations of conflict between aspects of a relatively solid and cohesive self. At the psychotic or borderline end of the spectrum, on the other hand, the self has never attained any degree of cohesiveness. Narcissistic disorders, for Kohut and his followers, represent discrete, structural deficits in the self, related to an *arrest* in development brought about by the failure of caregivers to respond with empathy to developmentally appropriate needs.

Kernberg (1970, 1975) distinguishes differently between normal and pathological narcissism. He conceptualizes the narcissistic personality as a specific distortion in development: the fusion of the ideal self, the ideal object, and the actual self. The resulting pathological formation, the *grandiose self*, according to Kernberg, is a defense against intense early conflicts, particularly conflicts involving envy, aggression, and dependence. The defended-against self-image—the aspects of the self that the grandiose self is meant to conceal—is that of a "hungry, enraged, empty self, full of impotent anger at being frustrated, and fearful of a world which seems as hateful and revengeful as the patient himself" (Kernberg, 1975, p. 233).

Although a predominance of aggression plays a central role in Kernberg's formulation, he leaves open whether pathological development is caused by constitutionally determined excessive aggression or by severe frustration during the first years of life. For Kernberg, the designation "narcissistic personality" refers to a specific instance of borderline personality organization rather than to a broad range of disorders, as Kohut and his followers suggest. Expanding on this notion, Rinsley (1989) and Adler (1985) proposed the concept of a spectrum of disorders in which the narcissistic personality represents a "higher level" manifestation of the borderline personality.

DSM-IV includes narcissistic personality disorder among the Cluster B personality disorders. It lists diagnostic criteria that bear a considerable resemblance to Kernberg's description of the clinical manifestations of pathological narcissism but pay scant attention to the more quietly grandiose, hypersensitive individuals identified by Kohut and captured by Gabbard's (1989) notion of "hypervigilant narcissist."

According to Gabbard (1994), Kohut and Kernberg drew their theoretical models from the observation of different types of patients: Kernberg was exposed to less well adjusted people, more closely approximating the oblivious type, while Kohut worked primarily with better functioning people, with more overtly vulnerable self-esteem. I believe that Gabbard's differentiation between oblivious and hypervigilant types is very useful, yet might require some additional elaboration to discriminate better between the narcissistic disturbances that are part of the Cluster B of dramatic personality disorders and the narcissistic problems affecting individuals with other types of problems.

"Obliviousness," for instance, can be linked to the pervasive "blindness" (Baron-Cohen et al., 1995) to other people's mental states and associated lack of empathy that characterize even the milder forms of pervasive developmental disorders and Asperger's syndrome. Likewise, the oblivious type of narcissism is characteristic of highly obsessional individuals whose rigid perfectionism betrays their inner sense of grandiosity, and whose chronic disconnection from their own affect handicaps their ability to connect emotionally with others and makes them come across, instead, as pedantic and controlling.

On the other hand, "hypervigilant" can refer to shy, clumsy, and anxious children who are perennially pained by fears of shame and humiliation. Eager to comply with the wishes and expectations of peers and other people, they readily sacrifice themselves for other people's sake. Their lives are burdened not only by their secret efforts to meet ideal standards of perfection but also by their terror—revealed only by their blushing—and their inhibition of being exposed as inferior, ugly, or inadequate.

I suggest that two features differentiate the narcissistic problems of children with Cluster B personality disorders from the narcissistic difficulties that mark other children's maladjustment. First, children with severe personality disorders are trapped in a pattern of discontinuity— or splitting—of experience. Some aspects of their lives and experience of their sense of self and others are *not* organized by integrated implicit–

explicit models guided by reflective function. Instead, they are organized by nonreflective modes of processing. Internal states or external
cues linked to an increased need for attachment trigger a defensive inhibition of reflective function and the activation of the nonreflective models. These children live in a state of hypervigilance, anxiously scanning
both the external environment and their own internal states for clues of
states that may render them vulnerable.

Nonreflective models *replace* the normal process of narcissistic regulation. The normal process is a dialectical one in which, on the one
hand, people strive to match the actual self with the ideal self, while, on
the other hand, they engage in an ongoing modification of the ideal self
on the basis of intersubjective exchanges. This double dialectical process optimally links enhanced mastery and self-regulation with interpersonal adjustment and the subjective experience of narcissistic well-
being or self-esteem.

In contrast, nonreflective models provide affective–perceptual–
motor strategies designed to reactively disown helplessness, pain, and
vulnerability, thus generating an *illusion* of safety, control, and effectiveness. Such illusion comes at the expense of disregarding aspects of both
internal and external reality.

The second key feature of the pathological narcissistic regulation
associated with severe personality disorders is indeed the *externalization*
of the nonreflective models into these children's interpersonal world.
The *dramatic* quality ascribed to these developing personality disorders
stems precisely from children's reliance on a coping strategy that consists of coercing others to respond to them according to their internal
model's rigid and unreflective script. It is only in the ensuing drama
generated around them that these children find a semblance of intimacy
and human connection.

GRANDIOSITY AND THE FALSE SELF

One consequence of the splitting or fractionation of experience described in Chapter 4 is a corresponding discontinuity of the sense of
self. The subjective sense of continuity and coherence of the self—what
Erikson (1959) called a sense of "me-ness"—stems from the intersubjective exchanges that allows infants to find their internal states
reflected in another person's mind. Through such reflective processes,

internal states can be elaborated in their implicit and symbolic features and integrated into an evolving autobiographical narrative.

Winnicott (1967) beautifully described the predicament faced by children who *fail* to find their internal state in the mind of the caregiver when he asked: "What does the baby see when he or she looks at his mother's face? . . . Ordinarily, the mother is looking at the baby and what she looks like is related to what she sees there" (p. 29). In other words, babies find *themselves* in the reflection of their caregiver's face and behavior. But, added Winnicott, what of "the baby whose mother reflects her own mood or, worse still, the rigidity of her own defenses? They [babies] look and they do not see themselves. . . . What is seen is the mother's face" (p. 29).

The lack of caregivers' reflective function, however, is rarely continuous. Instead, the path to a narcissistic–antisocial organization, as we saw earlier, is paved by caregivers who *intermittently* retreat from reflective function *in response to their children's bids for attachment*. As the dependency and vulnerability overwhelm them, these caregivers become abusive, and may ridicule and/or avoid their children's display of the very traits of vulnerability and wishes for closeness that the caregivers find intolerable in themselves. Arguably, the resulting inability of children to organize at a reflective level the dependent, vulnerable, striving-for-attachment aspects of the self and subsequently integrate them into their evolving sense of self are key factors in narcissistic–antisocial development.

As recipients of the projection of their caregivers' disowned vulnerability, these children suffer from a double developmental insult: the caregivers' lack of attunement to the children's needs for attachment, coupled with relentless efforts to instill in the children their own rejected self-aspects. The unreflective strategies that a caregiver utilizes to coerce a child to "own" aspects of the caregiver's self set the stage for the construction of split-off, unreflective models. These models, in turn, are the "ghosts" threatening to intrude "at unguarded moments," ensuring in due time the transgenerational transmission of abuse and insensitivity.

But the coercive cycles of caregiver–child interaction also carry other connotations. Caregivers often respond to their disowned dependency needs with subtle (or not so subtle) maneuvers to turn their children into caretakers, as the following vignette illustrates.

Pete was adopted when he was 6 months old. His adoptive mother remembers that he smiled easily and seldom cried when she first began caring for him. He would even resist her efforts to feed him, insisting at a very young age on holding the bottle himself. Pete's growth only intensified his demands to be in charge of his own and everyone else's affairs. He reacted with terrible temper tantrums to any effort to set limits on his demandingness.

When Pete was almost 2 years old, his adoptive father walked out on the family, shortly after the mother gave birth to a baby girl. The newborn suffered from a congenital heart malformation and her physical needs and demands for care and attention left the mother drained and exhausted—just when her husband had abandoned her. Pete, on the other hand, seemed to become more cheerful, more helpful, and better adjusted. He became quite protective of his baby sister and talked of now being his mother's boyfriend. The romance, however, came to an end a year and a half later, when Pete's mother remarried. Pete began to throw even more furious tantrums when limits were set on him. Limit setting, however, became more urgent as he devised increasingly more cruel schemes to hurt his sister, the same child he had sworn to care for and protect a few months earlier.

Pete's nursery school teacher described him as a provocative and exhibitionistic youngster who acted and talked like a miniature adult. His remarkable skill at picking out people's vulnerabilities betrayed his heightened awareness of interpersonal nuances. Interestingly, as Pete's treatment got under way, and as his mother formally "fired" him from the "boyfriend" position, he responded with panic. He found comfort only when he began to steal articles of clothing from other children, and he poignantly insisted on dressing like his peers and imitating other people's gestures and expressions.

This vignette raises several distinct points about the sense of self and the narcissistic disturbance of children with a severe personality disorder. These children feel both internal and external pressure to become self-sufficient. They distance themselves from experiences of pain and vulnerability, thus failing to achieve a psychologically integrated self-experience.

First, the pressure to develop competence in manipulating the environment and to achieve an appearance of self-sufficiency for children in the antisocial and narcissistic end of the cluster seems to come both from within and without. Brutality, neglect, misattunement, and early loss are common experiences in the lives of many of these children. These circumstances lead them, as we saw earlier, to disown dependence and to turn their attention to controlling the environment and achieving a sense of self-reliance and numbness to pain and vulnerability. Innate resourcefulness promotes self-reliance and pseudomaturity as the only coping responses available. Survival is predicated on propping up depleted caregivers who, like Pete's adoptive mother, are in need of far more love, comfort, and protection than they can provide to a needy child.

Adopted children like Pete and Elliot (described in Chapter 6) face the need to integrate into their evolving autobiographical narrative the fact of their adoption. They can never ignore the reality that their biological parents "gave them up." These children are at particular risk for developing the mixed disorganized/avoidant attachment and dismissiveness of vulnerability and dependence previously described, while turning instead to unreflective strategies to ensure a sense of control. For them, nothing is more crucial than to "control" the helplessness and devastation of abandonment. Some children become hypervigilant to cues that signal abandonment and proficient at actively coercing others to enact the very rejection they fear having to suffer passively.

Adoptive parents, on the other hand, must contend with the narcissistic injury of their infertility, the long wait for a child, and the scrutiny required to demonstrate their adequacy as parents. Until the adoption is finalized, parents and children often feel "on probation," which naturally handicaps the development of smoothly reciprocal, mutually reflective exchanges. Attunement *may* be further disrupted by the absence of the experience of having a baby. Although it is questionable how much gestation contributes to the maternal ability to attune to a baby, the adoptive mother, as Reeves (1971) suggests, "got a baby, but has not 'had a baby'" (p. 167).

Adopted children thus appear at greater risk than nonadoptive children for setting in motion ever-spiraling cycles of rejection-seeking behavior that compounds parents' feelings of inadequacy and narcissistic vulnerability. As adoptive parents recoil, even in subtle ways from their children, this withdrawal further fuels these children's expectation of abandonment—and triggers a defensive retreat from reflective function and the deployment of unreflective models to ensure control. But the development of reflective function can also suffer in a more insidious way in adoptive children. As Brinich (1980) points out, the concrete reality of an abandonment that has already happened inhibits adopted children from freely experimenting in their minds with "as if" scenarios such as finding new parents or creating a different identity within a different family. These fantasies greatly enrich children's ability to consider different points of view and to adapt their mental representations more flexibly while negotiating the challenges of development. Instead, adoptive children are drawn to nonreflective responses that haunt them particularly during adolescence (Chapter 6), a time that calls for substantial reorganization and integration of the multiple aspects of the representations of self and others.

Second, children with a severe personality disorder often feel no pain, which fuels an illusory sense of power—a sense of grandiosity—that is reinforced by the children's capacity to control their feelings and their environment. Their grandiosity receives additional support from the coercion they experience either directly or indirectly to turn into their caregiver's caretaker. Indeed, these resourceful youngsters are called on to play special roles in their family's adjustment: to hold the family together, or to serve as a companion or protector to one of the caregivers. They are then rewarded for their performance with a sense of specialness.

The grandiosity of these children thus holds hostage any desire they may have to assert their own separate needs and characteristics, particularly wishes for care and dependence. According to Rinsley (1980a, 1984, 1989), future narcissistic children are enmeshed in interactive patterns that convey an encouragement—indeed, a demand—to develop competence, resourcefulness, and self-reliance—individuation, in the terms of Mahler and colleagues (1975)—while precluding any real separation. Children and caregivers become enmeshed in a tight web of mutually coercive, procedural cycles that prevent *everyone's* independent functioning, as first the caregivers, and subsequently the children themselves, are trapped by their mutual need to control the disowned aspects of themselves that they project onto each other. Children experience this entrapment as an unspeakable dread that a catastrophe will follow any effort to escape the family's coercive cycles.

The third characteristic of children with a severe personality disorder is that they experience a psychological void regarding aspects of self-experience, coupled with relentless externally and internally generated coercion to embody disowned aspects of someone else's experience. This tendency leaves a devastating legacy, a sense of a lack of authenticity or completeness, and a haunting feeling that something is wrong or missing, or not quite real inside. This feeling is best captured by Winnicott's (1965) concept of the "false self," a sense of self that serves defensive purposes (i.e., denial of dependence, helplessness, and vulnerability) and that accommodates environmental demands and expectations (i.e., becoming a parent's caretaker or the recipient of a caregiver's disowned vulnerability).

But a sense of identity organized around a false self, no matter how impressive, is built of psychological cardboard because it is not anchored in an internally coherent, reflectively processed sense of self that is open to intersubjective exchanges. This false identity centers on mental states that preclude taking into account and integrating children's changing emotional and cognitive states, and their ongoing assessment of other people's minds. When challenged, as Pete could attest, such constructions prove brittle. At best, they leave children deprived of the feelings of purpose, vitality, and authenticity normally derived from a coherent sense of self. Instead, these children feel like "phonies," bent on deceiving others yet dependent on external responses and the control of others to define themselves and to feel worthy and safe.

6

Histrionic and Borderline Children and Adolescents

Whereas narcissistic–antisocial children are alienated from dependence and vulnerability, a different form of narcissistic disturbance affects a group of youngsters edging toward the borderline end of the cluster: the narcissistic–histrionic patients. These children's early lives are *not* marked by gross misattunement to their bids for attachment. They are far less likely to encounter malevolent and abusive intentions in their caregivers' minds in response to dependence and vulnerability. Instead, they find a distinct coercion to display those features best suited to match the caregivers' own narcissistic ideals and thus regulate the caregivers' self-esteem. These children soon find out that their accomplishments are important primarily as a source of their caregivers' pride, gratification, and narcissistic regulation.

Special attributes make it more likely that a child will be chosen to play such a special role in regulating caregiver self-esteem. Unusual beauty, precocious development (particularly language development), and uncommon artistic, intellectual, or athletic gifts greatly increase the odds that children will be invested with their caregivers' narcissistic aspirations. Such gifts fuel the caregivers' hopes that their children will serve as receptive vehicles to carry forward their own often unfulfilled fantasies and ambitions.

Particular circumstances surrounding birth also endow such children with special meaning to their caregivers. Gifts and singular meanings become heavily invested by caregivers, who perceive their children as a sort of appendage, a source of pride and gratification, the providers of the goodness and appreciation that caregivers feel entitled to themselves but have been denied. Thus, while inflating children's grandiosity with exaggerated attunement, responsiveness, and subtle coercion to display the "brilliant," "perfect," "beautiful" aspects of themselves, these caretakers tightly control the children's performance. These children are the apple of their caregivers' eyes, but they dare not fail or disappoint, because the caregivers' self-esteem has become entangled with the children's magnificence. At the same time, such caregivers ignore, reject, or ridicule characteristics of the children that fail to match their ideal. The case of Elliot, a gifted boy of 10, epitomizes this developmental trajectory.

Elliot was adopted when he was 1 week old. His adoptive father, Mr. B, an enormously successful investment banker, already felt burdened by the demands imposed on his lifestyle by his two daughters. However, Elliot's mother, Mrs. B, was determined to replace the baby boy she had lost when she had given birth to a stillborn child.

From the outset, Elliot's mother felt drawn by the appeal of this bright and very alert baby. She marveled at his ability to keep track of people's comings and goings, and his sensitivity to other people's moods. She felt, in fact, that she should shield this exquisitely sensitive baby from the onslaught of her pushy, aggressive husband. Thus, Mrs. B anxiously held Elliot in a tight embrace that kept her husband at bay. Soon the baby cried if his father even approached him. Mrs. B, in turn, could hardly disguise the pride she derived from both the boy's precocious achievements and the uniqueness of her relationship with him. She felt that the boy was her creation, one that had not even required a contribution from her husband.

Mrs. B had Elliot evaluated at age 1 and enrolled in speech therapy by the time he was 18 months old, because she was worried that his speech was less fluent than she had hoped it would be. Before long, Elliot was talking in adult-like expressions, to everyone's amazement and his mother's delight.

As Elliot grew, he became increasingly more controlling and demanding. In particular, he demanded constant attention and seemed determined to turn every situation, from a family dinner to an English class, into an opportunity for frantic exhibitionism. He responded to any efforts to set limits, particularly by his father, with vicious, mocking disparagement. But when he was calm, he relished opportunities to display his many talents, particularly his ability to impersonate show business personalities and other celebrities.

When Elliot was brought for consultation at age 10, he conceded that his problem was his inability to "stop living in the future." By this, he meant that he could not stop thinking that he was 25 years old. When I asked what it meant to be 25, he quickly replied that, among other things, it entailed watching over his mother, whose life he had saved when he found her unconscious after she overdosed with sedatives.

Elliot reluctantly agreed that some form of treatment might be of interest to him, if it could focus on helping him become more organized. He was concerned, he said with an impish grin, that his chronic inability to concentrate on tasks that did not place him at the center of attention could interfere with his grand design to become a Nobel Prize–winning nuclear physicist, the best neurosurgeon in the world, *and* a future President of the United States. His mind, he suggested, was like an ill-fitting puzzle. (I discuss further in Chapter 8 how I *mistakenly* then proceeded to inquire whether the piece that did not fit might include his feeling at times somewhat baffled or uncertain about which way to go.)

Prefacing his remarks with a sarcastic comment about my Julio Iglesias–sounding accent, Elliot contemptuously replied that his life had been devoted to achieving control of mind over matter. Like pain, bafflement was an alien experience to him, he said smugly. With a straight face, he proceeded to tell me that "everyone knows" that babies only learn to feel pain and cry, and then become wimpy and dependent, when they have a mother who gets all frantic and worried after they hurt themselves. Without such maternal antics, he thought, babies do not learn to feel pain or become dependent. Instead, Elliot declared, they grow like himself, always thinking clearly about their path and where they are headed.

One anecdote, he thought, would sum up his experience: When he was 6 years old, he cut his foot, which bled profusely. He did not notice what had happened until his older sister—who was subsequently sent to a finishing school in Switzerland, where she later committed suicide—brought to his attention the trail of blood he was leaving behind. When he asked his mother what he should do, she responded, he said, in typical fashion: "Oh, gosh, you should be careful not to stain the Oriental rug. Blood is very hard to clean. And, yes, you may go to the drugstore across the street. They can help you. . . ."

However factually accurate Elliot's account of his mother's response might be, it captures some crucial features of the psychological and intersubjective landscape of the development of these children: They experience their caregivers as self-absorbed rather than attending to their needs. What they find in the caregiver's face and behavior is not, as Winnicott suggested, a reflection of themselves, but rather that of the caregiver's own predicament. Elliot perceived his mother as having "acquired" him as a companion, a source of pride and self-esteem, a protection against depression and despair, a precious extension of herself, capable of shining and impressing others, and a weapon with which to attack her husband. Assigned a special role in his mother's life, he was loved in direct proportion to his capacity to meet the demands of that role. She rewarded and demanded the boy's sense of uniqueness, his exhibitionistic display of talent, and his parroting of adult-like language. His pain or vulnerability, however, led to maternal withdrawal and disgust, giving him the message that he would have to find reflection of those messy and bothersome aspects of himself on his own, or with someone else's help.

This child's skill in picking up interpersonal cues not only made him aware of what would bring his mother close and what would drive her away, but it also made him realize that he himself had to be perfect. After all, if he failed to attend to his mother's distress—as opposed to his own—and if he did not respond in ways that would distract her, lift her spirits, and repair her despondence, she might commit suicide.

THE PLIGHT OF BORDERLINE CHILDREN AND ADOLESCENTS

Borderline personality disorder (BPD) is the paradigmatic severe personality disorder. Antisocial, narcissistic, and histrionic personality disorders present a number of overlapping features and are often defined in relation to BPD. The disparity in the number of male and female patients diagnosed with BPD—over 75% of the total are female (Gunderson, Zanarini, & Kisiel, 1991)—may be caused by cultural bias, since male patients with similar features are often diagnosed as antisocial or narcissistic. On the other hand, the difference in gender ratio may result from differential exposure to specific risk factors, such as sexual abuse, or from the interaction of environmental and biological risk factors, with differential patterns of development and distinct psychosocial demands placed on boys and girls (e.g., difference in the expression of aggression or the importance of body image). Yet regardless of the explanation for gender ratio differences, the significance of both maltreatment and biological vulnerability in the development and pathogenesis of BPD is now clear (Goldman, D'Angelo, DeMaso, & Mezzacappa, 1992; Gunderson & Links, 1995; Siever & Davis, 1991; Zanarini et al., 1999).

In contrast to the apparent toughness and self-sufficiency of narcissistic–antisocial children, borderline youngsters openly display their vulnerability. Seductively, often manipulatively, and at times poignantly, they strive to keep others engaged with them while they anxiously search for the slightest hint of abandonment. But plain engagement fails to comfort them. Instead, they try mightily, by hook or by crook, to coerce those involved with them to take part in what feels to others like a tightly choreographed dance, a script with rigidly defined roles.

Cory, for example, is a girl of 8, adopted in Taiwan at 10 months of age by a white Midwestern couple. As she grew, her vulnerability to separations became increasingly more pronounced. Even the possibility that her adoptive mother would leave her for the day triggered what appeared to be dramatic disruptions in Cory's reality contact, as well as outbursts of rage and misbehavior in school. She pleaded with her mother to care for the many aches and pains that plagued her. If her mother stayed with her, they could both enjoy the girl's favorite game: the mother playing the part of an Asian queen, with Cory as her beloved princess. Yet the girl's demandingness, including the requirements of "royalty," were so exhausting that the mother would at times seek relief at her own mother's home in a nearby town.

Such "abandonment" would more than perturb the idyllic fantasy of the queen and her princess. Without the love, protection, and presence of the "queen," Cory herself changed, turning into a "Chinese bitch." Later, in therapy, she could discuss how a vivid fantasy would come to her at times of separation. In this fantasy, a witch, a vicious vixen of mixed Caucasian and Asian features, taunted Cory and threatened to drag her down into a bottomless pit.

Cory hated this witch nearly as much as she hated the "Chinese bitch" she herself became. She hated, in particular, the rage and anguish that overwhelmed her. To punish the "bitch," she would hit herself and poke at her skin until it bled. Cory illustrates some of the characteristic features of borderline children, specifically, (1) an unstable sense of self and others, and (2) subjective dyscontrol, self-victimization, and hidden omnipotence.

UNSTABLE SENSE OF SELF AND OTHERS

Borderline youngsters alternate between blissful contentment and elated feelings of power and pleasure on the one hand, and moments of utter despair, anxiety, or rage on the other. Whatever safety and stability they experience is often contingent on the presence and the specific responsiveness of a particular person or persons. The absence of this person precipitates utter terror and rage. Alternating experiences of self and other can take various shapes and forms. For Jay, age 6, whose case I review in a subsequent section in this chapter, separations (or even the merest hint of conflict with those to whom he was attached) not only triggered fits of screaming, spitting, kicking, and tearing of clothes, as well as banging his head, scratching himself, pulling his hair out, or biting his own hands, but also evoked an alternate identity, "Cinderella," who embodied his intense desire to be the protagonist of the fairy tale and coyly sought to convince other boys to become "her" prince, marry him, and give him a baby. A key feature of borderline children is a fragmented, highly unstable sense of self, not anchored in a taken-for-granted conviction of the stability, continuity, and coherence of the self.

This fragmentation of the self appears to be on a continuum with the "alters," distinct identities or personality states that are the hallmark of the dissociative identity disorder. These "personality states," relatively organized subsets of mental schemas of the self and others, are formed unreflectively and developed initially as rather desperate coping strategies.

Kluft (1998) describes how a 5-year-old girl, Lois, developed an array of alters to cope with molestation. The following are some of the coping strategies and alters employed by Lois: Her coping strategy, "This did not happen," led her to create one Lois who knew and another who did not; Lois translated the coping strategy, "I must deserve it," into the creation of a "bad" Lois, whose badness would explain the molestation as a punishment; the coping strategy, "I can control it better if I take charge," led her to an aggressively sexual alter, Vickie; the strategy, "I would be safe if I were a boy," produced Louis, Lois's male "twin," while the wish to feel nothing created Jessie, who endures all yet feels nothing.

Although dissociative identity disorder may represent an extreme, or perhaps a qualitatively distinct subtype of BPD, cases such as Lois's serve to illustrate the unstable, kaleidoscopic nature of borderline children's and adolescents' sense of self and others. The subsets of self–other schemas appear to be organized in an unreflective manner, comparable to the schemas contained in the "proto-narrative envelopes" (Stern, 1995) described in Chapter 3. These envelopes "open up," that is, are activated, in response to particular internal or interpersonal cues (e.g., feelings of distress or interpersonal conflict) that are specific reminders of the intolerable experiences that gave rise to self-fragmentation in the first place.

The activation of unreflective models leads inevitably to coercive efforts to compel other people to "fit" with the script contained in the proto-narrative envelope. Thus, Cory, the princess, seeks to evoke the protective embrace of a queen just as surely as the "bad" Lois is bound to elicit punitive responses that confirm her badness. These coercive efforts give an oppressive feeling to these children's relationships and almost inevitably lead to the very rejection they strive so mightily to avoid. Yet the drama, intensity, and even poignancy of the scenarios they seek to enact can also be strikingly alluring.

Clinicians (e.g., Leichtman & Nathan, 1983) have long described not only how vigorously borderline children seek to control the agenda of all interactions but also how convincingly they create vivid scenarios that powerfully summon others to play their prescribed roles. Cory, in her incarnation as an Asian princess, indeed compelled her therapist to join her in a magical world of royalty and privilege, while the "Chinese bitch" evoked visceral responses of hatred and wishes to punish and get rid of her—indeed, to treat her like a rabid animal. Jay was equally compelling in evoking strong desires to become his Prince Charming and rescue him from a life filled with loss, hurt, and unfairness.

Chethik and Fast (1970) have spoken eloquently about the arbitrariness that borderline children introduce in their treatment of reality and of other people, to whom these children react as if they were mere props in a predesigned drama. Such arbitrariness gives an "as if" quality to these children's interactions with others: a sense that *both* participants must behave as if they fully believe a shared falsification of reality.

Arguably, one of the roots of such an "as if" quality may be found, as Coates and Wolfe (1995) discuss in reference to the origins of gender identity disorder, in the "highly reactive" (Kagan, 1994) constitution of many future borderline youngsters. As I speculated earlier, the high reactivity of children born with a lower threshold for limbic–hypothalamic arousal to unexpected changes in the environment (Kagan, 1994) may also be a marker of their *exceptional* sensitivity to social cues and their innate facility for mind reading. They employ these skills as a coping strategy in their often remarkable capacity to manipulate others. Thus, future borderline children seem, from the outset, more vulnerable to disruptions of attachment (e.g., separations, insensitivity, neglect by their caregivers), particularly when such misattunement happens intermittently and seems linked to changes in the children's own internal states.

For these children, the loss of a reflective caregiver is a catastrophe, because their hypersensitivity makes them need (even more than ordinary infants) the presence of an attuned caregiver. Yet exceptional mind-reading abilities also give these children a terrifying glimpse of the destructive internal states that their caregivers can periodically harbor toward them, prompting them to retreat from mind reading. I suggest, again speculatively, that the responses of these children to the loss of a reflective caregiver is a desperate effort to restore, through unreflective means, a replacement of the lost relationship, albeit one that not only appears less terrifying and more under their control but that also creates an illusion of perfect attunement—thus, the compelling need to coerce the other person into fitting precisely with a preordained script. These efforts to restore a "perfectly contingent" relationship through coercion are powerfully reinforced by a particular pattern of interaction with their caregivers. As discussed earlier, the caregivers of future borderline children often alternate between neglect and abuse of their children and anxious, guilt-driven overinvolvement with them. This pattern reinforces the splitting or fractionation of self–other experiences and forms the basis of the "traumatic bonding" described by Allen (2001), in which a victimizing or traumatizing relationship appears to be the prerequisite for any sustained attachment.

Borderline children thus seek to restore relationships lost to caregivers' insensitivity and their own defensive retreat from reflective function through the organization of a self–other scenario built on the basis of unreflective, instrumental aspects of the self and the caregiver—a selective imitation, so to speak, that draws on the children's innate capacity to pick up interpersonal cues. The resulting scenario indeed feels like an act, because it replaces genuine intersubjectivity with a scripted actualization of the *likeness* of the self in relation to the other in a controlled and predictable fashion. Such mechanical imitation of the caregiver is subsequently reflected in children who appear as caricatures of their caregivers and assume pseudoparental roles in their families.

The case of Frederick offers a glimpse into the process of replacing attention to reality with an alternative, more manageable, defensively driven reality. The somewhat controlled suspension of reality contact— what Cain (1964) calls "playing crazy"—allows borderline children to monitor reality. Frederick, on the one hand, was clearly aware of the reality of his stepfather's beatings. On the other hand, his suspension of reality contact enabled him to disregard his own awareness of what was happening and to behave as if he believed his own falsification of it. In Chapter 8, I review the treatment problems generated by these excursions into reality distortion.

The instability of the sense of self and others in borderline youngsters includes some of the most basic aspects of the self, namely, gender identity and the body self. One case example serves as an illustration: Thirteen-month-old Jay, a healthy yet sensitive infant who adjusted slowly to changes and had trouble digesting milk, was faced with a brutal change when his mother died suddenly of a stroke. Her death also devastated the boy's father, an airline pilot, who was overwhelmed by the impossibility of meeting both his son's needs and the demands of his job. His solution was to place the child in the care of the maternal grandparents.

Jay's grandmother assumed his care with extraordinary fervor. Still grieving, she kept her daughter alive in her only grandchild and sole link to the memory of her daughter. She could do so by encouraging Jay to dress in his deceased mother's clothes and to play with her childhood dolls and toys. Gradually, Jay and his grandmother were drawn together in a tight web that significantly limited their independent functioning. Jay was his grandmother's "only reason to live" and "the apple of her eye." He became the ruler of the household and the recipient of his grandmother's most tender ministrations.

Yet a new loss lay in store for Jay. When he was 3 years old, his father remarried. Removed from his grandmother's care, Jay was reclaimed by his father and returned to the house they now shared with his father's new wife.

Jay did not wait long to show his anger and distress. He openly rejected his stepmother's affection and defied all her attempts to set limits on him. When anyone frustrated his efforts to be in control, Jay would throw terrible temper tantrums—furious fits of screaming, spitting, kicking, tearing his clothes, and destroying furniture. A self-destructive aspect of his behavior also became increasingly prominent, particularly when he felt threatened by the possibility that his father would abandon him. He would then resort to banging his head, scratching his arms and legs, pulling his hair out, biting his hands, or refusing to eat. Poor eating and disrupted sleep became prominent problems, along with verbalizations of self-hatred and a desire to die so he could join his mother.

When Jay was 5, his nursery school teacher described him as a sad yet provocative and destructive youngster, with unusual skill in picking out people's weak spots. At home, Jay's parents became alarmed by his compulsive masturbation and preference for feminine dress and play, behaviors that escalated whenever Jay was stressed. He certainly became distressed when his parents, exhausted after several failed attempts at outpatient treatment, arranged for his admission to a children's residential treatment unit.

Jay impressed the unit staff with his generous supply of intelligence, charm, and shrewd awareness of the right buttons to push to elicit the responses he wanted from other people. A short, slender, elfish-looking boy, Jay appeared much younger than his stated age of 6. Yet in contrast to his fragile appearance, he was never at a loss for words or ideas, and his adult-like expressions and sophisticated language made him sound like a miniature grown-up. But Jay was mostly subdued and brooding, generally unhappy and lacking in appetite.

Jay's heightened awareness of interpersonal nuances and his exceptional charm made him a most effective manipulator. However, when things did not go his way, he became anxious, provocative, and aggressive, and he escalated his insistence on dressing and acting like a girl.

After Jay had been on the residential unit for 2 months, his enormous vulnerability to separations became apparent. His cautious attachment to a preschool teacher came to grief when he had to move from preschool to elementary school. Such a move marked the beginning of a predictable pattern: Real or threatened losses of people that Jay depended on were followed by marked deterioration of his behavior and adjustment, and, particularly, a driven, flamboyant display of pseudo-femininity in the form of painting his nails, tying batteries to his shoes to pretend he was wearing high heels, and desperate requests for other boys to marry him and get him pregnant.

Jay illustrates how gender identity disorder (GID) may develop in boys. According to Coates and Wolfe (1995), boys with GID resemble the inhibited children described by Kagan (1994); that is, these children have a constitutionally lower threshold for limbic–hypothalamic arousal to unexpected environmental changes or threats and thus are highly vulnerable to early disruptions of attachment bonds.

Jay's GID arose in the context of the loss of his mother, an attachment figure whose disappearance was magnified by his father's frequent absences. For Jay, the loss of his mother's emotional availability and capacity to regulate his hyperactive psychophysiology was, as Coates and Wolfe (1995) point out, a catastrophe. Without an alternative caregiver, he had become overwhelmingly dependent on his mother's attunement to regulate his affective balance.

As Coates and Wolfe (1995) note, when these children lose the intersubjective connectedness with their primary attachment figure, they lose more than a love object. They lose also the ability to retain the reflective capacity with which to conceive of their own self and experience their own affective core (Emde, 1983). The "solution" Jay attempted is well articulated by Coates and Wolfe:

> Massive separation anxiety in the child is then defended against by a restitutive self-fusion fantasy with the mother. In essence, the child substitutes an identification for a relationship and comes to confuse being mommy with being with mommy, this during a period when he lacks stable internal representations of self and others and when his cognitive understanding of the permanence of gender classification is still immature. (p. 9)

Jay's cross-gender identification was massively reinforced by his grandmother's efforts to turn the boy into the link between herself and her dead daughter. By "becoming" his mother, Jay turned into the apple of his grandmother's eye and became her "only reason to live." He could thus acquire the illusion that he had the power to keep his grandmother alive and prevent the loss of yet another caregiver. Cross-gender identification not only helped Jay forge a tie to an available attachment figure, but it also provided him with reassurance against further losses and their associated catastrophic states of dysregulation and loss of self.

Identification with his lost mother gave Jay a sense of specialness, power, and self-reliance that countered threats of abandonment, deprivation, vulnerability, and helplessness. Overvaluation of this identification thus came from within and without. As Anna Freud (1960) and

Furman (1974) recognized in reference to the normal process of mourning, this overvaluation serves not only as an effort to accept the loss of a loved one and a bridge in the gap between the loss of one attachment and the formation of a new one, but also as a consistent disposition to organize Jay's sense of self, his coping mechanisms, and his relationships, based on an illusion of power and control predicated on denial of loss and the assumption of a false-self identity. Cross-gender identity succeeded in stabilizing Jay's sense of self and in reviving his attachment figure—his mother—in himself.

His illusory control and his attachment to his grandmother were both greatly strained by his father's remarriage when Jay was 3 years old. He lost, along with his grandmother, an environment that supported his omnipotence and cross-gender identification. Jay responded with an intensification of the one coping strategy that had given him a sense of control and connection: cross-gender identification. His identification with his mother also took a new direction: Jay became the new wife's oedipal competitor for his father's love. One can only speculate how much Jay's stepmother became the repository of his unexpressed rage at all the abandoning mothers of the past.

Jay's situation attests to Coates and Wolfe's (1995) statement:

> The contribution that cross-gender identification makes to the child's management of anxiety is such that the child experiences it as a "solution." As development proceeds, however, the child's creativity and spontaneity become increasingly consumed in the repetitive, stereotyped and joyless false-self enactment of the cross-gender identification while his social adjustment becomes increasingly precarious in the face of continued peer rejection. (p. 9)

At the time I saw him in treatment, when he was 6, Jay seemed well on his way to the consolidation of a GID and borderline–narcissistic personality organization. Paradoxically, the very hypersensitivity that made him so vulnerable to a disruption in attachment is arguably related to his increased ability to connect empathically and to "read minds." As Emch (1944) has proposed, the perceptual–affective resonance associated with special sensitivities can be employed in the service of identification and mimicry. Emch described this process in connection with some children's astonishing capacity for mimicry in response to otherwise unassimilated experience.

Such an "as if" quality pervades borderline children's experience of self and others. Paradoxically, they feel more real and alive when fulfilling—and coercing others to fulfill—one of their unreflective scenarios. In contrast, when other people refuse to play their assigned parts, borderline children panic or become enraged, increase their coercive efforts, and, in the process, betray their internal fragmentation and the extent to which they rely on enacting unreflective scenarios to rid themselves of intolerable internal states and to anchor, however precariously, a semblance of a sense of self and others.

SUBJECTIVE DYSCONTROL, SELF-VICTIMIZATION, AND HIDDEN OMNIPOTENCE

As previously noted, the first and most basic function of the attachment system is as a regulatory system. Humans are, of course, born without the autonomous capacity for psychophysiological regulation and can achieve such regulation only as part of a dyadic, transactional system. Normal infants are biologically prepared to signal distress and to enter into reciprocal relationships with caregivers who are disposed to understand, give meaning to, and respond to their infants' signals. The development of the capacity for reflective function is an outgrowth of these interactions.

Reflective function acts as a buffer when other people's behavior is unexpected or threatening, or when one experiences distressing internal states. The possibility of raising an alternative hypothesis to make sense of one's own or other people's responses turns inchoate affective–procedural experiences into more modulated ones that can be contained, integrated, and shared. For example, a 6-year-old can intuitively grasp that his mother's irritation might be related to her having had a hard time at the office, or having had a fight with dad, or feeling annoyance about the child's bickering with a younger sibling. Just as importantly, a child appreciates—without needing to think consciously about it—that mother's current state of mind is bound to change as she gets some rest, makes up with father, or is charmed by the child's cuteness.

By inhibiting reflective function, borderline children deprive themselves of these containing and modulating effects at the very time when they need them the most, that is, when they feel threatened, lonely, vulnerable, or overwhelmed. When they activate an unreflective mode of functioning, borderline children can only view the world as being without alternatives or potential for change: for example, as consisting of hateful, attacking caregivers whose behavior cannot be influenced by changing their state of mind. In other words, these children are thrown into a state of hopeless vulnerability, without much realistic possibility of "turning around" their helplessness and vulnerability, and of restoring coherence and control to their experience. Such states only reinforce their need to replace realistic self-righting efforts with attempts to gain a semblance of control through the arbitrary treatment of reality. More specifically, such states drive them to ever more relentless efforts to coerce others, through threats, manipulation, or seduction, to conform to arbitrary scenarios.

In the throes of a nonreflective mode of operation, borderline children are psychologically disconnected from their own emotional states because they are unable to represent these internal states in a psychological fashion compatible with their representational world and the world of meaning they share with others. One outcome of this disconnection is a state of subjective dyscontrol, a state of psychological void congruent with their experience of other people's behavior as occurring without the mediation of mental states. Just as they experience others as a kind of automaton without a mind, they also feel that their own emotional states and behavior "happen" to them. Thus, the inhibition of reflective function leaves children intermittently overwhelmed and helpless in regard to their emotional experience. In these states of subjective dyscontrol and emotional dysregulation, borderline children feel totally at the mercy of the soothing and regulation provided by others. Such reliance is perhaps based on the convergence of constitutional vulnerabilities to hyperarousal and psychophysiological dysregulation on the one hand, with a caregiving pattern that alternates frightening misattunement with anxious overinvolvement on the other. The combination of constitutional vulnerability, trauma, and intermittent misattunement arguably lies at the heart of the inability of borderline children to achieve a consistent capacity to soothe and comfort themselves, and to regulate their affect in the presence of threatening internal and interpersonal cues. They require, instead, something or someone to regulate them.

In the state of inhibited reflective function to which they retreat, borderline children can count only on the concrete, instrumental presence of another person for self-regulation, because they are unable to access the reflective–symbolic aspects of a relationship that normally ensures psychological continuity even in the physical absence of the other. These internal and interpersonal conditions may shed some light on the vulnerability to separations that is one of the hallmarks of borderline psychopathology. A number of typical features of BPD results from the strategies children evolve to cope with such states of subjective dyscontrol and their associated vulnerability to separation.

First, these children develop what Shapiro (1965) calls an *impulsive style*. Borderline children are often constitutionally prone to bypass reflection (e.g., considering the possible meanings of a given situation, the consequences of a particular response, or the implications of momentary states of need or desire for longer-term relationships, goals, or personal aspirations) due to attentional problems or difficulties modulating arousal. This constitutional proneness, however, is reinforced by an active defensive effort to *avoid* the recognition of unbearable mental states.

When reflective function is "turned off," children can respond only to the concrete outcome of other people's behavior, rather than to assumptions about the mental states that underlie behavior. Likewise, only through physical or quasi-physical action can they conceive of having an impact on other people. Fonagy (1999b) describes a dramatic example of such action-oriented nonreflectiveness: A boy confessed to his father that he had accidentally broken a lamp. The father reassured the boy that he understood that accidents happen. However, on seeing the broken lamp, the father became so enraged that he broke his son's arm when the boy raised it to protect himself from the father's vicious blows. The father is modeling a disconnection between a reflective stance (e.g., appreciating that the boy's actions were *not* the result of a malevolent intention) and his subsequent brutal behavior.

Second, these children actively provoke the very vulnerability, dyscontrol, and helplessness they fear will befall them. Clinicians can attest to the uncanny power of borderline children to evoke visceral desires to get rid of them or beat them up. These experiences are quite comparable to those reported by teachers, caregivers, probation officers, protective service workers, and others who come into contact with borderline youngsters and find themselves compelled to engage in impulsive, thoughtless, or even cruel treatment of these children that they subsequently regret and view as "out of character."

I concur with Novick and Novick (1996) that behind the capacity of borderline children to evoke destructive responses often lies a "fixed fantasy" or, in the framework discussed in this book, a rigid, nonreflective scenario of self-induced pain, abandonment, and victimization. At the core of this scenario lies a "delusion of omnipotence" (p. 48), which, following Freud, may be seen as "the essence of masochism" (Freud, 1919/1955, p. 189).

The omnipotence betrayed by the "fixed fantasy" underlying self-victimization or other forms of self-defeating behavior refers to an illusory form of "self-righting" or congruity attainment that borderline children create as a way of coping with the impossibility of achieving real control, secure attachments, and successful integration of experience. This self-righting scenario serves a function similar to that of the more obvious omnipotence and disavowal of pain and vulnerability of narcissistic and narcissistic–antisocial youngsters: It creates the illusory sense that they are actively producing the abandonment, pain, vulnerability, shattered security, and even outright trauma that would otherwise happen to them. The beatings or the abandonment may still take place, yet children can fortify themselves with the illusion that they are producing their own misery.

Just how important this secret sense of control is for children's sense of self becomes apparent when anyone attempts to stop these self-victimizing and self-defeating patterns. Cory tenaciously held on to the most provocative and annoying aspects of her behavior, even when it was clear to her that they inevitably led to the very rejection she so dreaded. Such tenacity, a striking feature of self-victimizing patterns of behavior, suggests that, in the course of development, these patterns acquire multiple adaptive functions. In particular, these children's maladaptive behavior patterns become the currency of relationships (the traumatic bonding discussed earlier) and serve as a key organizer of their sense of self.

Novick and Novick (1996) advance the hypothesis that one additional root cause of self-victimization, particularly the induction of beatings or other forms of abuse, can be found in the reduction of channels in the caregiver–infant relationship that occurs in severely disturbed early attachments. According to Novick and Novick, skin contact may be the *only* channel of stimulation and contact that is not dependent on emotional attunement, as are, for instance, eye contact, talking, and smiling.

Caregivers who "lose" reflective functioning in the face of their infant's distress may become incapable of attunement and responsiveness to their infant's mental states, yet they cannot avoid physically handling the infants, however mechanical such handling might be. The Novicks' premise is that, under those circumstances, infants come to regard some form of physical contact—even a painful one—as the only path to attachment with their caregivers.

The link between painful physical sensations and attachment is reinforced by the usual sequence of events in these children's attachment history: Caregivers "turn off" reflective function in response to their infant's distress and become abusive or neglectful. Yet the infant's increased distress, particularly physical pain, which is removed from the emotional pain that reminds caregivers of their own traumatic past, eventually leads caregivers to respond in an anxious, guilt-ridden, over-stimulating fashion. Actively seeking pain thus comes to signal for these children the most effective way to retain or reestablish a connection with caregivers. The privileged position of pain seeking and self-victimization as the main currency of any relationship grows as these children reach school age and later enter adolescence. Their capacity to coerce others into either victimizing or seeking to rescue them becomes more sophisticated and effective as they grow up.

But self-victimization and pain seeking are more than simple adaptations that secure a sense of control and attachment. Throughout childhood and adolescence, self-victimizing, self-defeating, and pain-seeking behaviors acquire additional functions that entrench them as core features of the sense of self and others.

One such function of self-victimization is a way of expressing aggression while avoiding assertive self-expression. The root causes of this maladaptive pattern of dealing with aggression and assertiveness are arguably found in the early childhood and preschool years. In normal development, children emerge from infancy with a core sense of self (mostly implicitly, procedurally processed) and with the trustful (Erikson, 1950) expectation of relatively smooth reciprocity with distinct others to whom they feel securely attached. Feelings and intentions become the focus of sharing and attunement, which allow the creation of a world of shared meanings.

The development of explicit–symbolic capacities and myriad maturational accomplishments, such as independent locomotion, bring about a critical reorganization of self–other representations. This domain is what Mahler and colleagues (1975) described as the practicing subphase of the separation–individuation process. During this phase ("the world is the toddler's oyster"), Mahler and her collaborators note that children partly shift their interest from close exchanges within the attachment system to the exercise of their rapidly growing capacity for exploration and more autonomous functioning. Describing the elation associated with this investment in autonomy, Mahler and colleagues state that "the child seems intoxicated with his own faculties and with the greatness of his own world. Narcissism is at its peak" (p. 71). Self-assertion involves some degree of aggression in the service of both denying vulnerability and protecting self-boundaries from the impingement of others.

A similar convergence of defensive needs to deny vulnerability, and maturational and psychosocial pressures toward greater autonomy, predictably occurs at other stages of massive developmental change, such as adolescence. At that point, this convergence prompts a similar surge of self-assertion and rebellion, mixed with profound narcissistic vulnerability (to be discussed subsequently).

For children on the path to development of a borderline personality, management of those developmental stages of self-assertion and associated aggression is enormously problematic. Typically, they are unable to process aggression or self-assertion in a reflective fashion because the hostility they experienced in their caregivers felt raw, unmetabolized, and associated with the "loss" of the caregiver. Their anger and self-assertion, particularly when triggered by feeling abused or abandoned, foreshadow a catastrophic outcome for them.

Thus, they turn their hostility into even more desperate coercive efforts designed, in part, to control what they experience as the unleashing of destructiveness—their own and that of others. In a typical sequence, 15-year-old Judy would become enraged if her boyfriend of the moment displayed any insensitivity to her. However, her rage acted like a match in a tinderbox. Soon engulfed in self-denigration and self-hatred, she felt that she was a disgusting, whiny, and needy baby, deserving only contempt and humiliation. Her tirades would escalate in viciousness until she resorted to self-cutting and ended up with an addiction to the self-inflicted scars that crisscrossed her arms like a grotesque game of tic-tac-toe. Rage, in effect, finds expression in self-inflicted pain and abuse, as borderline youngsters torture their attachment figures while protecting their own boundaries and asserting themselves via self-abuse and victimization.

Ultimately, borderline children develop the means to regulate temporarily the states of hyperarousal and affective dysregulation that haunt their lives. The model of such regulation is the dissociative state of numbness to which they seem constitutionally predisposed. But over time, they also discover that, through several other means, they can greatly "improve" the numbness they can achieve through self-hypnosis alone. Food, drugs, alcohol, and promiscuous sexual relationships become favorite "regulators" of internal states of hyperarousal and dyscontrol.

As noted earlier, a genetic disposition to addiction seems linked to the D_2A_1 allele, which is associated in turn with a decrease in dopamine D_2 receptors, and with the so-called "reward deficiency syndrome." It is plausible that the deficiency in the capacity to experience reward results from the convergence of active efforts of self-numbing brought about by dissociation and self-hypnosis and from a genetic predisposition to low levels of dopamine D_2 receptors in the mesolimbic and mesocortico-limbic pathways. The result is a heightened risk to develop one or a combination of addictive patterns that crystallize into comorbid Axis I disorders, particularly substance abuse and bulimia.

These syndromes lead to further maladaptation along several mutually reinforcing paths. First, the increased psychophysiological dysregulation produced by addiction and withdrawal, including the putative "addiction" to carbohydrate loads seen in bulimic individuals, and perhaps the addiction to endorphins released during self-mutilation, increases the sense of subjective dyscontrol and aloneness, thus exacerbating these children's need to coerce and manipulate others and numb themselves.

Second, addictive behavior, particularly substance misuse and promiscuous sex, increases these children's drift toward deviant peer groups (Fergusson & Horwood, 1999). Involvement with antisocial peers leads to further alienation from better adjusted peers and the adaptive opportunities offered by school and other prosocial alternatives. Such children's association with deviant peers, by reinforcing the escalation of antisocial behavior and conflict with authority (Dishion et al., 1995), leads caregivers to feel increasingly immobilized and incapable of providing effective care and control (Solomon & George, 1996). This experience escalates the coercive cycles previously described.

Thus, the reinforcement of maladjustment for these children comes both from within and from without. In a tragic transactional process, the youngsters' efforts to cope with loneliness, subjective dyscontrol, and unstable identity lead to responses from their environment, caregivers, schools, and peers that increase their alienation and their need to cling, ever more tenaciously, to their very maladaptation. A brief comment about suicidality and parasuicidal behavior that recapitulates the

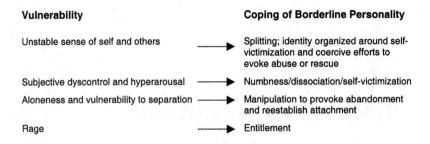

Vulnerability

Coping of Borderline Personality

Unstable sense of self and others ⟶ Splitting; identity organized around self-victimization and coercive efforts to evoke abuse or rescue

Subjective dyscontrol and hyperarousal ⟶ Numbness/dissociation/self-victimization

Aloneness and vulnerability to separation ⟶ Manipulation to provoke abandonment and reestablish attachment

Rage ⟶ Entitlement

FIGURE 6.1. Vulnerabilities and coping strategies in borderline personality disorder.

points made throughout this section: No other aspect of these children's maladjustment brings as much misery to caregivers and clinicians and is as clearly indicative of their inner torment as is their incessant threats and attempts at self-destruction. Undoubtedly, suicidal and parasuicidal behavior is a multidetermined phenomenon.

First, suicidal and parasuicidal behaviors often represent a desperate attempt to stave off physical abandonment or coerce another person into reestablishing a relationship. Second, self-destructive behavior also serves actively to produce the trauma one expects to suffer passively. A different way of formulating this function of self-destructive behavior is to view it as a form of unreflective, procedural identification with an abusive other that results in treating one's own body and self as it was treated by an abuser. Third, self-destructive behavior allows children to torture, attack, defy, and get back at their caregivers while masking their overt aggression. Fourth, some borderline children become "addicted" to parasuicidal behavior, perhaps to the endorphins released during self-mutilation. As clinicians have long noted, in children afflicted by numbness, cutting serves to terminate the state of feeling dead inside and make them feel alive again. Fifth, self-mutilation and suicidal behavior become important elements of an identity built around self-victimization. As such, they create a sense of self-worth based, among other things, on the transformation of feelings of rage and despair into the entitlement that the world owes them something because they suffer so much.

In summary, constitutional vulnerabilities and traumatic states lead to a borderline personality, as illustrated in Figure 6.1.

7

Beginning Treatment

Creating a Secure Base and a Representational Mismatch

In his classic essay *The Yogi and the Commissar and Other Essays*, Arthur Koestler (1945) described two competing views about how to achieve change. The yogi's approach is based on the notion that internal changes lead to a transformation of the world. The commissar, in contrast, believes that internal transformation follows changes in outside reality.

Faced with the challenge presented by youngsters with severe personality disorders, treaters turn both to yogis and commissars in search of guidance. The clinical literature reflects these competing perspectives: "yogis" are invested in exploring and making sense of children's subjective world as the basis for promoting changes in coping strategies and relationship patterns, whereas "commissars" target children's symptomatic behavior or environment through the use of medication, behavioral approaches, or family interventions. In this section, I present a treatment model that involves the integration of these two approaches and aims to achieve both intrapsychic change and modifications in children's interpersonal context using attachment and the development of reflective function as an organizing principle. Before describing the model, however, it is worth reflecting on the current status of the "yogi" therapists as viable providers of care to children and adolescents with severe personality disorders.

BASIC PRINCIPLES AND GOALS

The therapeutic focus on the subjective experience and internal world of children and adolescents with severe personality disorders has produced a rich and evocative literature (Bettelheim & Sylvester, 1948; Rinsley, 1980a, 1980b). Such practice is rooted largely in the psychoanalytic tradition's claim to legitimacy, which relies heavily on case reports that, however moving or dramatic, tend to resist objective assessment and controlled scrutiny. As the old quip goes, psychoanalytically oriented clinicians have failed to realize that the word "data" is *not* the plural of anecdote.

This quip, of course, ignores the vigorous efforts in the past quarter-century to bring methodological rigor to the assessment of adult psychodynamic psychotherapy (e.g., Crits-Cristoph et al., 1988; Hartley & Strupp, 1983; Luborsky, Crits-Cristoph, Mintz, & Auerbach, 1981). Nonetheless, psychodynamic child psychotherapy research lags behind (Barrnett, Docherty, & Frommelt, 1991; Kazdin, 1993) and still asks global questions such as "Is psychotherapy effective?" instead of addressing the more focused inquiries of contemporary research: "Which set of procedures is effective when applied to what kind of patients with what kind of problems as practiced by what sort of therapists?" (Barrnett et al., 1991, p. 2).

Several limitations have rendered individual psychoanalytic psychotherapy and long-term residential treatment models based on a psychoanalytic framework (e.g., Bettelheim & Sylvester, 1948; Noshpitz, 1962, 1975; Rinsley, 1980b) vulnerable to being dismissed as impractical, nonscientific, and uneconomical—if not counterproductive—enterprises:

1. Lack of operationalization in descriptions of technical interventions.
2. Inadequate specificity regarding technical interventions appropriate for children with a particular diagnosis.
3. Limited evidence of efficacy, especially evidence derived from randomized, controlled studies.

4. A rather loose relationship between theories of psychopathology (in turn, poorly supported by empirical data), theories of technique, and techniques as actually carried out in clinical practice.
5. Lengthy—and thus expensive—treatment aiming at rather global goals.
6. Absence of reliable procedures for evaluating ongoing clinical progress.

These limitations feed into the notion that long-term, psychoanalytically oriented approaches to the treatment of children and adolescents with severe personality disorders are not only expensive and ineffectual but also actually damaging, because they allegedly promote regression and dependence, induce false memories of abuse and victimization, and, more generally, exacerbate the maladjustment of these children and their families. Such accusations resonate in managed care organizations focused on short-term treatment and short-term cost savings. As managed care has expanded its control over reimbursement, psychoanalytically based approaches for youngsters with severe personality disorders appear to stand on the brink of extinction.

Some child analysts have argued that empirical research is antithetical to the very essence of analytic or analytically informed interventions. A growing consensus, however, proposes that it is possible and, in fact, essential to investigate systemically which aspects of psychoanalytic child psychotherapy techniques are effective for which types of clinical or developmental disturbances.

A major effort in this direction is the chart review and detailed examination of 763 case records of children and adolescents in psychoanalysis and psychodynamic treatment at the Anna Freud Centre (Fonagy & Target, 1996). These studies reveal that psychodynamic treatment was, as expected, particularly effective for children whose diagnosis included an emotional disorder. However, children with a diagnosis of only one emotional disorder and relatively high levels of adaptation appear as likely to benefit from nonintensive therapy (one session per week) as from intensive treatment (3–5 sessions per week). More surprising, however, is the finding that intensive treatment was remarkably effective for children with severe, long-standing, and complex psychosocial problems, including conduct disturbance, given the presence of at least one emotional disorder diagnosis (e.g., anxiety disorder, dysthymia). This group of children with complex psychopathology seemed to benefit little from nonintensive, once-a-week psychotherapy. The most helpful interventions for them, however, differed from those previously described as central to psychoanalytic approaches. In particular, interpretations of unconscious conflict aimed at promoting insight, which have been the centerpiece of psychoanalytic technique, appeared to be of limited value to these youngsters. On the other hand, less severely disturbed youngsters with emotional disorders seemed to benefit from an interpretive approach. The question raised by these findings, however, is whether a more intensive and expensive treatment program can be justified when the data point to similar effectiveness with one session per week.

This study, although limited by its retrospective nature, raises fundamental questions about the proper indications for, and the nature of, the therapeutic elements of, psychoanalytically oriented child psychotherapy. My basic premise is that, even though not recognized as such by psychoanalytic theories of technique, the crucial therapeutic aspect of psychoanalysis and psychoanalytic psychotherapy, particularly for youngsters with the complex problems associated with severe personality disorders, lies precisely in their ability to activate people's capacity to find meaning in their own behavior and that of others.

Psychoanalytically oriented child psychotherapy has always aimed at strengthening children's capacity to recognize and monitor mental states. The enhancement of this capacity helps them to manage their own behavior and to understand other people's feelings and reasons for acting the way they do. I propose a treatment program for youngsters with severe personality disorders that is centered on a systematic effort to help them regain reflective function in the face of the internal and/or external cues that trigger its inhibition. A focus on reflective function allows for a clearer definition and evaluation of the key interventions and a more specifically tailored approach to the particular developmental and adaptive problems of children and adolescents with severe personality disorders.

Focusing on enhancing reflective function also permits a fruitful cross-fertilization between psychoanalytically oriented psychotherapy and other, more empirically supported therapies, such as cognitive-behavioral therapy and interpersonal psychotherapy. These approaches boast of robust data documenting their usefulness in ameliorating specific symptoms of children (e.g., Kendall, 2000) and can even demonstrate normalization of brain functioning in neuroimaging studies following a course of treatment (Schwartz, Stoessel, Baxter, Martin, & Phelps, 1996).

Cognitive-behavioral therapy, interpersonal psychotherapy, and the psychotherapy approach I discuss in this book all aim to effect a change in how people organize and structure experience. Cognitive-behavioral therapy and interpersonal psychotherapy are both more active and directive, and more narrowly focused on specific maladaptive processes, for example, the particular cognitions underlying low self-esteem. These features are major factors that explain the success of these therapies in resolving specific symptoms. In contrast, a model focused on enhancing reflective function, although more targeted and active than traditional psychoanalytic approaches, seeks to promote a broad set of capacities that underlie a complex pattern of experiencing, coping, and relating rather than attempting to correct a specific cognitive or social deficit.

More fundamentally, a psychotherapeutic approach focused on enhancing reflective function benefits from its psychoanalytic heritage. Child analysts have always assumed that children's symptoms, and how children organize their subjective world, represent a largely unconscious adaptation to the demands of both their internal world and external reality. Thus, psychoanalytically oriented therapists anticipate children's attempts to resist therapeutic interventions, to fight change, and, from time to time, to sabotage efforts made on their behalf. This knowledge is crucial when embarking on the treatment of youngsters with severe personality disorders: Change, however well intentioned, threatens a painstakingly achieved adaptation. The clinical experience accumulated by child psychoanalysis and psychoanalytically oriented therapists has primed them to appreciate and deal with children's anxieties, which in this case include anxiety about sustaining a reflective stance—thus arousing potentially unbearable mental states in the children themselves and in those closest to them. But patients' anxieties are not the only potential problem. Training, supervision, and personal treatment sensitize psychoanalytically oriented practitioners to use their own emotional reactions better to understand their patients' subjective world, rather than to become entrapped in the quicksand of the rigid, unthinking patterns of experience and relatedness these youngsters are prone to evoke.

Recasting psychotherapy from a predominantly insight-oriented, conflict-solving modality to an approach based on enhancing reflective function also brings it closer to the mainstream of contemporary developmental research, which is centered on the interaction between risk and protective factors. This reshaping also aligns psychotherapy with contemporary views regarding the factors that promote resilience in vulnerable children and families.

A treatment program focused on enhancing reflective function also holds the promise of integrating the perspectives derived from the subjective–intrapsychic world of coping and experiencing with those that arise from the vantage point of the systems of family and social interaction in which subjectivity is always embedded. To paraphrase Minuchin and Fishman (1981), youngsters with personality disorders shape, modify, and reinforce their family's dysfunction every bit as much as their family's dysfunction shapes, modifies, and reinforces their maladjustment. Reflective function, the mechanism that links inner experience with interpersonal reality, offers a ready-made conceptual and clinical bridge between these two worlds. Standing at the convergence of neurobiological, psychological, and psychosocial perspectives, reflective function, and the attachment system from which it springs, can serve as the conceptual glue that joins pharmacological, cognitive, and family systems interventions into a coherent and integrated treatment program. From this conceptual vantage point, it becomes apparent that the yogi's interventions aimed at children's subjective experience necessarily have an impact on family relational patterns, while approaches that target behavior or patterns of family interaction inevitably alter children's internal organization.

The basic principles underlying this treatment model are as follows:

1. Conceptual and clinical integration is essential.
2. Treatment must be comprehensive.
3. An intensive, long-term process is a precondition for the development of secure attachments.
4. Caregivers must be involved partners in the treatment.
5. The treatment program must be tailored to the family's cultural traditions.
6. The characteristics of staff members are crucial for good outcomes.
7. The overall goal of the therapeutic program is to enhance the reflective function of children and their caregivers.

CONCEPTUAL AND CLINICAL INTEGRATION

The treatment of severe personality disorders in children and adolescents requires an *integrative focus*. Discontinuity of experience or inability to create coherence and organization in both internal and external worlds is central to these youngsters' maladjustment and is the hallmark of the interpersonal context that maintains and reinforces their psychopathology. The goal of enhancing reflective function provides such a focus, guiding the sequencing of psychotherapeutic, pharmacological, educational, and family interventions. Conceptual integration in the planning and implementation of treatment is essential to restore the protective and healing power of reflective function. This function gives children the capacity to generate a coherent narrative of their experience and their world that is the outgrowth of intersubjective exchanges occurring in the context of meaningful human connections. Thus, even more crucial than the availability of a full spectrum of therapeutic interventions and a continuum of services is the integration and continuity of understanding and planning.

COMPREHENSIVE TREATMENT

Restoring reflective function and the interpersonal context that sustains it requires a comprehensive approach. Such an approach addresses the multiple factors in the child and the environment that conspire to produce vicious cycles that perpetuate and exacerbate the inhibition of reflective function. Thus, this treatment program targets biological vulnerabilities, the range of developmental dimensions (cognitive, social, emotional, physical, and moral/spiritual), and environmental domains (e.g., school, peer group, family/extended family).

Setting up a comprehensive approach is, of course, a rather formidable challenge. Beyond the compromises mandated by financial and other practical limitations, a multifaceted approach by necessity involves multiple agencies and providers of services. Given the fragmented nature of the funding and coordination of services for children and families in the United States, the prospects of poor communication, territorial disputes, turf protection, and just plain "falling into the cracks" loom large in the care of youngsters with these severe personality disorders.

their caregivers—sympathetically and believing that their behavior has meaning; trusting that one can be helpful; being prepared to persevere despite hints of frustration; and accepting the need for supervision or consultation.

In addition, certain characteristics are associated with effectiveness: good communication skills; warmth and empathy; openness and willingness to show flexibility and humor; and an inclination to act, take risks, and seek novelty.

THE GOAL OF ENHANCING REFLECTIVE FUNCTION

The treatment program for youngsters with severe personality disorders employs an array of technical interventions in various combinations and sequences designed to achieve the following essential goals:

- Address mental processes via representations of self and others.
- Verbalize and share internal states.
- Break down unmanageable experiences into manageable ones that the youngsters and their families can master.
- Develop internal representations of affects, leading to mastery of feelings.
- Facilitate thinking by reducing anxiety and linking different aspects of thought processes.
- Promote understanding of meaningfulness and intentionality of behavior in the context of attachment relationships.
- Become aware of others' mental states and the difference between "world-as-given" versus world of multiple-person-related meanings.
- Set limits to impulsive, nonreflective, coercive, and otherwise destructive and maladaptive behavior.
- Protect generational boundaries and identify the distance between individuals that best balances individual differentiation with maintenance of connections between individuals.
- Develop adaptive coping strategies based on the ability to anticipate stress while relinquishing maladaptive defenses prompted by shame, loss of control, and cues that signal danger.
- Encourage an "as if" attitude that promotes play, fantasy, flexibility, and humor.

- Work through past and present disappointments.
- Develop a blueprint for an achievable future that matches real talents and opportunities to ensure achievements that anchor a realistic sense of self-worth.

Such a list of goals may appear imposing and even daunting. As I discuss in subsequent chapters, however, they are achievable in the context of a structured therapeutic program designed to mobilize the most powerful protective and healing mechanisms available to human beings. In other words, this program provides guidance that encourages growth in children and their caregivers, to free them from mutually reinforcing cycles of despair.

PROMOTING A REPRESENTATIONAL MISMATCH

How can the yogi's and the commissar's perspectives become integrated so as to break the vicious cycle of defensively driven, intrapsychic models reinforcing dysfunctional interpersonal patterns and vice versa? Clinical experience suggests that meaningful engagement in treatment is unlikely unless there is movement in the children's interpersonal context in a direction that creates what Horowitz (1987) called a "representational mismatch." In Horowitz's formulation, used to describe the grief following the loss of a loved person, a representational mismatch arises when external reality challenges or contradicts the expectations generated by internal models.

In the case of youngsters with severe personality disorders, a representational mismatch is created when caregivers and treaters demonstrate effectiveness and consistency as limit setters, maintain generational boundaries, competently nurture and support children, and invest in extricating these youngsters from the special roles they play in their families. These roles may include deflecting one caregiver's hostility against the other, holding the parents' marriage together, maintaining the caregiver's self-esteem, serving as the receptacle for the despised aspects of the caregiver, preventing parental suicide, or serving as the sexual partner of a caregiver.

For narcissistic and narcissistic–antisocial children, a representational mismatch challenges their claim to omnipotence and their insistence that others are worthless, weak, and incompetent. For borderline youngsters, a mismatch results from the caregiver's capacity to provide protection from maladaptive activities (e.g., involving sex, drugs, food) that give these youngsters a momentary sense of well-being, control, and connection with others. Thwarting children's self-defeating and self-destructive behavior challenges their view of caregivers as unreliable, indifferent, and mean at best, or as brutal and exploitive at worst. In the absence of such a representational mismatch, even powerful yogis are unable to counter the reinforcement of reality.

Inpatient or residential treatment settings offer the optimal option for certain youngsters with a severe personality disorder. Putting aside financial constraints, the clinical considerations in deciding whether an inpatient or residential placement is indicated are (1) the capacity of the youngster's caregivers, with therapeutic support, to stop their own destructive behavior—such as maltreatment—and to move in the direction of greater competence, more effective limit setting, and better maintenance of generational boundaries; (2) the availability of community resources and services such as in-school support services, in-home crisis stabilization, and office- and home-based family treatment that can be mobilized to support the caregiver's competence; and (3) the extent of the youngster's need for containment and structure to prevent behavior dangerous to self or others.

Youngsters with severe personality disorders respond to changes in their environment with desperate and often destructive efforts to recreate a context characterized by the caregiver's ineptitude, inconsistency, and unreliability. In short, a representational mismatch generates anxiety because it challenges patterns of experience and relationship that, while painful and maladaptive, were also often felt to be lifesaving and to provide a measure of safety, coherence, control, and attachment. In turn, the intensification of anxiety is a powerful trigger of the unreflective models that mobilize pathological defenses and coercive interpersonal maneuvers designed to reestablish a reality supportive of the children's unreflective internal organization. Such maneuvers can be so destructive that effective containment surpasses the "holding" (Winnicott, 1965) ability even of well-functioning caregivers. A range of services midway between outpatient and inpatient care offers the best combination of cost-effectiveness and clinical efficacy. Without removing the youngster from the family, day treatment involving high or moderate management, sometimes combined with school-based and after-school services, can effectively create a representational mismatch.

Unfortunately, reimbursement patterns limit access to these midrange services.

Treatment in specialized residential centers is indicated for some children, particularly those with intricate combinations of learning disorders, ADHD, substance abuse, or mood disorder, along with a severe traumatic history and a predominance of dissociative or antisocial tendencies. Brief hospitalizations are necessary when an acute crisis puts such youngsters in danger of harming themselves or others. Finally, a group home or specialized foster care setting may be required for youngsters who need to be removed from profoundly disturbed or destructive home situations or whose exhausted caregivers need additional support. (For a discussion of the issues that arise in the inpatient and residential treatment of these youngsters, see Chapter 10.)

Regardless of whether the setting is inpatient, "midrange," or outpatient, treaters can anticipate an onslaught of blatant or subtle efforts from *both* the youngsters and their caregivers to reestablish the previous patterns of coping and relationship, particularly in response to the introduction of a representational mismatch. The following vignette provocatively illustrates the principles and potential problems of introducing into the lives of youngsters with severe personality disorders and their families a way of functioning that allows caregivers and treaters to be more competent, sensitive, and controlled.

The late Donald Rinsley, a gifted and controversial adolescent psychiatrist, once described in the following fashion his first encounter with a 16-year-old girl with a mix of narcissistic and borderline features, just admitted to the long-term residential unit he directed (D. Rinsley, personal communication, February 25, 1980). On entering Rinsley's office, the girl responded to his greeting with an outburst: "You fucking shrink, who the fuck do you think you are? . . . I don't have to listen to you!" Calmly, yet with as much flair as he could muster, Rinsley proceeded to extract an impressive-looking gold pen from his breast pocket. "Do you see this pen?" he asked the girl. "I don't give a shit about your fucking pen or anything you have to say!" came the reply. Rinsley persisted, until he ultimately managed to capture the patient's attention: "All right, what the fuck about your stupid pen?" she finally asked. "Well," Rinsley said, "with this pen, I can send you to your room for 1 hour, for 3 hours, or for 24 hours. With this pen, I can prescribe medication for you today or next week. With this pen, I can order that you start school this Monday or 2 weeks from now. With this pen, I can order that you visit with your parents this weekend or a month from now. With this pen . . . I can discharge you from this center today . . . or next year." As he ceremoniously put his pen in his pocket, Rinsley made his grand exit from the office, leaving the girl perplexed and, for once, speechless.

Two years later, as the girl was about to be discharged and she and Rinsley reminisced about her treatment and what she had found most helpful, she said, with a beaming smile: "Do you remember that pen of yours, Dr. Rinsley? I think that's what did it."

This vignette epitomizes the therapeutic style of a creative clinician with an uncanny capacity to connect with seriously troubled adolescents. It also illuminates the subtleties and potential pitfalls in the initial gambits of treatment that, as in the often-repeated analogy to a chess game, are so critical to the unfolding and eventual outcome of the therapeutic process.

Rinsley's response to the girl's provocative and devaluing "greeting" firmly conveyed a capacity to contain her hostility, bravado, and impulsivity. Arguably, the presence of an "all-powerful" caregiver, capable of holding (Winnicott, 1965) and containing (Bion, 1962), is a crucial precondition for infants to develop a secure attachment based on the trusting expectation of effective responsiveness to their needs for nurturance and regulation. These experiences with a holding and containing caregiver in turn serve as the blueprint for the performance of self-regulating functions. Using the mental representation of the holding and containing caregiver as a model for the self, children can begin to approximate the model and thus "internalize" the caregiver's regulating functions (Kohut, 1971).

But Rinsley did more than provide a statement of his power of containment. He ascribed that power not to himself per se but to an object that stood squarely between the concrete person of the doctor and the symbolic realm of rules, ideas, and values: the pen. A pen, of course, is an instrument whose power derives from its capacity to create symbols. Rinsley thus introduced his young patient to the perspective that genuine power and effectiveness do not come from empty bravado and efforts to coerce others to enter a world that admits only one interpretation. It comes instead from the use of reflective–symbolic capacities that open the door to a life with options and possibilities "today" or "next month"—options that can be considered on the basis of information gained through intersubjective exchanges of personal meanings. Implicit in Rinsley's message was that the patient herself was not without choices: How she chose to respond to him and his pen would determine, in turn, how "the pen" would respond to her.

The crucial point in introducing a representational mismatch lies precisely in finding the balance between the capacity to convey holding, support, and containment of destructive and self-destructive behavior on the one hand, and in leaving both youngsters and their caregivers with a sense of control over the choices they face on the other. Treatment founders when the treaters become intimidated or paralyzed by the youngsters' unreflective onslaught. But therapeutic failure is also the likely outcome when treaters react with defensively driven responses of their own to counter the pressure to experience the helplessness, vulnerability, or despair engendered by the deflating "greetings" of youngsters with severe personality disorders. Under such circumstances, treaters are driven to adopt an omnipotent stance of pseudo-control that is every bit as hollow as that of the youngsters themselves. This "omnipotence" only succeeds in reinforcing the unreflective coping strategies of their patients. Chapters 8 and 9 examine the unreflective land mines that dot the landscape of clinical encounters with these youngsters, setting the stage for predictable patterns of transference and countertransference.

What separates Rinsley's statement from a defensively driven statement is this: First, his message bears the hallmarks of a reflective communication. Delivered with just a touch of playfulness, and with a keen eye on the girl's moment-to-moment verbal and nonverbal responses, it was carefully calibrated to balance firmness and clarity with empathy for her sensitivity to threats to her illusory sense of control. Second, in those pre-managed-care days, Rinsley was quite capable of delivering on all the possibilities he outlined. He was convinced that the treatment of choice for children and adolescents with severe personality disorders required extended and intensive residential care focused on reinstating them to a normal developmental path, and that other, less intensive approaches were as irresponsible as aspirin or antibiotics would be for the treatment of appendicitis. Thus, he did not hesitate to claim that "with this pen" he could order the visit of the girl's parents in a week or a month, because he was fully prepared and capable of providing her with a parenting function for several years to come.

Nowadays, clinicians would be hard pressed to claim the level of control over the treatment process that Rinsley enjoyed. Obviously, it is hard to argue against the need to monitor the cost of psychiatric services for troubled children and adolescents, particularly in light of the enormous growth in psychiatric and substance abuse treatment services and the explosive increase in the use of inpatient adolescent services that preceded the surge of managed care.

Thus, it is imperative to establish empirically exactly which children should be treated with extended residential treatment—children for whom less intensive approaches may be ineffective or actually counterproductive. Yet for most children and adolescents with severe personality disorders (including those who require inpatient or residential treatment), the most effective—and cost-effective—way to create an optimal context for treatment entails supporting the caregiver's competence and well-being (Liddle & Hogue, 2000). In so doing, a representational mismatch results not from the verbal pyrotechnics of a brilliant clinician but instead from the steady efforts of treaters and caregivers to work collaboratively and with mutual respect, in order to provide the caregivers with more effective tools to support, nurture, and protect their children. At the same time, the caregivers are spared the implied assignment of blame for their children's failures and are not themselves placed explicitly in the role of patients.

AN IMPLICIT REPRESENTATIONAL MISMATCH

Lee Combrinck-Graham (1990) points out that unless we as treaters are prepared to adopt our young patients—a practice she strenuously discourages—we would be well advised to focus our interventions on helping families to advocate and care for themselves and their children. In other words, we should seek to enhance caregivers' competence rather than to reinforce their helplessness. Such an approach could be construed as a rejoinder to the capacity of Rinsley's pen to dictate the frequency of his patient's parents' visits. This rejoinder stems not only from increased conceptual sophistication but also from a pragmatic need to arrive at a more compassionate view of the interactional struggles of families. Such a view can provide the basis of a more effective—and more economical—way of engaging the caregivers in a collaborative therapeutic process that minimizes their dropping out of treatment and improves overall outcome.

Attachment theory and the disruptions in reflective function associated with dysfunction in attachment offer a framework to facilitate the caregivers' alliance with treaters by minimizing their experience of being blamed, shamed, or made to feel guilty for their children's problems. From this vantage point, treaters first discuss with the caregivers an assessment of the youngster's problems. This assessment examines the problems in the context of the youngster's perceived threats to the continuity and safety of attachments that lead to a retreat from reflective function. Caregivers are thus introduced to the perspective that the inhibition of reflective function is a maladaptive coping strategy. Although borne of efforts to retain some semblance of control and connection, inhibited reflective function is doomed to give rise to rigid, unreflective schemas of the self and the world, and to coercive patterns of behavior.

The notion of coercive patterns of behavior driven by unreflective models of self and others helps caregivers appreciate the transactional context of their children's—and their own—behavior. Such a perspective is essential to shift the discussion from behavior that needs to be managed or eliminated to relationships and internal states that can be altered once they become meaningful and shareable. *Implicitly*, the caregivers are invited to consider their own role in maintaining and reinforcing coercive cycles of unreflective behavior. First, by making clear to the caregivers that they are essential to the treatment, treaters help them to appreciate the links among their own well-being and competence, their effective communication, and their youngster's adjustment. By not explicitly confronting the caregivers' own dysfunction, treaters can help them to hear such formulations without excessive defensiveness and thus with a greater appreciation of how the process of treatment can indeed be helpful. Caregivers can best be enlisted as partners in treatment when they experience the process as an attempt to enable all of the family—children as well as caregivers—to sustain conceptualizations of each other as intentional beings, even in the presence of cues they associate with threats to their relationships or to their very survival as individuals and as a family.

From this vantage point, treaters can point out the active role that children's unreflective behavior plays in shaping the overall family context. Caregivers find particularly helpful those formulations that recognize the power of biological vulnerabilities (e.g., attention-deficit/hyperactivity disorder, mood disorder, chronic physical illness) and other risk factors (e.g., early disruptions of attachment in adopted children) that shape the family's emotional and interpersonal patterns of interaction.

It is helpful to use a storytelling format when asking questions to access narrative detail (Liddle & Hogue, 2000) or, alternatively, to identify the points at which the caregivers' capacity to retain narrative coherence breaks down. These points represent important cues about the areas of experience and interaction that trigger a breakdown of reflective function.

As Liddle and Hogue (2000) propose, asking questions in a storytelling format tends to elicit autobiographical accounts of personal or historical connection among family members. Examples include the following:

> "When you first held your child, what dreams did you have for him or her as an adolescent or adult?"
> "Describe some of the happiest—and some of the hardest—times you have had as a family."
> "How did your parents let you know when they were proud of you?"
> "How do you let your child know that you are proud of him or her?"
> "How has parenting this child been different than you expected?"
> (p. 271)

Questions such as these allow exploration of how family members think about themselves in relation to their family and one another and introduce the perspective of understanding behavior in the context of underlying meaning.

This is an important juncture to assess the knowledge that the caregivers possess about their youngsters' lives. Such questions—Who are the youngster's best friends? What do they do together? What is happening in school?—serve not only to evaluate the caregivers' knowledge about their children but also to direct caregivers' attention to the broader context of their children's lives and to the notion that understanding this context helps make children's behavior intelligible.

Helping caregivers to see their youngsters' difficulties as a manifestation of maladaptive attachment and reflective function sets the stage for two important processes. First, the treaters present the formulation that mutually reinforcing patterns of unreflective experience and coercive behavior are at the heart of the unrewarding cycles of anger and despair in which caregivers and children find themselves stuck. From this perspective, the central therapeutic task is to promote a shift from coercive and unreflective exchanges—for example, the "dialogue of the deaf" between caregivers who bemoan their children's "out-of-control" behavior, while the children bristle and reject their caregivers' efforts to control them—to a genuinely reflective dialogue that enables all family members to grasp each other's point of view and convey their own experience. Second, treaters and caregivers together can examine how particular experiences or interpersonal transactions in the family's developmental history have become signals of danger and triggers of a defensive retreat from reflective function. These experiences typically concern issues of safety and trust, commitment and loyalty, protection and love, and long-standing problems of betrayal, abuse, abandonment, neglect, and misattunement. Unreflective modes of experience and interaction become coercive patterns that give rise to particular hypersensitivity and to a readiness to respond rigidly and unreflectively to specific forms of perceived threat. Such patterns—unreflective modes of experience and behavior that evoke unreflective responses in other family members in a circular, self-reinforcing manner—render families less able to respond adaptively to developmental pressures for change. These patterns also shape family transactions, which are then transmitted from one generation to the next. Exploring the multigenerational context of transactional problems, however, is a task of the middle phase of treatment, because it first requires a reasonable working alliance between caregivers and treaters.

Breaking the cycle of unreflectiveness rekindles empathy, mutuality, and a sense of agency in children and caregivers. But empathy does not preclude limit setting. An attachment framework recognizes that reflective function is built on the foundation of effective and responsive caregiving. As Diamond and Liddle (1999) point out, family members must have "a fundamental basis of trust and attachment before they are willing to learn communication skills and seek mutually supportive solutions to problems" (pp. 7–8). Such trust, in turn, grows out of children's repeated experiences with strong, reliable, and responsive caregivers who are capable of regulating the children's arousal, nurturing them, and ensuring their safety. For children and adolescents with severe personality disorders, such caregiving entails practices that combine continued connectedness and support with appropriate containment of destructive, self-destructive, or otherwise maladaptive behavior—a combination associated with a decrease in adolescent deviance and substance abuse (Fletcher, Darling, & Steinberg, 1995; Schmidt, Liddle, & Dakof, 1996).

Framing the goals of treatment along these lines focuses the therapeutic process on first assisting the caregivers in achieving the skills they need to remain calm and in control even when facing the internal or interpersonal cues that have so far signaled their own retreat from reflective function. In Chapter 8, I discuss how to tailor interventions to enhance caregivers' competence in sustaining reflective function in the caregiver–child relationship.

Yet before treatment can begin, the caregivers need the opportunity to agree—or disagree—about whether the formulation of their children's problems and the goals of treatment make sense to them. Such agreement can be facilitated by a thorough examination of the problems that might be associated with an attempt to change. My approach to Elliot's parents (see Chapter 6 for a detailed case description) serves to illustrate this process.

Elliot's father, Mr. B, a powerful, take-charge business executive, began the first meeting by launching a bitter tirade about Elliot's misbehavior and his wife's inability to discipline him. Mrs. B, as if on cue, wasted no time in mounting a spirited defense of her child. She viewed the boy as a sensitive and gifted child, brutalized by his father's pushiness and aggressiveness. Previous treatment efforts had collapsed when one parent invariably felt blamed by the treater for the child's problems, while the other parent felt vindicated. For example, Mr. B discontinued a 2-year psychotherapy process when he felt that Elliot had become "too attached" to his therapist. Mr. B believed that this therapist ascribed the boy's difficulties to the chronically conflictual father–son relationship and to Mr. B's unavailability. Unsurprisingly, Mrs. B found a subsequent therapist, chosen by her husband, to be not only incompetent but also an instrument of her husband, hired by him to blame her for the boy's problems. She fully expected that therapist's efforts to be directed at disrupting the close tie between herself and her son.

The forces impinging on this family and giving shape to their interactions became available for therapeutic intervention only after months of work with both Elliot and his parents. This family perceived the world as a hostile jungle. They expected to find loyalty only in their immediate family, but even there they were suspicious of any signs of tenderness and intimacy.

As the oldest son of a poor family that had perished in the Holocaust, Mr. B had immigrated to the United States and forged a new life for himself. The theme of brutal uprooting ran deep in Mr. B, who held the strong conviction that survival required permanent vigilance. Yet a guilty hue colored his view of the world: He had survived, while his family had been destroyed.

Mrs. B grew up in a family that, although settled in America for a generation, had been unable to fulfill the immigrant's dream of prosperity and security. She experienced her father as weak and ineffectual. His ineffectualness was dramatized in her mind by her experience as an adolescent of being sexually molested by one of her father's drunken friends.

Guilt, fear, mistrust, and ambition joined Mr. and Mrs. B together, along with a desperate need for security and belonging. They succeeded, by some measures, beyond their wildest dreams and became powerful and wealthy. Yet they were crippled in their ability to support one another when feeling threatened or vulnerable, and particularly when experiencing failure, sadness, or weakness. Weakness, after all, led to death or victimization.

The developmental forces of separation and autonomy buffeted this family, and such vulnerability became tragically evident when their 19-year-old daughter, Jessica, killed herself while she and the family struggled with the demands involved in her going abroad to attend an exclusive finishing school. Jessica's suicide both expressed and triggered a family crisis. Marital conflicts became unmanageable: Mrs. B became involved in an extramarital affair as Mr. B became even more emotionally distant. Eventually, Mrs. B tried to kill herself, an attempt that failed only because of Elliot's intervention—a rescue that reinforced his conviction that he should try to act like a 25-year-old rather than a boy of 10.

It was in this context that Elliot's bossiness and provocative behavior at home, and his temper tantrums and clownish, exhibitionistic, and disruptive behavior in school, pushed his parents into seeking treatment for him and, incidentally, forced them to talk to each other. Early disruptions in attachment might have sensitized Elliot to turn away from dependence and vulnerability, but his illusory sense of power or control received enormous reinforcement after he prevented his mother's suicide. His sense of omnipotence was fueled by his ability to keep his mother alive, careful attunement to her moods, and his apparent ability to keep his parents together by uniting them in shared concern about his misbehavior.

Pointing out to the parents *their* role in sustaining and exacerbating Elliot's maladjustment would confirm their expectation that outsiders—particularly authority figures such as clinicians—would only expose them to abuse, shame, or hurt. For both Mr. and Mrs. B, as for most caregivers of children with severe personality disorders, the world in general, and treaters in particular, came across as hostile and frightening. Thus, they had to maintain constant vigilance and never let their guard down.

My initial formulation was designed to invite the parents to experience treatment as a collaborative enterprise, first with each other, and then with the treatment team. I stated that each parent was strongly connected with one aspect of Elliot. The father recognized the angry, demanding brat in need of discipline and limits. The mother was keenly aware of the sensitive boy, desperate to avoid being ignored or abandoned and afraid to lose face or feel out of control. Elliot and each parent had become locked in a vicious cycle that continuously reinforced expectations yet prevented any reflection on the other's internal state. Being stuck in this way reinforced Elliot's conviction that he could connect with his father *only* by engaging him in a constant battle and that he could sustain an attachment to his mother *only* by making her proud, preventing her from feeling depressed, or keeping her and his father engaged with one another.

At this juncture in a case, the therapist might redirect the discussion from "behavioral problems" to concerns about relationships related to internal states. For example, I asked Mr. B to consider what might make it difficult for Elliot to accept his rules and instead resent him and his authority. Therapists often "lend" caregivers inner states that are not readily available to them (Minuchin & Fishman, 1981). When asking Elliot's father about the boy's inability to reveal his "weakness" and dependence, I suggested that it might be frightening to expose those aspects of the self if one anticipates ridicule or risks even greater vulnerability. Months later, Mr. B was finally able to speak openly about his own unmet needs for dependence and his reluctance to expose his own vulnerabilities.

Both parents struggled with the notion that they could reach a common view of Elliot that would provide a basis for exploring alternative ways of interacting and trying to solve problems. They were helped in this effort by the partial validation of their points of view: that they each had an accurate perception of an aspect of Elliot that formed the basis of an intense yet problematic attachment. They were also helped by the affirmation that, however much strain they experienced in their marriage and however much they disagreed about their perception of their son, Elliot's treatment could begin only when they reached a sufficiently shared and mutually supported view of him, his problems, and the strategies necessary to help him. Caregivers are better able to reach such a shared perspective—though, typically, they will subsequently seek to sabotage and reverse whatever "agreement" they may have reached—when the treaters acknowledge the care and love most caregivers feel for their children and the desire most people have to help their children live freer and less painful lives than their own—a desire not actualized because of the unreflective cycles in which caregivers and their youngsters find themselves trapped.

Elliot's parents appreciated the boy's struggle to integrate his own experiences of himself—his vulnerability and dependence, his anger and need to stay connected, and so on. They also realized how much they could assist him in breaking loose from unreflective modes of functioning by presenting him with consistent rules and expectations (see the section on basic principles and goals).

The first obvious place to introduce coherence is in caregivers' perceptions, expectations, and responses to their children. Such a process begins by helping caregivers align their expectations of their children with the children's strengths and weaknesses. Legitimizing Elliot's dependency needs and vulnerabilities in no way negated the expectation that he adhere to realistic limits and constraints. In particular, early interventions with this family introduced the notion of boundaries within the family as a way of helping Elliot to disentangle from coercive cycles "inadvertently" reinforced by his conviction that he played a special role in the life and adjustment of the entire family. Thus, family sessions focused initially on preventing Elliot's attempt to solve his parents' difficulties, particularly his efforts to become responsible for ensuring his mother's safety.

Elliot's parents required frequent reminders of our agreement that they would bring their questions, worries, and disagreements to the family sessions for discussion, often in the boy's absence. The implicit message is that conflicts between the caregivers are their business and theirs alone to solve.

As Mandelbaum (1971) observed, the therapist directs the family members to "become clear and real to each other, consistent and dependable individuals who could be counted on to protect personal

space, to give empathy, to express affect, to balance all good with some bad and all bad with some good" (p. 437). In other words, a collaborative relationship with caregivers is built around an invitation to adopt a reflective stance. In so doing, caregivers and treaters create a new interpersonal context that implicitly challenges the children's unreflective mode of experiencing, coping, and relating. By producing an implicit representational mismatch, the alliance between caregivers and treaters can become a creative crisis that, in the words of Minuchin and Fishman (1981), takes a family "stuck along the developmental spiral . . . and pushes it in the direction of its own evolution" (p. 26).

To summarize: Treatment of children with severe personality disorders requires the "secure base" (Bowlby, 1980) of a collaborative relationship between caregivers and treaters. Such alliance can be optimally secured by the following:

1. Minimizing the caregivers' experience of shame, blame, guilt, helplessness, and incompetence.
2. Emphasizing the unreflective transactions or cycles in which caregivers and youngsters are stuck.
3. Defining as a crucial task of treatment the breaking up of coercive cycles that prevent secure attachments and a sustained reflective perspective.
4. Redirecting the discussion with the caregivers from behavioral problems to relationship concerns tied to internal states, in an effort to promote the caregivers' reflectiveness.
5. Introducing the goal of building the caregivers' sense of competence and control as a prerequisite for helping children deploy reflective function.
6. Recognizing that treatment can proceed only when caregivers agree with one another and with the treater on their understanding of the problem, the goals of treatment, and the approaches to achieve such goals.
7. Anticipating problematic areas, including, in particular, the caregivers' experience that treatment will take control away or threaten the connections between family members. Contrasted with this concern, treatment should be defined as an effort to find the optimal distance between protecting caregivers' personal space and maintaining sustaining attachments with one another.

8

Early Stages of Treatment
Forming the Alliance and Enhancing Reflective Function

THE THERAPEUTIC ALLIANCE

Achieving a sense of collaboration in individual psychotherapy with children who have severe personality disorders is hardly a simple task. Therapists typically contend with an opening phase in which the patient's behavior is marked by ruthless tyranny, aloofness, suspiciousness, demands for control of the sessions, or attempts to reduce the therapist's role to that of captive audience for an elaborate show.

Faced with even the hint of collaboration between treaters and caregivers, youngsters with severe personality disorders typically react with efforts, either blatant or subtle, to sabotage adult competence and undermine their collaboration. In so doing, they seek to recreate an interpersonal context in which their caregivers—and other adults—are seen as inept, inconsistent, and unreliable; it is a world in which the youngsters can count only on their own efforts to maintain an illusion of control and attachment. Open defiance and contempt, threats, assaults, or attempts to run away are the most obvious expressions of these children's attempts to instigate chaos in their environment, ultimately in the service of preserving the status quo.

Indications of collaboration between caregivers and treaters (e.g., expressions of support for the treatment plan or a concerted effort by

174

caregivers to set limits, provide structure, support one another, and maintain better generational boundaries) create a mismatch with the youngsters' expectations and convictions about caregivers' incompetence and unreliability. This mismatch paves the way for achieving the initial goals of treatment: (1) to establish adults, particularly caregivers, in a position more conducive to the creation of a "secure base," the prerequisite for secure attachment and reflective function; (2) to challenge the youngsters' maladaptive coping mechanisms enough to promote their capacity to enter a collaborative relationship and explore sharing some aspects of their experience and the possibility of finding help via a relationship with another person—through better understanding their own internal states; and (3) to enhance self-control through more adaptive, less harmful means.

Narcissistic and narcissistic–antisocial patients often present themselves as hotshots filled with bravado and pretentious self-sufficiency, bent on demeaning the therapist. Yet they may also appear grateful and seemingly compliant, brimming with intellectual insights or seductively communicating to the therapist that they find him or her exceptionally sensitive, brilliant, and attractive. Borderline youngsters can fall madly in love with their therapist and are eager to declare their good fortune in having found the perfect person to love—and to be loved by them. For example, Sam, an impish-looking boy of 6, insisted on the therapist's silent admiration of the elaborate fortified castles and walled cities that he built with a Lego set. His constructions were indeed meticulous and rather impressive. Whenever the therapist attempted to shift his role from admiring spectator to active participant, Sam would immediately pretend to be a skunk, whose fetid odor would keep people away.

These initial gambits provide a window into the range of interpersonal experiences and internal states that serve as cues to inhibit reflective function: In Sam's case, the possibility of spontaneous give-and-take seemed to require that he initiate an immediate distancing maneuver, not open to reflection or modification. The unreflective model with which he sought to coerce the therapist crystallized into a pattern in which what was wonderful and admired rarely concealed what was fetid and flawed.

The fundamental goal of the initial phase of treatment is to transform the sterility of coercive and unreflective exchanges into at least a modest sense of mutuality. This step promotes these children's dawning realization that some areas of their subjective experience can be safely shared and subjected both to private as well as to interpersonal scrutiny.

Creating the conditions to transform disorganized attachment into secure attachment is implicit in the concept of therapeutic alliance. The importance of the establishment of a positive alliance early in the treatment, as opposed to an alliance established later, as a predictor of a good outcome is well documented empirically (Horvath, Gaston, & Luborsky, 1993; Horvath & Symonds, 1991; Safran & Muran, 2000). The capacity or incapacity to form an alliance appears to be the crucial distinction between those individuals with narcissistic–antisocial features who can benefit from treatment and those who are unlikely to improve (Gerstley et al., 1989; Woody, McLellan, Luborsky, & O'Brien, 1985). Arguably, these findings serve to differentiate those youngsters with severe personality disorder for whom comprehensive treatment, including psychotherapy, would be useful. The centrality of the progression of the attachment relationship from insecurity and disorganization to security and reflective function is highlighted by Gunderson (2000). Gunderson argues that a review of the clinical and research literature supports the notion that the therapeutic alliance provides a framework to evaluate the progress of treatment.

Gunderson (2000) distinguishes three forms of therapeutic alliance that occur sequentially in therapy: the contractual, the relational, and the working alliance. The contractual alliance is the initial agreement among the patient, the patient's caregivers, and the therapist on treatment goals and their respective roles in achieving them. The relational alliance refers to the patient's experience of the therapist as mostly caring and understanding. The working alliance is the stage in which the patient can join the therapist as a reliable collaborator in the task of making sense—or deploying reflective function—in the service of understanding the patient's and other people's behavior.

The contractual alliance involves, as described earlier, first an agreement between the caregivers and the therapist about goals, treatment plan, and the roles of the therapist and the caregivers in the process. This agreement includes practical issues such as fees, attendance, and confidentiality, and also an understanding about the caregivers' responsibility to ensure the youngster's and their own safety, and the means to ensure such safety. According to Gunderson (2000), the creation of this alliance establishes a frame for the treatment that represents the therapist's professionalism and boundaries, and implies that the work ahead involves discipline, expectations, and restraint.

A number of experienced therapists of adult borderline patients (Akhtar, 1992; Clarkin, Yeomans, & Kernberg, 1999; Yeomans, Seltzer, & Clarkin, 1992) insist on formalizing a "contract" with the patient that is explicit about the roles and responsibilities of the patient and the therapist and establishes the minimal conditions under which treatment can be conducted. The therapist's use of the contract as a framework to be referred to when problems arise in the course of treatment decreases the therapist's appearance of becoming arbitrary, reactive, or punitive. Linehan, Heard, and Armstrong (1993, 1994) also insist on establishing a contract before starting dialectical behavioral therapy for borderline patients. The contract emphasizes, among other key issues, setting clear goals and making a commitment to attend sessions regularly. Yeomans and colleagues (1992) make explicit the limits of the therapist's responsibility out of a conviction that the therapist's involvement in the patient's life outside of the sessions is a frequent cause of treatment failure and invite the patient to engage in a dialogue in which problems are anticipated based on the patient's history (e.g., coming to sessions intoxicated, having a crisis during breaks in the treatment, dropping out after a few sessions).

I believe that the concept of a "contract" with the patients and caregivers is generally helpful. It clearly has drawbacks as well: Most caregivers, let alone most youngsters with severe personality disorders, are in no position to negotiate a meaningful contract. Contracts that define a priori the conditions that will bring treatment to an end set the stage for the patient's testing of limits and then outright efforts to actively destroy treatment—rather than wait for the therapist to declare that the contract has been breached.

I agree with Gunderson (2000) that a more useful clinical stance is to limit the "contractual" alliance to an agreement about practical issues, such as fees and frequency of sessions, and to add a few simple statements about the therapist's role and the nature of the treatment process. The therapist can say that these sessions are set aside to play with younger children, to talk, and to think, in order to make sense of what bothers them or causes them problems, and to help them change. The purpose of such a statement is to make explicit that treatment has a goal, and that in this particular type of treatment, the path to addressing problems is in "making sense" of what underlies behavior. I underscore some of the problematic issues that arise during the evaluation sessions, particularly those that seemed to trouble the patient, and point out that I foresee these problems as amenable to change. I always stress that I will keep confidential what we talk about in the individual therapy sessions, but I will give the caregivers a general report of progress. The only exception to this rule would be if the patient's behavior endangers him- or herself or others, or the continuity of treatment. Yet I emphasize that even under such circumstances, I plan to share with him or her whatever I discuss with the caregivers.

On the basis of clinical experience, two or more individual psychotherapy sessions per week are required to help transform disorganized attachment into a secure relationship in which reflective function serves to negotiate stress and conflict. This premise, however, has not been tested empirically. Clinical experience suggests that psychotherapy processes carried out at a frequency of once per week or less will generally revolve around providing direction, advice, education, limits, and crisis management rather than creating the conditions that allow youngsters to regain the capacity for secure attachment and reflective functioning.

Even at an optimal frequency of sessions, the difficulties in creating such conditions are formidable. The case of Robert illustrates such difficulties.

A 15-year-old adolescent in a residential treatment unit, Robert began therapy with a superficial eagerness to solve his problems. Such therapeutic zeal soon gave way to rather flamboyant expressions of contempt for the residential center, its staff, and the therapist. He had expected that "a famous clinic" would provide him with a therapist perfectly suited to treat him—a "perfect match." Robert had some hope when he first met me because he noticed that we both had blond hair and blue eyes. He was quickly disappointed, however, when he heard my obviously foreign accent. He could not understand why he had been subjected to the ignominy of having a "spic" for a therapist.

I commented that—if I heard him right—he seemed to experience my accent as a putdown that would embarrass him by association. "Not bad for a spic," Robert replied, quickly turning to his doubts about whether "spics" could understand the concerns of someone of obvious Nordic descent. I said that, if I heard him correctly, he seemed to be saying that if we were not identical, not only in looks but also in background, I would not be able to understand and appreciate him. "Not bad for a spic" was again his response. Yet I could detect a budding relatedness in his mocking compliment.

Such relatedness, of course, was only tentative. Nonetheless, in a subsequent session, Robert confided that if he trusted me, I might find a way to sabotage his plans to "behave appropriately" and maintain "a positive attitude," in order to convince his parents and the treatment team that he was ready to return to his beautiful northern state instead of rotting in dreadful Kansas. This comment, of course, was meant to show me how clever and in control he really was, as well as how little he valued my home state and anything Kansas had to offer him. It might also, however, betray his own questions about how effectively manipulation and pretense could solve his problems. Not picking up on any of these issues, I commented instead that, if I heard him right, he was concerned about what would happen if, indeed, I heard him right and he got to trust me even a bit. Would it help him or derail his plans and get him to lose control?

This vignette illustrates the principle of creating a context of safety (where children can share some aspects of their subjective experience) by focusing initial interventions on clarifying the patient's intended communication, perceptions, and feelings of the moment ("Let me see if I understand what you are saying—am I hearing you correctly?"). This stance only makes explicit the therapist's assumption that *all* of the patient's behaviors convey meanings based on internal states that give such behavior purpose—including a communicative purpose. In so doing, the therapist seeks to strike a careful balance between "too much" empathy, which these children experience as overwhelming (because it threatens to expose to themselves, as well as others, their hidden vulnerabilities), and "too little" empathy, which promotes despair and reinforces the conviction that relationships lead only to frustration, hurt, and misattunement.

What the therapist avoids doing is at least as important. At no point during the initial phase will the therapist point out the patient's envy, sadness, vulnerability, or rage, nor the related defenses of grandiosity, dissociation, denial, or projective identification. Linking the patient's current feelings and thoughts to events or feelings in the past is bound to create the same response as that given to a premature confrontation of vulnerability or defensiveness: an exacerbation of maladaptive defenses and an increase in the need for distance, control, or devaluation of the treatment and the therapist.

An indication that an area of tentative attachment is being established occurs when the child eagerly uses the therapist as an audience. Robert, for example, proceeded to fill our sessions with lengthy dissertations about his multiple areas of expertise, namely, nautical history, gourmet food (he prided himself on his culinary skills and wished to become a famous chef), and old movie stars (he fancied himself a connoisseur of classic films). In a cautious way, he seemed to invite me to share at least some aspects of his life.

Seeking out the therapist to share an aspect of his or her experience is a signal that the treatment relationship is progressing from what Gunderson (2000) calls "contractual" to a relational alliance, a process that can take anywhere from 1 to 3 months.

Elliot, whose history I reported in Chapter 6, illustrates the problems that arise when a therapist prematurely probes vulnerable spots. He responded to my inquiry into his feelings of sadness or loss, an inquiry that, in retrospect, was triggered by my annoyance at his haughty denial of vulnerability and his contempt for me, by frantically denying any dysphoric experience. He then launched into a tirade, explaining how "babies only feel pain when their mothers get all worried" after a cut or a scratch. Without such antics, he claimed, babies are unaware of their own hurt and do not feel pain. His claims became so desperate that he began to lose his grip on his usually outstanding reality contact. He sought to convince me that his power derived from having dedicated himself to achieving control of mind over matter. He illustrated this power by telling me how he had, when younger, fallen asleep wishing that he could fly. He woke up on the floor, yet he did not remember falling out of bed—and it was out of the question that such an occurrence could have taken place without his awareness. The only explanation, he concluded, was that his wish to fly had been so powerful that his mind had been able to overcome the laws of gravity. Then, he grew anxious, keenly aware that maintaining an illusion of omnipotence required from him an ever more arbitrary treatment of reality.

Helping Elliot at this juncture presented me with a dilemma. To acknowledge my "mistake" in addressing his vulnerability before he was ready would only add the insult of implying that he was not "tough enough" to handle the exposure of that vulnerability in the first place. Offering a compromise, I asked: "Are you saying that when you really put your mind to something, no matter how difficult it may seem, you believe you can accomplish it?" He at first dismissed this formulation

("No, that's not it.") but then agreed with it: "What I really mean is that when I put my mind to it, I can accomplish just about anything. I may even learn to fly an airplane." Elliot was thus able to save face, regain his grip on reality, maintain his sense of omnipotence relatively unchallenged, and use my help without ever having to acknowledge it.

INTERVENTIONS TO ENHANCE REFLECTIVE FUNCTION, STRENGTHEN IMPULSE CONTROL, AND CREATE AWARENESS OF OTHERS' MENTAL STATES

Interventions that help these youngsters save face can pave the way for a therapeutic or working alliance, that is, the dawning conviction that they stand to gain from the relationship with the therapist and collaboration in the therapeutic process. Face-saving interventions help youngsters with severe personality disorders maintain a sense of control and connection even when confronted with the deflating "blow" of their caregivers' growing capacity to set limits. Thus, such interventions help patients "survive" the anxiety generated by the representational mismatch, as well as the implicit humiliation and increased vulnerability brought about by entering treatment.

As the case of Elliot illustrates, therapeutic face saving—as opposed to these youngsters' usual maladaptive efforts to maintain an illusion of power and control—involves a delicate balance between fostering more adaptive responses to social demands, while maintaining a semblance of control, and keeping anxiety and shame within manageable limits. For example, therapists can help their patients figure out how to respond to caregivers' limit setting. At this stage of treatment, three categories of overlapping interventions are particularly critical: (1) interventions designed to enhance overall reflective functioning; (2) interventions designed to help children strengthen impulse control and enhance self-regulation; and (3) interventions designed to help children become aware of others' mental states. Just as critical as these interventions is the therapist's capacity to be aware, to contain, and to take advantage of the countertransference. The following sets of interventions, aimed at enhancing reflective function, strengthening impulse control and self-regulation, and creating awareness of others' mental states, reinforce and blend with one another and are utilized simultaneously during the early states of therapy.

Enhancing Reflective Function

How does one go about enhancing the mentalizing capability of children? They first need to learn to observe their own emotions, initially *not* in the face of threatening internal states that prompt them to retreat from reflective function. Therapists can suggest that children may still retain a sense of control even when those around them do not follow the old rules. They can do so by understanding the relationship between their own behavior and internal states, for instance, between frustration and anxiety.

As part of this process, therapists help children observe, label, and understand their emotional states, including the associated physiological and affective cues. The therapist thus introduces a mentalizing or reflective perspective that focuses on children's minds, as well as on the mental states of people who are important to them.

Anne Alvarez (1992) described her treatment of a young borderline girl who suffered from asthma. One day the girl came to the session with a slight shortness of breath and said anxiously that she was having an asthma attack. Alvarez described her approach: "I tried to show her that she seemed very frightened, as though she thought she was going to die" (p. 115). The girl's panic and breathing got worse following Dr. Alvarez's comment. She realized that her intervention had escalated the girl's anxiety and finally said that the girl "didn't seem able to tell the difference between a big asthma attack and a little one" (p. 115). Alvarez realized that this girl responded to anxiety with a loss of reflectiveness that made her hear the comment about her fear of dying as an expression of the therapist's conviction of her imminent death. With this same girl, Alvarez realized that rather than saying something terrible would happen during separation, she instead had to turn the idea around and talk to the girl about her difficulty in believing that both of them might make it through the separation.

During the initial stage of therapy, before a strong therapeutic alliance has been established, the therapist keeps the focus on simple mental states, such as belief and desire, rather than on more complex ones, such as conflict or ambivalence. Likewise, early in the process, the therapist refrains from linking the child's feelings to dissociated, repressed, or past experiences. Working with current, moment-to-moment changes in a child's mental state within the sessions, the therapist can focus the child's attention on the circumstances that lead, for example, to aggression in situations in which the child feels misunderstood, blocked, confused, or made anxious by others. At the same time, the therapist can point out how gaining control over automatic reactions may actually help these children feel more in charge of their own lives and behavior.

In this respect, the approach recommended during the beginning stage of psychotherapy requires a reversal of classic psychoanalytic techniques. Child—and adult—analysis opens paths to children's experience of repudiated affect. In contrast, children with severe personality disorders are likely to inhibit reflective function and thus require help in the opposite direction: to learn how to use their ideational capacity to modulate their emotional experience. Such children need help understanding which thoughts, ideas, and circumstances—both internal and environmental—make them feel certain things. Likewise, they need help learning to recognize what they say to themselves that aggravates or modulates their emotional experience. The parallels here with cognitive therapy techniques for children are obvious.

Robert, the boy described earlier in this chapter, followed my clarifications—"Let me see if I hear right what you are saying"—of his disparaging remarks about me, my heritage, The Menninger Clinic, and the State of Kansas, with an acknowledgment that he found it utterly demeaning to be "incarcerated" and in an abject state of deprivation of control and dignity, and in a hick town such as Topeka to boot. He could only imagine what his friends back home would be thinking of him. He blushed as he said this.

With this statement, he seemed to demonstrate a capacity to respond to a therapeutic stance aimed at recognizing him as an intentional being who communicated his mental states through his behavior. I proceeded to remark that, if I heard him right, it was an image in his mind of his friends looking on disapprovingly, perhaps mockingly, that seemed to trigger painful and angry feelings in him.

This inhibition of reflective function turns children's experience of thoughts and feelings into something akin to bodily states (McDougall, 1989; Sifneos, Apfel-Savitz, & Frankel, 1977). Megan, an 8-year-old girl, was totally overwhelmed by the rage and anxiety she experienced when her mother left her. In the early sessions with Megan, I drew attention to her flushed face and wide-open eyes and then wondered aloud if she found me threatening.

Several sessions later, as she had become more comfortable expressing and verbalizing simple mental states, she confided that when her mother was not around, she was overcome with anger and dread fueled by thoughts that her mother was going to be abducted or dismembered in a horrible car wreck. I was careful not to suggest any links between Megan's own anger at losing control of her mother and the thoughts about something horrible happening to her mother. We focused instead on devising ways to chart her worry and anger in order to identify the point at which she lost the capacity to think clearly and feel that she had control over her own mind. Megan discovered a method to accomplish this task by posting on the refrigerator door—in proximity of both a "cooling" presence and nurturing supplies—a "worry chart" and an "anger thermometer," where she could record the extent of her angry feelings or worrisome thoughts.

In summary, the therapist aims to enhance the reflective process by encouraging children to observe and label their somatic and psychological experiences. Key aspects of this intervention involve helping children focus on states felt in the immediate therapy situation and encouraging verbalization as a way to increase children's sense of control and lessen their feelings of vulnerability and shame.

Strengthening Impulse Control and Enhancing Self-Regulation

Children with severe personality disorders, particularly borderline youngsters, require considerable help in curbing their impulsivity. Rosenfeld and Sprince (1963) described a 6-year-old borderline child, Pedro, who frequently urinated on the therapist and her possessions. Other features of this child's behavior led the therapist to understand his urination as a crude attempt to coerce her into maintaining a connection to him in the form of a victim–victimizer mutuality. Neither interpretations nor physical restraint proved successful in reducing this misbehavior. The therapist then devised a way to address Pedro's need to stay connected (and avoid a disruption of attachment): She told him that she would continue whatever activity in which they were jointly engaged while he went to the restroom, and that she would give him a running commentary of what she was doing while he was in there. Since he seemingly felt able to maintain contact with the therapist through her voice, Pedro stopped urinating in the treatment room.

Mayes and Cohen (1993) pointed out that, for some children, the very process of developing imaginative play—or fantasy, pretending, and humor with adolescents—represents the critical therapeutic intervention. A good deal of the work, according to these authors, centers on helping children address the issues that create obstacles to entering the imaginary world. As noted in Chapter 3, the emergence of an appreciation of the difference between the subjective mental world and directly perceivable experience paves the way for enhanced symbolic thinking and, along with that, imagery, guessing, hoping, experimenting, planning, revising, and working through.

Indeed, the capacity to take a playful, humorous, or "as if" stance may be a critical step in the development—or the ability to maintain—reflective function, because it requires simultaneously holding in mind two realities, the pretend and the actual, in synchronicity with a moment-to-moment reading of the other person's state of mind. Therapists often need to create a context in which an attitude of pretense or humor is possible. For example, they may exaggerate their actions to mark for children the pretend nature of interactions, or they may choose objects that are clearly incapable of adopting an intentional stance (e.g., crude toys) in a way similar to how caregivers' "mark" their attuned responses to their children's internal states (see Chapter 3). Children who are confronted with intolerable anxiety when they genuinely try to take on the point of view of others may find it acceptable to imagine pieces of wood (or finger people) thinking and feeling. Under the section on becoming aware of others' mental states, I discuss the implications (beyond strengthening impulse control) of learning to play with objects and persons. During the beginning of therapy, however, the central message is that play, fantasy, and humor offer a way to "step back" from overwhelming or unmanageable experiences and instead break them down into more manageable bits that children can master.

Tooley's (1973) "Playing It Right" is a beautiful account of how therapists can attempt to align the behavior and play of impulsive children with the constraints of reality. Children are nudged to introduce small modifications gradually in their play or behavior so that it better encompasses the complexities, limitations, and frustrations of reality. Borderline youngsters, in particular, create such elaborately vivid and absorbing play themes that they—and, at times, their therapist—can no longer differentiate between fantasy and reality. In their play and fantasy life, these youngsters literally come to life, and they fight mightily against reality intruding and questioning the arbitrariness they impose on their life and relationships. In the magic of play—and in the fantasy world they inhabit—these children create an illusion of perfect relation-ships, while safely keeping away threatening aspects of their self and others.

By "playing it right," therapists can introduce children to the very idea of control. Pedro took on the role of a powerful but uncontrolled mechanical object—the most awesome train engine in the world. He proved his strength by climbing and jumping on the windowsill, whis-tling like a train, pulling the curtains down, and threatening to jump out the window. His therapist suggested that really powerful vehicles have brakes and that a true demonstration of strength consists of the ability to start and stop at will. Pedro took eagerly to the game of stop-ping and starting, allowing more space for the therapist to speak. She subsequently brought up the idea of a very clever mechanic who under-stood how the train worked and what could go wrong, and was thus able to figure out how to prevent breakdowns and damage. Pedro was able to use this bridge between psychological and physical reality to gain greater recognition and control of his feelings.

In the following section, I describe how play, fantasy, and humor provide a transitional space (Winnicott, 1953) where, during the mid-dle stage of therapy, children can try out new identifications, practice imagined solutions to life's dilemmas, explore new ways of being in the world and relating to others, and test behaviors that promise greater mastery, more effective coping, and increased pleasure and adaptation. In particular, play, fantasy, and humor offer a bridge between automatic, unreflective, and coercive models of self and others, and the world of re-flective intersubjectivity. But before those bridges can be built, it should be noted that as these youngsters' attachment to their therapist grows, their impulsivity—at least during the sessions—will actually be exacer-bated, because attachment brings about the very internal states of vul-nerability, fear of abandonment, and dependence that trigger for them a retreat from reflective function.

In the throes of unreflective models, borderline youngsters often require help to manage suicidal, parasuicidal, and other self-harming behavior, such as substance abuse or binge eating. The use of an addic-tion model involving groups and psychoeducation is helpful and effec-tive (Chu, 1998). These approaches are woven into the comprehensive treatment offered in residential and day treatment programs that are dis-cussed in Chapter 9.

Improved self-care and symptom control can be supported in the individual sessions with psychoeducational approaches and "grounding" strategies (Chu, 1998). Psychoeducational interventions emphasize communicating to the patient that symptoms such as flashbacks, dysphoric mood states, or overwhelming anxiety or panic, which contribute to feeling out of control and to hurtful, impulsive responses to blot them out, can in fact be controlled. Helping patients achieve improved self-control is indeed a key goal of treatment. For youngsters with a history of physical or sexual abuse, it is often helpful during the beginning phase of treatment to acknowledge the effects of early traumatization, including the adaptive function of their symptomatology, as crucial attempts to stay in control and maintain attachment. But this acknowledgment should be made without embarking on a detailed exploration of the traumatic events or the feelings associated with them.

Grounding techniques are approaches that seek to identify concretely the moments when these youngsters feel unsafe during the sessions and what they can do to counter such unsafe feelings (e.g., maintaining eye contact). In addition, the therapist helps them define the concrete circumstances when they are more prone to feel overwhelmed, such as when they are tired or alone at night. Then, the therapist helps design a "crisis plan" to deal with these moments when patients feel unsafe or out of control.

Contact with the caregivers gives therapists access to information about potentially disruptive events (e.g., divorces, hospitalizations, loss of employment). Anticipating how the caregivers are likely to feel promotes a reflective stance and introduces the idea that, in the face of certain internal or environmental events, they "lose" the capacity to retain reflective function and, with it, the ability to stay in control of themselves.

Sharing information about neuropsychiatric vulnerabilities (e.g., attention deficit, hyperactivity, mood, or reading disorders) provides a way to explain problems in self-control and opens the possibility for planning therapeutic responses to address these vulnerabilities. Such responses include medications, educational remediation, and cognitive strategies to compensate for deficits in attention or organization. Just as important, such discussion introduces the possibility of examining how these children experience their deficits and the implications of those deficits for their life, identity, adjustment, and self-esteem. This discussion is generally left to the middle phase of treatment, because it requires the protection of a more secure attachment to the therapist and a greater readiness on the part of the patient to explore areas of personal vulnerability.

To summarize, during the beginning stage of therapy, the therapist looks for strategies that children can learn for channeling impulsive behavior into socially acceptable forms of conduct, with increasing control over the expression of feelings in actions. Only later do therapists examine the specific cues generated in the attachment relationship between patient and therapist that trigger an intensification of impulsivity.

Creating Awareness of Others' Mental States

The therapeutic situation pushes children to become aware of the mental states of others. The aim is to show them that all may not be as it seems. Thus, the children begin to learn that their habitual thoughts and feelings are not the only way of seeing the world—or even, necessarily, the way that others see the world.

Children with severe personality disorders, however, actively resist such awareness. They find the mental states of adults confusing or frightening and oftentimes the trigger of threatening or overwhelming internal states. Clinical experience has shown that these children are best helped via interventions focused on their perceptions of the therapist's mental states, as a precursor to self-reflection. The therapist thus seeks to create a relatively safe environment where children can get to know how they are seen by others, mirroring the normal developmental process whereby reflective function and the sense of self and others arise from grasping how others experience them as intentional beings. Therapists, of course, do not necessarily reveal to these children what they actually experience; rather, they share with the children their perception of how the children might be experiencing the therapist's state of mind. Some therapists have used guessing games along these lines. Gifted therapist George Moran (1984) offered an illustration of this approach that serves also to show the limitation of a traditional interpretive technique.

A few days after his 10th birthday, David was found unconscious at school as a consequence of the hypoglycemia he suffered when he refused to eat breakfast. He had been hospitalized 12 times for multiple episodes of hypoglycemia after being diagnosed with diabetes at age 7. David was referred to treatment with Dr. Moran not only because of his

difficulty in controlling his diabetes, but also because of his violence and provocation of family and peers.

David had strained his mother's meager emotional resources. She was unable to feed him after he was born and, in fact, could not even see him for the first 2 weeks because she was crippled with depression. She was hospitalized for depression when David was 3 years old. Aggression seemed to be an accepted part of life in their household. In her fights with David, his mother "gave as good as she got," sometimes sitting on him, hitting him in the head, and pulling his hair. David's father, a conscientious provider who retreated to the sidelines after coming home from work, left his wife to handle their three children, then denigrated her for failing to control them.

After entering treatment, David wasted no time in provoking and launching vicious attacks on the therapist. He also insisted on playing a board game of his own invention. The game consisted of describing an alien culture of exceptional physical and intellectual powers. The therapist interpreted to David that the game helped him feel competent during the sessions, which felt frightening and alien to him. Such interventions failed to alter the boy's behavior. Subsequent interpretations about how David perceived the therapist as frightening and potentially violent did not curtail his attacks, which could only be contained by direct physical restraint. The therapist commented on David's uncertainty about his identity except when angry and fighting, his secret pleasure in his physical contact when fighting, his rebellion against authority, his lack of acceptance of his illness, and many other themes. Such interpretations only led to more abusive behavior. David claimed not to care about the therapist, whom he found stupid and irrelevant. The more the therapist tried to forge links in David's mind, the more hostile or withdrawn the boy became.

When David felt understood, the consequences were, if anything, more dire. About a year into the treatment, in an exceptionally lively session, David acknowledged feeling enslaved by his mother, his diabetes, and his therapy. This moment of therapeutic candor and trust was short lived. Soon afterward, David was hospitalized in a state of ketoacidosis. On returning to therapy, he appeared even more hostile and withdrawn.

David frequently accused the therapist of wearing a Darth Vader mask. At times, he would look at the therapist and ask, "What's the matter, do you want a fight?" Beyond revealing the boy's heightened fear of the therapist, these comments also shed light on the reason David could derive little help from traditional interpretations. Looking at a person—particularly when experiencing certain internal states or during particular interactions with the therapist—gave him no clear idea of the other person's mental state. He could only resort to a fixed, unreflective image of a cruel, vindictive other. At such moments, he could hardly conceive of his therapist as someone who was trying to understand him. In fact, the very perception of a caring, interested, and empathic therapist was arguably a trigger for David's increased desire for attachment, which in turn caused him to inhibit reflective function. Interpreting this state of affairs was of little help to David. George Moran, however, was a creative therapist. He invented a game in which both patient and therapist wrote notes on "What do you think I am thinking about you today?" David asked to repeat this game day after day for months.

Increasingly, David would call for a round of the game at times of heightened anxiety during his sessions. Taking his cues from David, the therapist focused on clarifications of David's current mental state, particularly in relation to him, rather than offering formulations of David's unconscious feelings about his past and present relationships.

Moran's account of one session shows the usefulness of interventions designed to help children become aware of the therapist's internal states. Such awareness is one way to facilitate an understanding of cause and effect in relationships and thereby establish at least a modicum of reciprocity in the treatment relationship.

Moran describes how, during one session, he and David engaged in a spirited game of "tennis" on the table. After David won, he showed the guilty anxiety he often manifested on such occasions. He became agitated and threw himself on the couch, shouting out the names of tennis stars. The therapist then said, "I wonder if you think that I would be less disappointed if I knew I had been beaten by a great tennis player, and then you would not have to feel so uncomfortable." Rather than replying, David stood up on the couch and tried to hit the therapist with his racket. The therapist moved out of harm's way but did not attempt to restrain David, who proceeded to shout, "You don't know me." The therapist then replied, "You don't want me to know you, because then I might not like how big and strong you feel." David spun around and around on his heels, making himself dizzy, and finally collapsed on the floor. He then said he had a headache, intimating that he was dangerously hypoglycemic.

Reflecting on the confusion he felt about David's possibly urgent need for food, the therapist said, "One can feel very helpless when one doesn't really know how someone else feels, but it is even worse when one doesn't know how one feels oneself. I think you feel very frightened that if you become strong and powerful, I will no longer want to help you and perhaps just let you die." David, without saying a word, emptied the contents of his pockets on the carpet. He then proceeded to stuff everything back so carelessly that a good deal of the material he had taken out did not fit anymore.

David snapped, "Why don't you just shut up?" The therapist responded, "By bullying me and shouting at me, I think you hope to get rid of all the thoughts and feelings that you feel we could not cope with." David looked at the therapist for the first time in a friendly way and suggested they play the "I think you think" game. He wrote "frightened" as his first guess about what the therapist thought David thought, then added, "Get lost." The therapist confirmed that he thought David was frightened because he somehow felt that his success would destroy the therapist, and then David would get lost.

This vignette mixes interventions appropriate for early and more advanced stages of therapy because it described sessions taking place more than a year after beginning the treatment. Moran sensed that in facilitating David's capacity to contemplate thoughts, fears, and wishes in himself—and in his therapist—he (the therapist) should *not* address the boy's experience of badness and vulnerability, which only triggered inhibition of reflective function. Instead he pointed out the boy's concerns about his strengths as a vehicle to help David gain some greater capacity to sustain a reflective perspective. He avoided commenting on the possibility that the hypoglycemic crisis, headaches, and dizzy spells might offer David a way to express his feelings of badness and vulnerability, to request help without acknowledging its need, to exact revenge against a threatening and tempting therapist, and to reconnect with experiences of pain and inadequacy, all the while leaving open the possibility of disowning such feelings.

Aggressive youngsters benefit from social skills and anger coping skills training (Bierman, 1989; Lochman & Wells, 1996), and particularly from problem-solving skills training (Spivak & Shure, 1978). Problem-solving skills training (PSST), the most systematically researched approach to the behavioral treatment of conduct difficulties, has demonstrated effectiveness in rigorously conducted studies, particularly in combination with parent training (Kazdin, 1996a; Kazdin, Siegel, & Bass, 1992; Webster-Stratton & Hammond, 1997). In this program, the therapist examines the habitual ways children address interpersonal situations, then encourages a step-by-step approach to solving interpersonal problems that includes "self-talk" to direct attention to aspects of the problem that may lead to effective and adaptive solutions. Modeling and reinforcing prosocial behavior are utilized, as are practice, feedback, homework assignments, and role playing in the context of structured tasks based on relevant, real-life situations.

PSST is a key component of the day or residential treatment of aggressive youngsters with conduct disorders and severe personality disorders (see Chapter 10). Individual therapy can take advantage of these approaches and reinforce their applicability in the context of discussing with these youngsters ways to focus on their distorted appraisal of social events and other people's internal states. Finally, the attachments cultivated in individual and family work with the youngsters and their caregivers seek to address the key limitation of cognitive-behavioral programs of known effectiveness, mainly the high risk of premature termination (Kazdin, 1996b).

USING COUNTERTRANSFERENCE

Not just the patient's reactions require careful attention, however. Perhaps the greatest challenge clinicians face when treating youngsters with severe personality disorders is their own emotional response. There is now considerable agreement in the psychoanalytic literature (Gabbard, 1995; Ogden, 1994) that the transference–countertransference relationship is a joint construction between patient and therapist, rather than the product of the patient's projections alone. The countertransference responses evoked by youngsters with severe personality disorders, however, place unique demands on the emotional resources, technical skills, boundaries, professional ethics, and personal integrity of treaters.

Therapists grow wary of the repeated alternation between reflective and unreflective modes of relatedness. As treaters, we enter into lives often marked by unspeakable despair and terror, and find ourselves responding to the sheer determination to survive that so many of these youngsters exude. Yet the very process of developing an attachment triggers in the patients a retreat from reflective function and the activation of coercive, unreflective modes of experiencing and relating.

As Gabbard (1995) points out, a common thread in contemporary psychoanalytic thinking about countertransference is that the mental contents of the patient are not somewhat mystically transported from patient to clinician. Rather, argues Gabbard, "interpersonal pressure is applied by specific patient behaviors that evoke specific clinician responses" (p. 7). The unreflective and coercive nature of the interpersonal pressures applied by youngsters with severe personality disorders is not only difficult to resist but also tends to evoke a predictable response in all people, including therapists: the momentary loss of the capacity to maintain a reflective mode of functioning.

The result of the activation of unreflective modes of operation in the therapist is an experience of an alien force disrupting one's sense of self and others. Certain patterns of response embody the therapist's efforts to contain and defend against this "alien" presence or, alternatively, result from the clinician being "taken over" by coercive pressures and responding in kind with unreflectiveness.

Therapists often grow to dread the sessions, anticipating the "loss" of the key personal and professional attributes that form the basis of their practice: a capacity to listen empathically to patients and then to respond flexibly, thoughtfully, and ethically. Instead, therapists feel "fooled" by borderline youngsters' pleas for relatedness that alternate with their coercive tyranny. Narcissistic and antisocial youngsters, bent on evoking helplessness and vulnerability in the therapist, often evoke boredom, irritation, or rage when they deny dependence or turn the therapist into an admiring audience. Therapists' defensive reactions against being subjugated and victimized throw them into a fight-or-flight mode that translates into open rage or pressure to demonstrate power and control. Alternatively, the unremitting devaluation and disparagement of attachment by narcissistic and antisocial youngsters evoke paralysis in the therapist, who feels as drained, defeated, worthless, and helpless as these patients would feel without their defensive grandiosity and projected vulnerability.

Borderline and histrionic youngsters seduce therapists by attributing to them perfect empathy, extraordinary power, or unique wisdom. Therapists are vulnerable to experiencing this coercive pressure to become an idealized rescuer (i.e., one who can heal the patient's wounds). The compelling notion of such unreflective models plays a significant role in leading to the destructive outcome of violations of professional boundaries—including therapists' professing love for or engaging in sexual relations with their patients—with tragic consequences for all involved.

Borderline youngsters who threaten suicide, who injure themselves frequently without intending to die, and who make serious suicide attempts from time to time stir up powerful reactions in those who treat them. These patients often threaten their therapist with the implicit message: "If I die, it will be because of your failure." The "failures" in question involve feelings that the therapist has in fact been coerced to experience—but against which he or she typically struggles. These feelings include "not giving a damn anymore," hatefulness, loss of hope, and the secret—or not so secret—desire for the patient to die.

Struggling against these coercive patterns of experience, therapists may experience a number of problematic reactions:

1. They feel more responsible for the patient's survival than the patient or the caregivers themselves (Hendin, 1981). As the frequency and potential deadliness of the suicide threats escalate, therapists rush to the rescue in an unthinking, unreflective fashion. When they do so, they deprive both the patient and the patient's family of responsibility for the youngster's living or dying—and his or her own destructiveness.

2. They alternate between desperate efforts to assume responsibility for the patient's psychological and physical survival, and subtle efforts to reject the patient and even induce the dreaded suicide.

3. They fall into full-blown activation of distancing, rejecting, and plainly sadistic patterns. Maltsberger (1999) reports a vignette that exemplifies the rejection these patients can evoke—and the deadly consequences of the mutually reinforcing cycles of rejection and rejection-inducing behavior.

A borderline patient was assigned to a tired and overworked psychiatric resident, who decided to "set limits" when the patient superficially lacerated her forearm: "She told the patient that no more wrist cutting would be tolerated and that if she persisted in it, the treatment would have to end. The patient cut herself again a few hours after the session ended and reported this at the next appointment. The therapist thereupon terminated the treatment, and the patient committed suicide" (Maltsberger, 1999, p. 36).

Countertransference reactions to youngsters with severe personality disorders are not shaped just by therapist–patient interactions. The therapist's responses shape and are shaped by the entire system of family transactions in which the patient's life—and the treatment relationship—is embedded. Thus, therapists find themselves reacting to the parents' behavior toward the patient and the treaters themselves, as well as to the responses of the patient to their caregivers' experience of the treatment. Again, several patterns of countertransference entrapment are common: (1) Therapists who unthinkingly seek to rescue caregivers from the cruelty and disruption inflicted on them by their children; and (2) therapists who compete with the parents, devalue them in overt or subtle ways, and find themselves compelled to "adopt" the patient and save him or her from abusive, unfeeling, exploitive, or self-centered caregivers.

Although the enactment of any one of these unreflective patterns of countertransference can derail the treatment, anticipating their emergence also opens new opportunities for therapeutic intervention. Carpy (1989) argues that the patient's observation of the therapist's ability to contain, tolerate, and reflect on intense feelings experienced in the therapeutic relationship is mutative in and of itself. Arguably, the therapist's capacity to manage in a reflective fashion the patient's barrage of coercive messages and feelings conveys that the feelings themselves are potentially manageable. Thus, the patient is offered a model of how to break the cycles of coercion and unreflectiveness, which can be demonstrated *in vivo* when the therapist follows—and comments on—a sequence of internal activities, not only focusing on diagnosing the patient's internal relations but also conducting self-examination and internal supervision (Gabbard & Wilkinson, 1994).

Diagnosis of Patients' Internal Object Relations

This step refers to an assessment of the aspects of the patient's internal world that are reflected in the emotions stirred up in the clinician. The self-observing therapist gains a window into the particular cues that evoke the patient's inhibition of reflective function and can profitably share with the youngster how, at certain moments during the session, something pushes the button and the therapist momentarily loses the capacity to think and understand what the patient may be thinking.

Self-Examination and Internal Supervision

Restoring the reflective space in the face of a barrage of coercion is, of course, a formidable task. One advantage of psychoanalytic training is that it requires an extended and intensive experience of personal treatment and supervision that sensitizes and prepares practitioners to observe and manage their own emotional reactions rather than become entrapped in the quicksand of rigid, unthinking patterns of relatedness and experience.

To reiterate, during the initial phase of individual psychotherapy with children and adolescents with severe personality disorders, the goal is to develop a working alliance. Children must be convinced that they can benefit from collaborating and forming a relationship with the therapist that will lead to enhanced self-control and adaptation. To this end:

1. Therapists must avoid confronting vulnerabilities and defenses linking past and present, or addressing repressed or dissociated experience. By minimizing regression, therapists can seek to balance "too much" with "too little" empathy.
2. Therapists can promote verbalization of internal states and differentiation of feelings—and implicitly convey their conception of the patient as an intentional being—by clarifying children's communication ("Let me see if I hear you right.").
3. Therapists can build a working alliance by helping the patient "save face." Interventions designed to help patients save face minimize feelings of shame and being out of control, and disconnected from others, all of which are brought about by the representational mismatch created by environmental manipulation and changes in caregivers (see Chapter 7).
4. Therapists can help their patients save face, regain control, and establish a sense of greater safety and connection by enhancing reflective function, strengthening impulse control and self-regulation, increasing awareness of others, and utilizing countertransference:
   a. Enhancing reflective function can be achieved by helping children observe, label, and understand their internal states—initially, the relatively simple states that arise on a

moment-to-moment basis in the sessions—and the circumstances that lead to automatic reactions as a way to feel more in charge of their behavior.

b. Helping to strengthen impulse control and self-regulation occurs by introducing a playful, humorous, or "as if" perspective as a way to "step back" from overwhelming or unmanageable experiences. Such distancing facilitates breaking down experiences into more manageable bits that children can master. "Playing it right" is one strategy for channeling a patient's impulsive behavior into socially acceptable conduct, with increasing control over the expression of feelings in action. When indicated, psychoeducational approaches, "grounding" strategies, and discussion of neuropsychiatric vulnerabilities can enhance self-control in highly impulsive youngsters.

c. Increasing patients' awareness of others can be achieved by helping them focus on understanding the mental states of their therapist and other people. In particular, it can be helpful for young patients to understand how therapists conceptualize the internal states that facilitate cause-and-effect relationships and establish reciprocity in the therapeutic relationship. In turn, reciprocity forms the basis for a reflective stance in the face of threatening internal cues. These approaches support structured programs designed to enhance problem solving.

d. Using countertransference becomes possible when therapists experience their own unreflectiveness as a window into the internal and intersubjective conditions that evoke inhibition of the patient's reflective function—and subsequently activate coercive models of relatedness.

9

Middle and Late Stages of Treatment

Using Connection to Move toward Integration

Youngsters signal their readiness to enter a more advanced phase of treatment by their capacity to use the therapeutic relationship as a trial base for more adaptive responses to environmental challenges. This capacity is demonstrated by how much youngsters can use the help of therapists to improve self-care, lessen self-destructive impulsivity, or, more generally, save face, that is, respond to the enhanced limit setting of caregivers—the "representational mismatch"—*without* an exacerbation of maladaptive defensive mechanisms. A child's ability to enter into pretend play without demanding that the therapist totally submit to a rigid script suggests a growing security of attachment to the therapist. Security of attachment is also implied by the capacity of adolescent patients to banter or enter into give-and-take exchanges with humor and playfulness. These indicators of attachment security may be subtle but they point to the children's desire for closeness with their therapist and the dawning conviction—fraught with uncertainty and fear of being abused, subjugated, abandoned, destroyed, or humiliated—that hope and help can be derived from this collaborative relationship. Therapists will need to test the readiness of children to enter this state of treatment by following the steps described here. Clinical experience suggests that 3 to 12 months of treatment are needed before reaching this stage.

The presence of an embryonic collaboration allows therapists to gently encourage youngsters to consider an expansion in the range of "shareable" experiences. Narcissistic youngsters are invited to share their experiences of vulnerability. Borderline youngsters are introduced to the notion of a continuity of self in relationships, including an opening for the exploration of traumatic events that disrupt such continuity.

For example, as Jimmy, a 10-year-old boy, gradually shifted from his initial efforts to exercise absolute control over his therapy sessions, various concerns began to creep into the therapy. He made a clay figure of a woman with large breasts, which he attempted to jam into the therapist's mouth. He also staged a game consisting of a gang led by a wicked woman, the "mother of the gang," whom he instructed the therapist to capture and kill.

The therapist, invariably the persecutor, commented how, in their pretend play, everyone seemed to have trouble getting what he or she wanted. Even mothers were involved in leading others into stealing. Jimmy then created a play theme involving his father, a role that he assigned to the therapist, who was to be the President of the United States. This "President," however, turned out to be a rather pathetic figure who could barely function without Jimmy's direction. The boy delighted in ordering his father–therapist–President around, while shouting directives for the country. The therapist began to point out how this play offered Jimmy a chance to share in the power of an exalted, yet secretly diminished, ruler. If he could be the real power behind the President, maybe he would not have to feel little or vulnerable, or afraid that others, envious of his power, might attack him. Perhaps, noted the therapist questioningly, Jimmy's insistence on placing himself in the position of the ultimate, yet secret ruler, betrayed how vulnerable he felt sometimes?

This line of intervention is similar to that used by Moran in his treatment of David. The therapist's comments first point out the patient's anxieties and defenses engendered by the *possibility* of closer contact with the therapist (i.e., in David's case, fear that his success would destroy the relationship, or, in Jimmy's case, concern that exposing vulnerability would lead to humiliation or even greater vulnerability). Only later, on the foundation of a more solid therapeutic alliance and a more secure attachment, can children be invited to contemplate a fuller range of fears, thoughts, feelings, and wishes in themselves and in their therapists—and in their relationships with important people in their lives.

Although the relationship between patient and therapist is clearly the central therapeutic arena, work with these youngsters is not aimed at "interpreting" the transference in the classic sense of expecting and commenting on how thoughts, feelings, wishes, and conflicts about caregivers are transferred to the therapist. Instead, the relationship with the therapist is central, because it is, first and foremost, the most effective route toward acquiring and sustaining a reflective capacity in the context of a significant attachment.

But the very stirrings of a growing attachment also trigger increased anxiety and defensiveness. Jimmy, indeed, became extremely anxious when his therapist pointed out his defensive need to cover up his fear of exposing his vulnerability. Similarly, the case of Joe, an 11-year-old boy with a history of brutal physical and sexual abuse at the hands of an alcoholic father, shows quite dramatically how unbearable it was for Joe to experience desires for closeness with me. Almost in spite of himself, Joe—spurred by face-saving "therapeutic" assistance with his challenging math homework—began to feel more comfortable in the sessions, but as he did so, he found himself hating his liking for me. He thus began to look for "mistakes" that would demonstrate how much I was a pedantic "know-it-all" who really knew little, if anything, about real life. According to Joe, I had learned everything I had in my "fucking rich shrink" collection of books, a source of knowledge that left me obviously unable to survive the mean streets of the big city, let alone able to help someone hardened by life on those mean streets. No longer willing to put up with me, Joe then declared his intention to run away from his residential treatment unit, locate my house, and set it on fire after raping my wife and murdering my children with intravenous injections of cocaine.

Joe's tirade spoke loudly of what his sense of a growing attachment to me had stirred in him: an intense fear of a painful invasion of his house–body; the penetration of his self, his body, and his bloodstream, leading to an initial rush of excitement followed by inner feelings of deadness; the envy of my possessions and relationships and his desire to deprive me of them all, hoping perhaps that he could more easily feel attached to me if we were both equally deprived, locked in a tight embrace of shared hatred, loneliness, and deprivation—once he had eliminated all rivals for my affection.

As I pointed out in the section on countertransference, the unreflective ways that these youngsters communicate their experience—once they have "turned off" reflective function—interferes with the therapist's own representational capacities, sometimes to the point of making it extremely difficult to think and function reflectively in the youngsters' presence. Yet a "check" of one's emotional reactivity can also provide helpful clues to guide interventions. While attempting to weather the storm of Joe's threats, I felt neither threatened nor cut off from him—the telltale signs of the activation of a fight-or-flight response in the presence of an unmodulated threat. I silently wondered if Joe wished to let me know that any more explicit discussion of our relationship was more than he could handle. He seemed to be provoking a change in our interaction from its focus on what gets in the way of greater closeness to more familiar, and thus safer, territory.

Sensing his desire to maintain a relationship with me while overtly disowning it, I commented on the meanness and cruelty of his imagery—without referring to either one of us or our relationship. He looked at me with mixed contempt and amusement, and proceeded to describe, in a wildly exaggerated fashion, the toughness of the neighborhood and brutal gang wars where he used to live. He was certain that a wimpy nerd like me had been sheltered from such roughness and would perish there in a matter of minutes.

Although his statement was richly seasoned with contempt and devaluation, I detected a distinctly teasing, playful invitation to join him in his account of gang adventures. In effect, I knew—and he knew I knew—that he had grown up in the far more sedate environment of an upper-middle-class community in New England. His interest in, and knowledge of, gangs had been acquired mostly through extensive reading. In earlier sessions, Joe had brought in magazines and tapes glorifying gangs.

I picked up (perhaps with more hope than conviction) on the implied teasing and replied with an even more fantastic account of my own heroic battles as a gang kingpin—a secret identity hidden behind my deceptively mild appearance. Joe seemed to enjoy this gambit and responded with mock disparagement. Over the next few sessions, we engaged in a good deal of increasingly good-natured bantering about the relative merits of his gang and mine. Only after this bantering had gone on for about 2 weeks was he able to initiate—in between denunciations of my Latin kings—a more serious discussion of how gangs helped by providing a sense of belonging and powerful protection. He asked me: "What do you do when you are upset?" I replied that his question was an excellent and very tough one to ask or answer. I added that I would only tell him *some* of the things I do; I said that I try to bring to mind memories of times when I have been similarly upset, ways I have managed to feel better, and people who have soothed me and provided comfort.

Joe seemed puzzled by my answer and, after a moment of hesitation, said: "But I don't have any memories like that." After thinking a bit more, however, he corrected himself: "No, wait . . ., " he said, and proceeded to relate, for the first time, how, when he was 6 or 7, he and his father would dance to the mellow tunes of soft rock music. These were the times when he had been sexually abused.

This vignette illustrates several principles that guide interventions in the middle stage of therapy with youngsters who have severe personality disorders, specifically, the importance of pacing and abreaction in the use of transitional experiences to face traumatic attachments and explore an alternative mode of relationships. Youngsters with severe personality disorders have fractionated their sense of relatedness. They carry forward an internal model of a cycle of interactions that involves emotionally intense, close relationships in the context of physical and sexual abuse or in the guilty, overinvolved aftermath of maltreatment. The alternative to this intense relatedness entails moments of painful neglect and emotional disconnection. The prospect of a benign, attuned, caring relationship fills them with panic. As Joe's case illustrates, connection happens for them only in intense, violent, abusive relationships. But such abuse also increases their need for comfort, security, and soothing, thus heightening their need to cling to the only model of attachment available.

However, internal states in these youngsters that are associated with attachment also signal danger, because they indicate that caregivers may be driven to frightened or frightening responses, resulting in traumatic experiences. Thus, the youngsters retreat from reflective function—from awareness of their own and their caregivers' internal states—and cling instead in a nonreflective, procedural fashion to coercive, rigid models of self–other interaction.

Rather than simply acknowledging how much the patient has been abused, the therapist can gradually help flesh out the many reasons for clinging to abusive models of relationships. Discussing traumatic experiences such as sexual or physical abuse is helpful when such experiences can be placed in a relational context. Such a context gives meaning to the patient's understandable reluctance to give up patterns of coping and relating that cause pain and maladaptation, yet are the only known sources of safety and connection.

Abreaction of traumatic experiences requires a careful, ongoing assessment of a youngster's security of attachment to the therapist and capacity to envision the self as someone other than a victim or victimizer. Without such capacities, these youngsters cannot be expected to give up a model of relatedness that evolved around trauma and detachment. Instead, they experience this possibility as a challenge to plunge into a total void, without their only source of identity, security, and attachment. Therapists find themselves struggling with the urge to cajole the patient into abandoning obviously self-destructive and maladaptive modes of coping, relating, and experiencing. Such a stance by the therapist only increases the patient's anxiety, suspicion of the therapist, and need to defeat the treatment.

At this juncture, youngsters in treatment often require a transitional area of relatedness, akin to Winnicott's (1953) transitional experience, as a safe place to test the possibility of secure attachments, mutuality, and reflective function. Play, fantasy, and humor offer just such transitional space. With Joe, the tall tales we exchanged about "our gangs" provided the threads that wove a jointly created story in which Joe could both own and disown feelings of dependence, belonging, security, and vulnerability. At the same time, he was testing out my attunement, respect, and responsiveness to the vulnerable, attachment-seeking aspects of his self.

Some young narcissistic children, such as Jimmy, introduce an imaginary twin as a transitional relationship. This "twin" typically embodies the weak, helpless, dependent experiences that such children find unbearable. Somatic complaints or somatic crises, such as the ones engineered by David, offer another version of a transitional experience of sharing feelings of pain and vulnerability while also asking for help without explicitly acknowledging such feelings.

The transitional sphere of shared play, fantasy, or humor, which can be structured as games (e.g., Moran's [1984] "What I think you think I am thinking about you"), provides a safe arena in which to create an illusion of secure attachment with the therapist. At the same time, threatening aspects of the self and others, and of reality constraints, can be kept at a safe distance.

As discussed earlier, Tooley's (1973) "Playing It Right" describes a process that uses play as a way of gradually nudging children to acknowledge and face the complexities, limitations, conflicts, and frustrations of reality, of themselves, and of their relationships. The transitional space of shared play, humor, or fantasy offers a stage on which to explore new ways of being in the world. It allows patients to relate to others—in Joe's case, this form of relating permitted him to ask openly for advice and help; it tested behavior that may promise greater mastery, pleasure, and adaptation; and it explored the bringing together of the split-off or fractionated aspects of Joe's internal world. Thus, Joe could examine his longing for security and belonging in the space provided by our shared construction of the "gang's" world. The magic of anonymity afforded by the transitional space is a function of an implicit agreement to treat these constructions as if they are real, yet clearly knowing that they are all—or almost all—pretend. Thus, in a transitional space, children can be invited to consider that a whole region of their experience stands unlived, so to speak (i.e., never processed in the reflective mode that allows for sharing, ownership, and integration). Kernberg and colleagues (2000) report on a 7-year-old borderline boy who, when told by his therapist that he seemed loving and friendly on Mondays and Wednesdays but whining and tyrannical on Saturdays (when he was brought to the sessions by his parents rather than the housekeeper), replied with a grin: "You don't know what I am like on Tuesdays and Thursdays" (p. 171). Such exchanges offer the opportunity to explore the advantages of—as well as the price exacted by—split or fractionated ways of experiencing, coping, and relating in different contexts.

To summarize:

1. Readiness to enter a more advanced stage of therapy is signaled by evidence of a collaborative relationship between patient and therapist. At this point, children demonstrate that they can utilize their therapist's help to enhance their adaptation.

2. The first set of interventions in the middle stage of treatment should be designed to address the anxieties and defenses that these children mobilize against a closer attachment with their therapist. The possibility of a closer attachment intensifies anxiety and thus triggers an exacerbation of maladaptive defense mechanisms—particularly evident in the relationship with the therapist.

3. Therapists must resist the urge to cajole their patients to relinquish maladaptive defenses and patterns of attachment, recognizing instead that these are the only source of identity, security, and connection available to these youngsters.

4. Patients can benefit from a transitional space provided by shared play, fantasy, and humor. This space allows them to explore more safely issues of attachment, the possibility of integrating split-off aspects of their internal world, and the use of alternative modes of coping and relating.

FACILITATING INTERVENTIONS AND THE THERAPEUTIC BARGAIN

The transitional space provides a relatively safe haven for beginning to examine systematically not only youngsters' maladaptive patterns of coping and relating but also the motives that underlie the perpetuation of such patterns. Not surprisingly, intense anxiety and intensified reliance on maladaptive coping mechanisms accompany every move in this process, as Joe's case illustrates. The Menninger study of change in adult borderline patient collaboration (Allen, Gabbard, Newsom, & Coyne, 1990) and detailed studies of successful therapies with borderline adults (Waldinger & Gunderson, 1984) confirm how rapidly patients with severe personality disorders alternate between a collaborative attitude and coercive, unreflective behavior within each session and from session to session. This alteration is even more dramatic in the treatment of children and adolescents.

Therapists can expect to be turned into transitional objects (Winnicott, 1953) by their patients' efforts to buffer the emotional storms that buffet them. Gunderson (1996) proposes a hierarchy of transitional options that therapists can offer patients with severe personality disorder to help them deal, in particular, with the panic, rage, and dysregulation brought about by interruptions in the treatment or other disruptions in their attachment with the therapist. At the end of the hierarchy, therapists make themselves accessible by telephone either as needed or on a prescheduled basis. In the middle part of the hierarchy, the therapist provides "therapist-associated transitional objects" such as handwritten notes that the patient can use for comfort and reassurance, cognitive directives to follow at times of distress, or items from the therapist's office to remind the patient of the support offered by the therapist.

A 15-year-old borderline girl, for example, became able to tolerate interruptions in treatment without feeling like a helpless infant, panicked about falling apart and disgusted at her own dependency, by keeping a "separation diary." She would ask me to write a few lines in her diary on the last session before an interruption so that she could then read the note when she felt lonely or anxious. A 16-year-old narcissistic boy became able to use the help of his teachers, without becoming defiant and demeaning, by silently repeating an "interpretation" I had made about how important it was for him to have all the answers and feel in control.

Alvarez (1992) illustrates the use of tall tales—such as Joe's "gang"—as a transitional space in which to facilitate a self-reflective stance. Carol, a girl, whose rude behavior had rendered her

> hard-to-place after her parents had declared their inability to care for her, brought one day a photograph of herself with someone whom she maintained was her "uncle." The therapist realized that this must be an uncle in one of the foster families who had neglected Carol and commented something like, "I think you would like me to think that is your uncle, but we both know the sad truth is he is probably an uncle from your foster family." (p. 181)

Alvarez suggests that behind the girl's story is the wish to be *conceived* of by the therapist as someone who would have a close family. Thus, she proposed that the therapist could say: "I think today I should see you as a person who could have a close family" or "You feel you and I are getting to know each other, a bit like family" (p. 181).

The use of these transitional activities offers a buffer that allows the youngster to tolerate a range of internal and interpersonal experiences, without entering into fight or flight and inhibiting reflective function, thus permitting the active exploration of the youngster's inner world. The therapist's acknowledgment of the utter terror that children must feel as they enter unexplored areas of self–other relatedness is often useful in preventing a therapeutic stalemate. Facilitating comments at this juncture may provide a needed therapeutic push. Only in the later stages of therapy can therapists utilize less-reality-distorting options in the hierarchy of transitional activities, namely, self-initiated options such as planning increased contact with friends or accessing other supports during therapists' absences, as examples of a more adaptive way to anticipate and cope with stress and vulnerability.

Pointing out the courage required to venture much further into this unfamiliar territory—for example, Joe's question about how to deal with distress—aligns the therapist with the patient's "proximal area of development" (Vygotsky, 1962, 1978), that is, with what Friedman (1982) calls "the person he is about to become" (p. 12).

In fact, as described earlier, such alignment is generally more effective when therapists point out the price—in greater anxiety and exposure to unfamiliar dangers and vulnerability—of giving up the maladaptive mechanisms that these children have found as their only source of identity, security, control, and attachment. Thus, after Joe related his experiences of abuse, I pointed out how understandable it was that he would want to dismiss any possibility of closeness with anyone, including a "fucking rich shrink" like me, and the tremendous amount of guts it would take for him to venture into exploring closeness. On the other hand, keeping people at a distance and afraid of him helped Joe feel safe and in control.

Such a stance can free these youngsters to examine the price they pay for relying on maladaptive patterns of coping, experiencing, and relating. At this point in treatment, therapists present to their patients in more explicit fashion the therapeutic bargain that the treatment represents: The patients can choose, if they are able, to relinquish pathological, maladaptive defenses and coercive patterns of relatedness—and the illusion and control, safety, and connection they derive from them—but such relinquishment requires the laborious and at times painful process of attempting real mastery and meaningful relationships. Youngsters call into play strong compensatory mechanisms in response to the "offer" of a therapeutic bargain. If both the therapist and the patient can withstand the onslaught of unreflective coercion that usually follows, then themes of dependence, safety, autonomy, vulnerability, body integrity, envy, and competition become available for exploration. Intermixed with these issues are the real joy, renewed hope, and genuine pride these youngsters experience as a result of their increasing capacity to conceive of themselves and others as genuine human beings. The crucial milestones at this stage in the treatment process are as follows: (1) Patients give evidence of a capacity to be aware of the implications of their thoughts, feelings, and intentions toward another person from the point of view of a third person, that is, a capacity to maintain a reflective stance that simultaneously encompasses several psychic realities; (2) patients give evidence that they can respond to stress, anxiety, and conflict with the development of defensive adaptations based on repression, thus not necessitating the suspension of reflective function and the loss of the capacity to consider various levels of meaning simultaneously; and (3) patients give evidence of restored hope—or "remoralization" (Bateman & Fonagy, 1999)—that is manifested by a resistance to the inclination to reject offers of help at moments of anxiety or conflict.

These milestones indicate youngsters' readiness to embark on the construction—more accurately, a co-construction in which the therapists participate—of a narrative of their lives and experience that offers them meaning and identity.

Robert's therapy process illustrates the unfolding of these issues. After 9 months of treatment, which Robert had mostly spent demonstrating his nautical, culinary, and cinematographic expertise, he began to worry about whether I found him interesting and considered him a good patient. He promised me that he would work very hard, and he fantasized that I bragged to my colleagues about my hardworking, interesting patient.

Clouds of doubt darkened this sunny scenario. Robert feared that he would fail to meet my expectations and that I would then wish to get rid of him. This was our first opportunity to gain access to Robert's so-far-disowned feelings of vulnerability and his concern that his plea for attachment would evoke rejection or worse. In fact, wishes for closeness were a signal to him to suspend reflective function. The result of such inhibition was a nonreflective scenario that turned me into a destructive force and him into a helpless, terrified infant.

Over several sessions, I pointed out to Robert how his interest in my thoughts about him seemed to trigger a shutdown of his capacity to think of me as a person who could understand him as a regular human being. He responded to these interventions by voicing great concern about his weight. He devised a system that he believed would allow him to lose weight: He was to report to me the first session of the week whether he had achieved the goal of losing 4 pounds during the previous week. If he succeeded in meeting the goal, I was to praise him for his success and encourage him to go on. More important, I was not to make any inquiries of the kind we therapists are so keen on, about the script we were to follow. He indeed experienced any invitation on my part to examine his plan as a cruel, unfeeling rejection. Clearly, I did not give a damn about him. I had the power to help him conquer his obesity and become attractive to girls, yet I callously let him become dangerously overweight. He felt totally out of control of his eating, particularly after the sessions that made him feel ravenously hungry and drove him to buy potato chips and doughnuts, which he thought of as evidence of my inability to control him.

I thus had an opportunity to comment on how frustrating and frightening it must be for him to feel that I had such control over his body and his appeal to girls. No wonder he also wished to show me that I was in fact impotent to stop him—even from doing something that he felt would hurt him. Yet hurting himself gave him at least a sense of some control—and the right to be mad at me for not taking care of him.

As we talked at some length about how much power I really had, I pointed out that, in fact, I could help him lose weight only as long as I followed a very tightly written script created by him. I suggested that feeling so out of control seemed better to him than to allow me to have my own thoughts and responses to him. Robert responded to these comments with memories of his favorite childhood play: More than anything, he liked to play by himself. He would set up a vast army of soldiers, who blindly obeyed his every command. He always wished to see himself as a puppeteer who could make people move according to his will. He had become attracted to movies because he loved to fantasize that he could script life like a movie. In real life, however, people refused to comply with his lovely scripts.

As we examined these issues over several weeks, he asked that we follow his weight-loss plan. For the next 8 weeks, we started the week with Robert proudly reporting that he had met the goal of losing 4 pounds. This ritual provided a transactional space to explore safely his efforts to assert his power and control and yet find help and regulation in me. As we did so, he spontaneously began to talk about how he had felt out of control as a child with his mother. Increasingly frustrated over her marriage, Robert's mother sought his companionship and comfort when he was barely 5. Robert remembered that his mother would appear half-naked and more than half-drunk in his bedroom. She would lie in bed with him, bitterly complaining about his father's insensitivity, while praising Robert for his understanding, until she would pass out. Such encounters left Robert with a tangle of feelings: sexually excited; proud of his power to comfort his mother and "beat" his father; enraged at the arousal and confusion she stirred up in him; terrified that she had died when he could not rouse her; afraid of his father's retaliation; guilty at his sexual pleasure and the special role he played in his mother's life; and embarrassed at his own arousal and feelings of being out of control. His father added insult to injury when, rather than finding him a worthy rival, he ignored Robert. That indifference, mixed with his father's disparaging remarks about Robert's body and his competence, left Robert feeling humiliated, angry, and confused, and longing for someone to guide and protect him. His "solution" had been a pattern of self-destructiveness and self-nurturance from which he derived a secret sense of omnipotence: He asserted his power by defeating and compelling everyone to comply with the scripts he devised. He may not have dared to display his masculinity assertively and become attractive to girls in front of either one of his parents, but he could surely defiantly display his obese body, his out-of-control eating, and his obnoxious and self-destructive behavior.

The effort to help Robert regain reflective function in a dyadic relationship opened the way for him to consider the implications of his feelings, thoughts, and intentions toward another human being (e.g., his feelings toward his mother) from the perspective of a third person (e.g., his father). This capacity marked a fundamental change in Robert's self-awareness, in his awareness of his own and other people's mental functioning, and in his capacity to represent self and others in a more complex, reflective–symbolic fashion. Such a transition marks the point at which treatment can shift from seeking to promote a way to process experience (reflective function) that is being inhibited to examining defensive maneuvers (e.g., repression, denial, reaction formation) that pertain to particular mental states that have been processed reflectively.

Robert's obesity, for example, symbolically represented a way of signaling to his father that he was retreating from sexual competition with him. His obese body, which so much annoyed his father—and which his father could not control—also represented a way for him to convey to his mother his defiance of his father—a sort of huge penis that he could safely display. At an even more deeply defended level, Robert also longed for his father—a father who could control him, comfort him, and give him strength, power, and a sense of direction. His "out of control" behavior was an ongoing challenge and invitation for his father to regulate him, soothe him, and comfort him—just as he asked me to take over his weight reduction plan.

To summarize, the task of facilitating interventions enables the therapist to explore the motives behind maladaptive patterns of coping, experiencing, and relating in the following ways:

1. By acknowledging the terror associated with changing and the advantages of not changing—and the courage required to entertain the "therapeutic bargain" of substituting illusory control for the effort to achieve real mastery and genuine attachments.

2. By freeing youngsters to acknowledge the price they pay for relying on maladaptive patterns of coping, relating, and experiencing. Such acknowledgment opens the path to a more systematic exploration of core beliefs and experiences that are at the root of maladaptive coping. In turn, this exploration allows for a shift from interventions designed to promote reflective function to the examination of defensive maneuvers against specific reflectively processed mental states.

FAMILY TREATMENT: ENHANCING CAREGIVERS' COMPETENCE AND SENSITIVITY

Enduring changes in reflective capacities and the readiness to relinquish rigidly held coping and relationship patterns are unlikely unless such changes are syntonic with changes in children's interpersonal context. Without an alignment of individual and family treatment, the "therapeutic bargain" offered by the therapist is unlikely to prove appealing.

The alignment begins with caregivers' capacity to support and promote their children's reflective abilities in the face of danger signals. Such a capacity, in turn, is predicated on the caregivers receiving help to become more competent and feel more in control, rather than feeling buffeted by the emotional and behavioral turmoil that they and their children generate. Thus, as described in Chapter 7, the first order of business with caregivers is to assist them in becoming more effective and consistent at setting limits, more capable of maintaining generational boundaries, and more invested in extricating their children from the roles they play in perpetuating the family's and the children's own maladjustment. Such roles may include deflecting one caregiver's hostility against the other; holding the caregivers' relationship together; or maintaining parental self-esteem while relieving the caregivers' own traumatic memories of pain, vulnerability, and helplessness.

There is strong empirical evidence that a number of structured approaches designed to help caregivers improve their parental effectiveness can also alter the destructive and self-destructive behavior of children and adolescents. As Fonagy (2000b) points out, however, in his review of the treatment of conduct disturbance, the most potent effects of parent training programs are obtained when the following conditions are present: younger children in the family; less comorbidity; less severity of conduct disturbance in the children; less socioeconomic disadvantage; parents who stay together and parental discord is low; more social support for the family; and absence of any parental history of antisocial personality.

Such findings certainly support the view that with any treatment approach, "the rich tend to get richer." Although the literature about the effectiveness of parent training is compelling, for a substantial number of these families (particularly for the most dysfunctional ones with the least support and the greatest disadvantages), the demands of structured parent training prove overwhelming. In addition to attending sessions, these demands include reviewing educational material, systematically observing children's behavior, implementing reinforcement procedures, and maintaining telephone contact with the treaters. Not surprisingly, a large percentage of families prematurely discontinue the treatment.

Arguably, the dropout range can be reduced if the therapists have first built a collaborative relationship. Such collaboration is fostered when the treaters and caregivers together carefully assess whether every aspect of the treatment makes sense to the caregivers, and when the treaters' consistent stance is that nothing that undermines caregivers' sense of comfort and control—or does not make sense to them—is likely to benefit the youngsters who are the primary focus of treatment.

Structured approaches to parent training can be incorporated in the treatment to help caregivers increase their parenting competence. Among those approaches best supported by empirical evidence of effectiveness, the following deserve special mention:

• *"Helping the noncompliant child"* (Forehand & Long, 1988; Forehand et al., 1979; Long, Forehand, Wierson, & Morgan, 1994) is a program that includes didactic instruction and models role playing and skills practice, with therapist feedback from behind a one-way mirror. Structured exercises are designed to ensure generalization beyond the clinical setting. The early phase of this program attempts to break coercive cycles of interaction by increasing caregivers' attention to their children and their socially appropriate behavior, and by teaching them to increase children's compliance using social attention as a contingency. In the second phase of the program, caregivers are taught how to communicate and monitor directions and limits, and how to use time-outs as a consequence for noncompliance.

• *Videotape modeling group discussion* (Webster-Stratton, 1996). This is a 9- to 10-week program that shows to a group of parents a standard package of videotapes showing vignettes of parents interacting "appropriately" or "inappropriately" with their children. After each vignette, the therapist leads a discussion, pointing out the relevant interactions and soliciting responses from the parents. Parents are taught to play and to use reinforcement for limit setting, as well as other nonviolent discipline and problem-solving techniques.

• *The Oregon Social Learning Center programs* (Patterson & Chamberlin, 1988; Patterson & Forgatch, 1995; Patterson, Reid, Jones, & Conger, 1975). These target a wide range of children (3- to 12-year-olds rather than the 3- to 8-year-olds in the two programs described earlier). During the initial phase of the program, parents learn to identify and track two or three of their children's noncompliant aggressive behaviors. They then learn to utilize positive reinforcement, such as points, treats, privileges, praise, and attention to increase desirable behavior, and time-outs, response cost (loss of privileges), and mild punishment (chores) to decrease aggression and noncompliance. The program also teaches problem solving and negotiation strategies to deal with marital difficulties, family crises, and caregivers' personal adjustment problems.

• *Parent–child interaction therapy* (Eyberg, Boggs, & Algina, 1995). This is designed to teach parents to build a warm and responsive relationship with their children. In the first phase, parents learn nondirective play skills similar to those used by play therapists. During the second phase, caregivers use the play interaction to learn to direct their children with clear, age-appropriate instructions, praise them for compliance, and apply time-outs for noncompliance. Therapists observe the interactions behind a one-way mirror and provide coaching in real time via earphones.

• *Modification of the Oregon model* (Bank, Marlowe, Reid, Patterson, & Weinrott, 1991). The Oregon model has been modified for application to the disturbance of conduct in adolescents. Modifications include targeting behaviors that increase the risk of delinquency (e.g., class attendance, affiliation with antisocial peers, drug use); increasing parental monitoring; and replacing time-outs with more drastic procedures (e.g., restriction of free time or restitution of stolen property). Parents are expected to report their children's offending behavior to the juvenile authorities and then to act as advocates in court. Adolescents are engaged in setting up behavioral contracts.

A number of adjunctive approaches described in the literature attempt to improve the effectiveness of parent training. These approaches include support with the caregivers' marital problems (Griest et al., 1982) and social problem-solving skills training for caregivers (Webster-Stratton, 1996). A significant issue left unaddressed by most parent training programs is the degree to which parenting styles and methods of communication and discipline are strongly culture specific. One exception is Strayhorn and Weidman's (1989) study, which describes an attempt at providing culturally sensitive parent training to multi-stressed, low-income (predominantly African American) parents. In this study, the treatment was delivered by African American paraprofessionals recruited from the community.

A more comprehensive recognition of the cultural–ecological determinants of child and adolescent dysfunction is embodied in multi-systemic therapy (MST; Hawkins et al., 1992; Henggeler et al., 1999; Offord et al., 1992). This structured approach has emerged as the most promising intervention for serious juvenile offenders. The program goes beyond parent training to utilize combined, multiple interventions as indicated by the clinical picture, in a fashion congruent with the flexible, comprehensive, integrated, and individualized approach proposed in this book.

MST utilizes techniques from systemic and structural family therapy (e.g., joining, reframing, assigning specific tasks), cognitive-behavioral therapy, parent training, marital therapy, supportive therapy, and social skills training, as well as case management. Therapists, who also act as advocates for the family to outside agencies, are available 24 hours a day, 7 days a week. The family, rather than the adolescent, is the focus of the treatment, and the sessions are held in the family home and in community settings.

The overarching goal of MST is to empower parents by providing them with the skills and resources necessary to cope with the strains of raising an adolescent, particularly one with conduct problems, while empowering the adolescent to cope with the adaptive challenges arising both within and outside the family. The treatment seeks to identify and mobilize the strengths of the various systems impinging on the adolescent and the family, and promotes responsible behavior among all family members.

While MST utilizes a range of techniques from a variety of treatment approaches, its greatest strength lies in its focus on the interrelationship among systems and its clear definition of interventions. These interventions are described in treatment manuals that still permit a flexible and highly individualized approach.

These structured parent training approaches can powerfully boost the effectiveness of the treatment of youngsters with severe personality disorders. The demands of some approaches—including the demands of MST on treaters—can be formidable, calling for a more flexible use of treatment program *components*.

Helping caregivers increase their parenting competence, however, is rarely a straightforward proposition. The very fact of being in treatment, and of being offered help, is often as much a signal of danger to caregivers and other family members as it is to the identified patient. Thus, involvement in treatment and evidence of the youngster's formation of a collaborative relationship with the treater characteristically mobilize caregivers' efforts, often not conscious, to undermine the treatment and the youngster's engagement in it. The unreflective patterns of interaction triggered by the cues of therapeutic engagement are powerfully coercive and carry the strongest affective load: guilt, anxiety, shame, and vague but overwhelming dread of ridicule, banishment, damnation, abandonment, and destruction of the self and the family.

Treaters can assist caregivers in regaining a reflective stance by exploring the historical and multigenerational context in which dysfunctional patterns of interaction have emerged. Several months into Elliot's treatment, it became possible to examine with his caregivers—after carefully determining that this exploration "made sense" to them in sessions with only the parents present—the history of how expressing "weakness" or vulnerability had become, over several generations, so unacceptable that emotional support within the family could neither be asked for nor given in a direct way. But at the same time that vulnerability had to be ignored or ridiculed, the family seemed to have developed the expectation that outsiders bring only hurt, shame, or abuse. Both caregivers became interested in learning how to express their own concerns more directly and how to give and receive support, because acquiring these skills was defined as something that would help Elliot in his struggles to express vulnerability more directly as he learned to fit together the "pieces of the puzzle" of his identity. Indirectly, of course, learning to express concern on behalf of Elliot helped the parents address their own unspoken and unacknowledged feelings of exhaustion and depletion.

To promote the caregivers' reflective functioning requires an acknowledgment that they are generally under enormous strain from a variety of sources. Many are single parents with other children and are entangled in bitter battles with the other parent or deeply resent his or her abandonment. Others struggle with relationships or are themselves riddled with depression or trapped in lives marked by despair, substance abuse, and/or financial hardship. Stressors on the caregivers precipitate coercive cycles in the family and symptoms resulting from the youngsters' inhibition of reflective function.

A significant focus of the work with the caregivers is thus devoted, as Liddle and Hogue (2000) recommend, to (1) identifying how these stressors affect their caregiving capability and the caregiving environment within the family; (2) determining how the children may be better protected from their impact; and (3) helping caregivers access supportive resources, including psychiatric assistance for themselves and other family members.

In focusing on these issues, it is helpful to examine the history of how the caregivers attempted to raise their troubled youngster while also coping with multiple stressors. The narrative that emerges from this account serves to point out how, under certain conditions, reflective function—and narrative coherence—are lost, undermining the caregivers' best efforts to be effective and helpful to their children. Caregivers often, either spontaneously or with the assistance of the treaters, place their parenting efforts against the background of the parenting they received in their family of origin.

Developing these narratives allows for a detailed discussion of the caregivers' unspoken or not fully conscious attributions that underlie their parenting as a preamble to focusing on parenting practices related to how to set and enforce rules, monitor behavior, and provide support, guidance, and recognition of the children's individuality.

These discussions with the caregivers alone precede sessions with the caregivers and the youngster—and other children—designed to create an interactional context in which families develop the motivation, skills, and experience to break coercive cycles, promote security of attachment, and interact in a reflective mode. As Liddle and Hogue (2000) suggest, caregivers and their children are asked explicitly to "evaluate their attachment bonds and the balance they achieved between autonomy and connectedness" (p. 273). The therapist's crucial goal is to find the optimal point at which specific family members can both be themselves and feel connected to one another.

The main approach to achieve this goal is to review interactions that either occur spontaneously during the sessions or are prompted by the therapist or family—specific care themes. The therapist first observes how caregivers and children communicate, how they recognize or ignore each other's individuality and intentionality. The therapist then proposes new modes of interaction in an attempt to interrupt coercive cycles and promote a reflective stance. This may require "translating" one person to another, ascribing meaning to an interaction as it unfolds—particularly, by pointing out when specific interactions trigger a loss of reflective function, or by heightening or lowering the intensity of the discussion.

Often, both the youngster and the caregivers need considerable individual coaching before they can engage in reflective interactions with regard to particularly emotionally loaded or conflictual topics. The coaching is carried out in sessions designed to help family members—whether the caregivers or the children—with "the content and style of what is to be said, prepare for potential reactions by other participants, and solidify a minicontract that challenges the participants to follow through as planned once the interaction begins" (Liddle & Hogue, 2000, p. 274).

The preparatory coaching often focuses on enabling family members to appreciate others' point of view and to become clearer about their own perspective and motivation, which encourages less extreme and rigid positions. By processing in advance interactions that habitually result in the loss of reflective function, family members can take a first step toward restoring it. The therapists can help the family recognize what a reflective interaction feels like by pointing out when it takes place either spontaneously or in a planned exchange.

A useful approach that promotes caregivers' reflective stance is to encourage one or both parents to tell their children stories about times when they themselves felt distressed, in circumstances comparable to those now faced by the children, and how they coped with such distress. I could, for example, point out to Joe's father, when, after years of estrangement he indicated a desire to reconnect with his son and share with him his success in conquering alcoholism and turning his life around, that Joe was courageously asking "What do you do when you get upset?" because he did not know how to grow up as a man facing distress, pain, and vulnerability. Could Joe's father help by sharing stories not only about his successes but also about his struggles? Storytelling serves to connect parents with their own vulnerability in the process of helping their children and collaborating with the therapist in a way that avoids the "patient" role.

Paradoxically, interventions that help caregivers attain a reflective stance and empathize with their children—and themselves—free them to "fire" their children from the role of functioning to maintain the family's equilibrium. Thus, Elliot's mother "fired" him from both his self-appointed—but enormously reinforced—role as the regulator of maternal self-esteem and the preventer of her suicide, and from the role, through his misbehavior, as rescuer of his parents' failing marriage. In reviewing these issues, both parents also felt freer to give Elliot explicit encouragement to form a relationship with the *other* parent, minimizing the intensity of the mother–child coalition that had served as such a strong reinforcement of the boy's sense of omnipotence. At the same time, Elliot's father became able, for the first time, to talk openly about his own unmet dependency needs and previously unexpressed fears of weakness—and to share with his son the harrowing details of his immigration to America and his helplessness as his family was destroyed in Europe.

Children, of course, observe, question, and test the encouragement and assurances offered by their caregivers. But changes in family interaction patterns and the growing capacity of the caregivers to sustain a reflective stance allow all family members to experiment with previously restricted behavior and modes of relationship. Not only do children find greater developmental opportunities but they also receive "permission" to bring to their individual therapy a host of important issues, with greater freedom from the binds of loyalty and concern about the implied rules of family life.

In summary, by doing the following, therapists involved in family treatment strive to enhance caregivers' competence and sensitivity:

1. Aligning the youngster's interpersonal context with the individual psychotherapy. The first step in helping caregivers retain a

reflective perspective involves enhancing parental competence. Several structured parent training approaches that can boost parental competence also place substantial demands on the most vulnerable families.

2. Recognizing that caregivers will mobilize coercive patterns in response to their children and to their own involvement in treatment.

3. Exploring historical and multigenerational interactive patterns associated with an inhibition of reflective function, thereby promoting caregivers' ability to retain a reflective perspective.

4. Acknowledging the stressors impinging on the caregivers and identifying how these stressors affect the caregiving environment.

5. Determining ways to protect the children from the impact of stressors that affect the caregivers.

6. Helping the caregivers access support and, if necessary, treatment for themselves and other family members.

7. Focusing on parental practices with regard to setting rules, monitoring behavior, and providing support, guidance, and recognition of individuality.

8. Evaluating explicitly the family's attachment bonds and the balance between autonomy and connectedness.

9. Reviewing interactions around specific core themes and planning new modes of interaction designed to break coercive cycles and promote reflective function. Individual coaching is often required before these interactions can take place.

10. Enhancing caregivers' reflective capacity by encouraging them to share stories about their own experiences of vulnerability.

11. Increasing caregivers' empathy, which enables them to "fire" the patient from the special role he or she plays in the family's dysfunction, and giving the youngster permission to connect with the other caregiver.

TOWARD TERMINATION: MOURNING AND RESUMING DEVELOPMENT

The harbingers of termination are found both inside and outside the treatment process. Naturally, a sustained amelioration of symptomatic and maladaptive behavior is an important sign. Perhaps even more significant is the achievement of nondelinquent peer relationships and interests. Changes in family interaction and school functioning are also particularly important. A child's growing ability to use caregivers and other nondelinquent adults as sources of protection, comfort, and regulation, and as models of identification, signals the end of the therapeutic process. When the youngster can approach caregivers and teachers for help in solving problems in reality, the beginning of termination is in view.

Within the treatment process, therapists recognize other clues of impending termination: youngsters' open acknowledgment of missing their therapists during interruptions and vacations; expressions of gratitude for help received; youngsters' accounts of how they use outside the sessions what they learned in treatment; and—perhaps the most sensitive clue—patients' reports in treatment of their sense of loss regarding missed or botched opportunities.

The final stage of therapy generally begins after 1 to 3 years of treatment and offers a chance to test children's readiness to relinquish pathological defenses. Discussing possible termination dates with patients and parents fuels anxiety and often brings about both a reactivation of symptoms in the patient and a resurgence of dysfunctional interaction patterns in the parents.

When Jill, a 10-year-old girl in residential treatment, began to attend public school, the move clearly meant that discharge from the residential treatment center and termination of psychotherapy were imminent. This narcissistic girl proceeded—as was characteristic of her before beginning treatment—to alienate her classmates with her petulance and manipulativeness, her tall tales about her extraordinary accomplishments, and her demand to be the center of everyone's attention. Along with this return of old patterns, Jill attempted to present in therapy a rosy picture of her adaptation to the world outside the residential treatment center. She was liked by her peers, she said, eagerly sought out as a playmate, and could count two or three girls as her best friends.

Only a school report brought home the true picture of the girl's struggles. Confronted with the discrepancy, Jill could speak at last of her fears of disappointing me, the staff in the residence, and her parents. She wondered whether her progress was completely contingent on the therapy and the staff's support, and she worried about whether she could sustain it without such a protective envelope. She was skeptical as to whether her parents and I would really appreciate her if she was anything less than a perfect, smashing success. Could she be loved if she were just a regular girl? Only after much additional work did another dimension of her regression emerge: Jill's difficulties in dealing with the sadness and loss associated with termination.

Mourning the anticipated loss of the therapy and the therapist is an essential task of the termination phase. Just as important is the opportunity for children to work through their disappointments in their own shortcomings, in the adults who never measured up to their expectations, in everything they could not achieve in therapy, and in the therapist's limitations.

Regardless of apparent regressions and symptomatic reactivations, the termination phase requires a relaxation of supervision and the provision of expanded responsibilities and increased privileges. Naturally, such a stance is not without risk. The following vignette illustrates the vicissitudes that can be encountered during termination.

Adam, a 12-year-old boy, found himself in the state's custody after his mother repeatedly deserted him. His unremitting destructiveness and defiance landed him in a residential treatment center. There he explained to his therapist, in the metaphor of his play, the reasons for his hatred: The therapist, the leader of the "Irams"—the treatment occurred at the time of the Teheran embassy hostage crisis—had kidnapped his mother. Adam naturally was bent on revenge and fully intended to rob all the banks in the world and kill people until his mother was released. Much work went into turning this play theme slowly around, until it could encompass the possibilities of maternal abandonment, Adam's rage at his mother, and the notion that his badness, greed, and neediness had damaged his mother and driven her away.

When discharge to a group home became a realistic possibility, Adam ran away. However, he returned on his own a few days later. He had traveled more than 100 miles and located his mother (a feat that had eluded the investigative powers of child protective services). Having found her, he said, he had made peace with this distraught and rather limited woman. Soberly, Adam told his mother that "he knew what she had done" and no matter what happened between them, he still loved her and would go on with his life. Anna Freud herself could not have stated more eloquently the criteria for termination: the child's experience of reinstatement on the path of growth and development.

10

Residential Treatment and the Continuum of Services

Although an integrated approach to individual and family therapy is the cornerstone to achieving long-term developmental objectives for healthy adaptation and secure relationships, it is clear that most children with severe personality disorders also require other forms of treatment. These interventions are part of a therapeutic program designed to respond to urgent clinical needs, to break the cycles that reinforce distress and maladjustment in these patients and their families, or to target optimally certain aspects of the youngsters' problems. For example, social rehabilitation (e.g., managing anger, giving and receiving feedback, solving interpersonal conflicts, showing attention) is more effectively addressed by partial hospital treatment or residential treatment that offers more systematic instruction, guided peer interaction, and social consequences. Behavioral therapy approaches, such as dialectical behavior therapy, appear more effective in curbing self-destructive and parasuicidal behavior. Medications can improve specific symptoms or associated Axis I diagnoses, such as ADHD or mood disorder, as well as personality dimensions that reflect trait and state vulnerabilities. Life-threatening crises, such as acute suicidality, can be an indication for emergency hospitalization. Finally, more severe forms of personality disorder, particularly narcissistic and antisocial disorders, may require residential treatment in the hope of averting a developmental trajectory with an ominous prognosis.

The different treatments required by children with severe personality disorders match the complexity of their problems and the intricate way that biological, psychological, and family systems factors combine to generate and reinforce their psychopathology. At the same time, the complexity of these children's problems and the diversity of treatments required in various combinations militate against the possibility of testing the treatment model presented in this book with the gold standard of evaluation research, randomized controlled trials (RCTs). The superiority of RCTs to evaluate the efficacy of a treatment approach objectively is unassailable. RCTs are thus held as the best response to the demands of payers of medical services and regulators of medical care for "evidence-based medicine" (Sackett, Rosenberg, Gray, Haynes, & Richardson, 1996). Evidence-based medicine has been embraced as the ideal foundation for treatment decisions. Clinical judgment, on the other hand, is no longer accepted as adequate justification for treatment recommendations.

The driving force behind the movement to scrutinize medical care through the lens of demonstrated efficacy appears to be less a concern with quality care and more a desire of payers and purchasers of health services to reduce escalating costs. This scrutiny naturally focuses more intensely on those services (i.e., inpatient services) and groups of patients (i.e., the "outliers") that consume a disproportionate share of available financial resources. As we discuss later, children, adolescents, and young adults with severe personality disorders figure prominently among the outliers, because they require repeated and/or prolonged hospitalizations as a result of their persistent suicidality, substance abuse, life-threatening eating disorders, or destructive and reckless behavior. Faced with mounting costs for the care of this group of patients, payers naturally demand greater accountability from clinicians and clinical organizations. An emphasis on evidence-based outcomes is the understandable social response to massive increases in the cost of health care services in general and of mental health and substance abuse services in particular.

Between 1970 and 1980, admissions of children under age 18 to psychiatric inpatient units more than doubled (Thompson, Rosenstein, Milazzo-Sayre, & MacAskill, 1986). An additional 400% increase in hospital days for adolescents between 1980 and 1986 (Weithorn, 1988) led cynics to wonder whether an epidemic of adolescent madness had descended on the United States. A more likely explanation for such explosive growth probably lies elsewhere. The decade of the 1980s saw a proliferation of inpatient facilities for adolescents, including a mush-rooming of investor-owned, for-profit units whose integrity and competence often failed to match their marketing savvy and willingness to engage in questionable, sometimes illegal, schemes to fill their beds. To cite only one example, a lurid television commercial depicted grieving parents at a child's graveside while the voice-over pointed out that such a tragic outcome could have been averted if the parents had only brought their child to a particular proprietary hospital. Well-publicized findings of children held in locked facilities until their benefits were exhausted, of bribes paid to referring physicians, and of "bonuses" bestowed on "bounty hunters" who channeled adolescents into certain inpatient facilities fueled the public's outrage, the payers' skepticism, and the authorities' intent to crack down on profit-driven practices. Arguably, as England and Goff (1993) noted, unjustified and even harmful hospitalizations resulted from unfortunate marketing campaigns.

The explosion of profit-seeking entrepreneurship likely contributed to the sharp increase in mental health and substance abuse costs that stimulated the development of managed behavioral health care. But the overutilization of inpatient services seemed rooted in the patterns of reimbursement that prevailed in the 1970s and 1980s. Typically, hospitalization was covered by both public funds and private payers. However, alternatives to hospitalization, such as day treatment, crisis resolution services, and after-school or in-school programs, were generally not funded. Thus, children were hospitalized because midrange services were not available or not funded, or they remained hospitalized longer than necessary for lack of aftercare services. Perverse incentives to increase the supply of expensive services and disincentives to develop and utilize less expensive alternatives undoubtedly played an important role in driving the alarming escalation of health care costs during the 1970s and 1980s.

Indeed, throughout the 1980s, health care inflation rose twice as rapidly as the consumer price index. The cost of mental health and substance abuse treatment increased at an even more staggering rate. Between 1986 and 1990, mental health and substance abuse expenditures in the United States increased by 50% (Iglehart, 1996). By 1990, Americans were spending an astonishing $85.1 billion, or about 10% of the approximately $900 billion of total health care expenditures, to treat psychiatric and substance abuse problems (Iglehart, 1996). The pressure to contain costs inevitably pitted, on one side, a health care system, with values and incentives aligned to maximize the well-being of individual patients and to reimburse the providers of care, against, on the other side, a payer system, with values and incentives aligned to protect the resources available to care for a growing—and aging—population. Suddenly, the realization that large profits could be made by reducing health care expenditures to payers in the private and public sectors drove venture capitalists and entrepreneurs from the psychiatric hospital business into the managed care business.

As a mechanism to reduce health care costs, managed care appears to be a resounding success—although the resurgence of double-digit health care inflation from 1999 to 2000 raises questions about whether such cost reductions will be sustained. Nonetheless, the numbers tell the story of how financial resources available for psychiatric treatment have been eroded. In their study, *Health Care Plan Design and Cost Trends: 1988 through 1998* (Hay Group, 1999), analysts with the Hay consulting group reported that the total value of employer-provided health care benefits, in constant dollars, decreased by 14% between 1988 and 1998. Using a standardized benefit value equivalent to the average premium for health care per employee for medium-to-large U.S. companies, the Hay Group estimated that, in 1988, the value of the average plan was $2,526.49 per employee. Of this amount, $154.48 (6.1%) was spent for behavioral or substance abuse treatment. By 1998, the benefit value was worth $2,168.55, a decline of 14.2%. During that same period, however, the portion expended for behavioral health and substance abuse care declined to $69.87 (3.2% of the total), a reduction of 54%. These numbers, in fact, underestimate the loss of funding for treatment because they fail to consider the percentage of resources captured by the managed behavioral health care organizations as profits, as well as the money these organizations spend to cover their marketing and administrative expenses.

As a result of these reductions, most corporations saw their mental health expenditures decline drastically. Battagliola (1994) reported that the introduction of managed behavioral health care reduced IBM's mental health expenditures from $97.4 million in 1992 to $59.2 million in 1993. Most of these reductions were achieved by restricting access to inpatient services, limiting the length of hospitalization, and "flexing" the benefits to pay for alternatives to hospitalization. Between 1987 and 1994, among Xerox Corporation workers, hospital admissions per thousand employees declined from 9.7 to 6.1; hospital days per thousand employees dropped from 327 to 61; average length of stay per episode of psychiatric hospitalization fell from 33.7 to 9.9 days; and average cost per episode of psychiatric and substance abuse services was reduced from $337 to $214 (Iglehart, 1996).

Corresponding with these funding declines, lengths of hospital stay, total number of hospital days, and reimbursement per hospital day have all plummeted at Xerox, and elsewhere, as managed behavioral health care targeted inpatient services to achieve cost reductions. Managed care organizations not only succeeded in reducing the number of inpatient days but were also able to use their clout as the managers of large numbers of covered lives to negotiate deep discounts in daily rates and in the reimbursement for all types of services.

Public funding for psychiatric and substance abuse services followed in the footsteps of the private sector. The treatment of dependents of military personnel covered by the Civilian Health and Medical Program of the Uniformed Services (CHAMPUS) was placed under the control of managed behavioral health care companies. The Balanced Budget Act of 1995 had a devastating impact on hospitals dependent on Medicare reimbursement, particularly academic hospitals. Public policy changes went beyond reimbursement reductions. Concerns about Medicare's future insolvency and the perception of widespread abuse by corrupt providers led the Health Care Financing Administration (HCFA) and the Office of the Inspector General to increase vastly their efforts to identify and prosecute fraudulent practices among health care providers. The zeal and aggressiveness displayed by these agencies prompted providers to engage in expensive and time-consuming corporate compliance mechanisms in order to avoid inadvertently running afoul of Medicare's convoluted rules.

The leading "centers of excellence" in psychiatric treatment were hit hardest by the combined onslaught of loss of revenue and increased regulatory pressures. One nationally recognized treatment facility reported a change in median length of stay from 33 days in 1989 to 9 days in 1994. Occupancy rates at this institution declined from 92% in 1989 to 55% in 1994 (Sharfstein & Kent, 1997). At The Menninger Clinic, reductions in length of stay, total number of hospital days, and occupancy rates were just as significant. Menninger's extended care units, which specialize in the treatment of patients with severe personality disorders, saw a reduction in length of stay from 134 days in 1984 to 21 days in 1999. Although the number of admissions increased from 564 in 1984 to 2,238 in 1999, the net result of the reduction in length of stay was a decline in total hospital days, from 75,081 in 1984 to 45,597 in 1999. Reimbursement per day dropped as well, by as much as 40–50%.

Funding declines have had a devastating impact on the hospitals that traditionally specialized in the care of patients with severe personality disorders. Yet a silver lining may be visible for organizations that can successfully respond to the challenge of managed care. Although the pressure to reduce costs has not abated, growing public resistance to further reductions in the amount and level of care has joined forces with governmental and regulatory concerns regarding lack of parity between behavioral and medical services, and the concentration of managed care on cost containment that neglects the goal of serving patient needs, particularly the needs of the outliers. A cost-containing focus naturally zeroes in on *avoiding* rather than serving those who consume a disproportionate share of financial resources.

As a result of this convergence of forces, an evolution in managed care appears to be taking place. Enlightened managed care organizations have shifted their emphasis from limiting utilization of inpatient services to improving access to the appropriate level of service, thus promoting the development and utilization of a full continuum of services for patients with complicated problems, including those with severe personality disorders (Sharfstein & Kent, 1997).

The next step in this evolution may resolve the conflict between the economic imperative to conserve scarce financial resources, and the social and clinical expectation of high-quality care for all, including people with complex problems. The key is the change in focus from pure cost savings to the search for the lowest cost to deliver care compatible with solid evidence of clinical effectiveness.

The availability of a full continuum of services makes possible the creation of systems of care designed to capture outcomes in a naturalistic fashion (Fonagy, 1999a). Rigorous outcome measurement, careful monitoring of quality of care, and experimental strategies to monitor the introduction of novel methods of treatment and service delivery may improve the internal validity of naturalistic approaches. Rigorous outcome measurement, in conjunction with the naturally occurring variability in service delivery, will yield hypotheses concerning both effective and ineffective components of care. A standardized battery of instruments that comprehensively evaluates individual patients' strengths and weaknesses, and that may be readily aggregated to describe specific patient populations (Clifford, 1999; Graham, 1999), such as children with severe personality disorders, can create the conditions to assess which procedures, as practiced by what kind of clinician, can effectively produce specific results for specific patients with specific problems, and for a specific cost (Barrnett et al., 1991).

In this chapter, I examine the indications of these various approaches, and the components and strategies involved in integrating inpatient and residential treatment for youngsters with severe personality disorders as part of a continuum of services.

NEED FOR RESIDENTIAL TREATMENT

Many youngsters with severe personality disorders will, at some point, meet generally accepted criteria for inpatient treatment: Their behavior is dangerous to self and/or to others; their symptomatology, which includes substance abuse, suicide attempts, life-threatening and out-of-control eating problems, runaway behavior, and other provocative, destructive, and self-injurious behavior, is not contained by outpatient interventions; and their problems are so complex, multifaceted, and fluctuating that intensive diagnostic assessment in a controlled environment becomes necessary. Last, their aggression, exploitiveness, and manipulation become such a burden, and elicit such destructive responses from the environment, that an inpatient admission may be sought in order to provide teachers and caregivers with much-needed respite (Strauss, Chassin, & Lock, 1995).

The inpatient treatment of children and adolescents, however, has come under savage attack from third-party payers. As described earlier, utilization reviewers routinely challenge the need for hospitalization and insist on prompt discharge except in instances when acute and immediate danger to self and/or others can be demonstrated concretely, such as by threatened or attempted suicide within the past 24 hours.

Clinicians who seek to justify a longer inpatient stay find themselves under intense, often hostile, scrutiny. Phone and record reviews challenge those who practice in inpatient settings. To add insult to injury, discounted and all-inclusive rates have drained the financial resources available to compensate clinicians for their efforts.

Inpatient facilities for children and adolescents have been particularly vulnerable to the effects of funding decline and increased regulatory demands. Psychiatric hospitalization of children and adolescents has always been controversial. The cost of hospitalization, particularly extended hospitalization, can be staggering. On the other hand, research validating the psychiatric inpatient treatment of children and adolescents is virtually nonexistent. Such lack of empirical validation stands in stark contrast to the compelling and extensive literature largely devoted to the psychodynamic–developmentally oriented inpatient and residential treatment of children and adolescents (Bettelheim & Sylvester, 1948; Noshpitz, 1962, 1975; Rinsley, 1980a, 1980b). Programs organized around these principles have been particularly tested by the challenges of managed behavioral health care.

The literature reflecting the experience of these psychodynamic–developmental programs has provided the conceptual basis of the understanding, assessment, and treatment of children with severe personality disorders. The basic premise in this literature is that youngsters with severe personality disorders and psychotic psychopathology have complex problems arising from pathogenic influences generally embedded in a dysfunctional family system. Underlying this view of psychopathology is the basic assumption that severe psychiatric disturbances must be optimally addressed at the level of psychological causation: The representation of past experience, its interpretation, and its meaning, both conscious and nonconscious, is believed to determine children's reactions to the environment and their capacity—or incapacity—to adapt to it. This emphasis on psychological causation does not imply inattention to other levels of intervention, such as biological or family interaction. Nevertheless, the psychodynamic–developmental approach to children's inpatient residential treatment sees the severe personality disorders as the evolving, meaningful organization of children's conscious and unconscious beliefs, thoughts, feelings, and coping and defensive strategies. This evolving pathological organization is seen as not likely to be significantly ameliorated by short-term, symptom-focused programs (Rinsley, 1980b).

The psychodynamic–developmental literature on inpatient residential treatment of youngsters with severe personality disorders does not present a homogeneous treatment model. Nonetheless, it emphasizes several common points:

1. It supports the belief that every aspect of the youngster's life—neurobiological, physical, educational, psychological, recreational, social, and familial—must be carefully integrated in a total treatment milieu.

2. It defines a milieu as a context of relationships and interventions designed to reinstate children in a healthier and more adaptive developmental path, in order to promote mastery-of-life challenges and to facilitate negotiation of developmental tasks.

3. It conceptualizes the essential element in the milieu as a set of relationships with members of the therapeutic team. The team members play various complementary roles and strive to offer supportive, empathetic, interested, nonexploitive relationships. The team seeks to be effective at providing youngsters with a secure "holding environment" (Winnicott, 1953) as a means (a) to protect against distress and psychological fragmentation, (b) to offer a limit-setting context ensuring that children cannot hurt themselves or others, (c) to create an attuned setting that respects and recognizes youngsters' inner experience and individuality, and (d) to serve as a facilitating environment (Winnicott, 1965) that pushes children in the direction of greater mastery and adaptation.

4. Treatment is seen as a process with (a) an initial phase, designed both to create a therapeutic alliance and to confront youngsters' resistance to engaging in treatment, (b) a middle phase, in which conflicts are addressed and the milieu's adaptive and regulating functions are internalized, and (c) a termination phase, which deals with the anticipated separation from the treaters and tests the youngsters' readiness for discharge.

This model of residential treatment typically is extended over many months and even several years. The inevitable clash with managed behavioral care organizations, bent on reducing costs and focused on behavior management rather than on interpretation of meaning, took psychodynamic–developmentally oriented residential centers on a downward spiral of "working harder and moving faster to stand still and even move backward" (Plakun, 1999, p. 246). Many of these centers were unable to withstand the challenge of managed care. Others adapted by utterly transforming their treatment programs into behaviorally focused approaches more compatible with managed care's demands. A few residential programs, however, recognized the opportunity the managed care revolution offered to promote the development of an effective continuum of services.

As discussed earlier, managed care has the potential to evolve into a system that emphasizes outcomes and promotes optimal access to the appropriate level of care along a full continuum of services. In this continuum, inpatient services are reserved for acute crisis intervention, which is designed to provide immediate containment of destructive and self-destructive behavior, to resolve the precipitating crisis, to identify supportive resources within the family and community, and to initiate long-term aftercare. Children with severe personality disorders require acute hospitalization when there is imminent danger of suicide, running away, or assault, or when eating problems have spiraled out of control, creating a life-threatening medical emergency. These crises are typically triggered by a threat to the youngsters' and their families' precarious attachment. The inpatient crisis intervention, however, does not address the psychological or family-interaction factors that underlie the crisis but instead focuses on returning the youngsters to community-based programs or, if necessary, referring them for residential treatment.

Residential programs can retain a meaningful role in an environment demanding fiscal restraint and demonstrated effectiveness if they address several fundamental issues: (1) provide evidence, based on outcomes captured in a naturalistic fashion, that documents what kind of youngsters with severe personality disorder require residential care because outpatient interventions will not suffice; (2) articulate what components of care in residential treatment (e.g., pharmacological, psychotherapeutic, educational), in what sequence, are effective for particular youngsters with severe personality disorders; (3) demonstrate what components of the continuum of services must be in place to sustain the efforts of residential treatment and to shorten the length of stay; and (4) describe how continuity of care, planning, and relationships is achieved between the residential and other parts of the continuum of services.

In the next section, I describe a model of focused residential treatment designed to be integrated into a continuum of services for youngsters with severe personality disorders.

A RESIDENTIAL TREATMENT MODEL
FOR CHILDREN AND ADOLESCENTS WITH
SEVERE PERSONALITY DISORDERS

Indications for Residential Treatment

Psychodynamic–developmentally oriented models of residential treatment have been challenged not only by the pressures of declining reimbursement but also by competing scientific and clinical models. Neurobiological paradigms embodied in more effective pharmacological interventions and more sophisticated neurobiological understanding of psychopathology present one challenge. Another comes from developmental and psychosocial formulations that include empirically supported methods of psychosocial treatment and a clearer understanding of the risk and protective factors underlying the developmental paths of adjustment and maladjustment.

These challenges, however, have introduced a creative tension that has fostered the evolution of new paradigms of briefer residential treatment. One such paradigm integrates residential care within a full continuum of services rather than conceiving of it as the site of the total treatment. This paradigm also integrates a psychodynamic tradition with neurobiological, developmental, and family systems models and approaches (Leichtman & Leichtman, 1996a, 1996b, 1996c).

Yet these new models of residential treatment also require the validation of evidence-based criteria documenting which youngsters with severe personality disorders require this level of care, because less restrictive approaches will be insufficient or counterproductive. Such validation is critical, because even the shorter, more focused version presented here carries a substantial cost per episode of care. Equally significant is the emotional cost to youngsters and families whose precarious equilibrium, tenuous personal connections, and rigid coping strategies are strained by the imposed separation and the implicit challenge that treatment introduces into the family "ecosystem" (Liddle & Hogue, 2000). The following case vignette illustrates this dilemma.

Eddie, a 13-year-old boy with borderline personality disorder, had been hospitalized four times when his mother, Mrs. D, brought him to the Menninger residential unit. Mrs. D had cared for Eddie by herself since his father had walked out on the family when the boy was just an infant.

Convinced that Eddie would find the treatment he needed only at a well-known residential program in another state, Mrs. D disparaged the "inferior" treatment to which she and her son had been subjected at various hospitals. She recalled how, when she had voiced her dissatisfaction with the shortcomings of Eddie's treatment, she had been told that she was "resisting" his engagement in treatment. She responded to such "interpretations" with demands for discharge and a renewed search for the "right" treatment for Eddie.

At Menninger, Mrs. D lavishly praised the competence and sensitivity of the staff, which, she conceded, might be almost as good as that of the program she had targeted for Eddie. The clinician who interviewed her commented that, as competent as the staff was, the "right" program was the one she believed was right for herself and her son. Thus, it would be important to evaluate periodically her comfort with the treatment that her son was receiving and to be prepared to consider a transfer if she felt that their needs would be better served elsewhere.

Sure enough, a month after Eddie's placement in the unit, when Mrs. D grew impatient with the treatment, she was reminded of the initial discussion and was again told that the most effective treatment for her son would take place at the facility that, in her view, was best suited for him. Perhaps enough had been achieved by giving her a respite and an opportunity to regain her strength. Now, it was time to seek help in the place she had long favored, while neither she nor her son felt frantic or in a state of crisis.

With the assistance of the doctor in the program, Eddie's transfer to the "ideal" residential facility was arranged. Three days before the scheduled date of transfer, however, Mrs. D walked into the principal's office of the school where she taught and threatened to kill him. She claimed to have discovered his plan to murder her and wished to beat him to the punch. Eddie's transfer came to naught as security guards dragged Mrs. D away to a psychiatric hospital.

The attachment between Eddie and his mother seemed to require a deep mistrust of anyone else's ability to soothe, comfort, or help. This conviction was strengthened by Mrs. D's assumption that the "good" attachment (a hallowed, saving paradise) remained eternally unreachable. Her belief in a murder plot against her, following the sudden availability of her long-sought ideal, betrayed her conviction that breaking the rigid, nonreflective pattern of attachment and experience would lead only to her own destruction—and perhaps that of her son.

The inhibition of reflective function at times of stress and vulnerability gives rise to coercive patterns of interaction, coping, and experience. Nonreflectiveness imposes extreme rigidity; enormous vulnerability to change from prescribed patterns of experiencing, coping, and relating; and a proneness to mobilize powerful forces to prevent change or violation of the implicit rules of interaction. Thus, separations in these families are experienced as a catastrophe.

Residential treatment is not only financially expensive and emotionally painful, but also costly in terms of missed normative social–developmental opportunities when the child is placed in a residential program for up to several months. There is also the potential to foster dependence, regression, and institutionalization, and the risk of stigmatizing children as seriously disturbed mental patients. Acknowledging these costs requires a careful cost–benefit analysis before a therapist recommends such an intervention.

In the absence of empirically based criteria, the clinical literature offers only general guidelines for determining which youngsters with severe personality disorders should be referred for residential treatment. Rinsley (1980a, 1980b), for example, offered the following criteria: (1) cases in which the youngster's behavior is so disruptive as to preclude outpatient treatment; (2) cases in which the home situation is so chronically difficult or disturbed that residential placement is necessary to relieve family tensions; (3) cases in which the children's behavior endangers them or others on a chronic basis, or is unacceptable in a nonclinical setting because of its bizarreness or failure to respond to the usual social controls; and (4) cases in which children exhibit progressive psychosocial deterioration to the extent that failure to admit will likely result in damage to their interpersonal relationships and make future rehabilitation efforts more difficult or impossible. Leichtman and Leichtman (1996a, 1996b, 1996c) claim, more simply, that residential treatment is indicated for youngsters with severe personality disorders who have not responded to adequate trials of outpatient treatment.

Ultimately, the clinical decision to recommend residential treatment is based on assessment of the balance between risk and protective factors. Strengths and psychosocial supports must be weighed against the weaknesses and psychosocial demands of both the children and their families.

As discussed in Chapter 7, the crucial factors in deciding between outpatient and residential settings are (1) the capacity of the youngster's caregivers, with therapeutic support, to provide a safe and consistent environment that can sustain treatment and contain the youngster's destructive and self-destructive behavior, and to stop caregivers' own destructive behavior, including maltreatment; (2) the availability of necessary resources and services—including financial resources—to support the caregivers in carrying out the treatment process and in providing a safe environment for themselves and the youngster; and (3) the extent to which these youngsters require, on an ongoing basis, more support, structure, and containment than even normally competent caregivers can provide in order to prevent behavior dangerous to self and/or others.

The following clinical constellations are common indications for residential treatment:

1. Borderline youngsters with an intricate combination of neuropsychiatric vulnerabilities, such as attention-deficit/hyperactivity disorder, mood and learning disorders, and a traumatic history and/or current maltreatment, who exhibit a predominance of dissociative, self-destructive responses to stress.
2. Borderline children with significant addictive problems and/or out-of-control eating disorders.
3. Borderline–narcissistic youngsters who become disorganized, impulsive, and destructive when their grandiosity or efforts to exert control over their relationships are challenged.
4. Narcissistic–antisocial youngsters whose depravation, mistrust, callousness, and lack of concern or remorse are so serious that they raise questions about treatability.

These children evoke destructive and alienating responses from others that reinforce the youngsters' reliance on antisocial peers and illegal drugs. For many of them, clinical experience suggests that only 2 to 6 months of residential treatment can break the vicious cycle by which their psychopathology evokes destructive responses from their environment, which, in turn, reinforces their maladjustment.

Characteristics and Components of the Residential Milieu

The concept of the "milieu" as a total therapeutic environment is the foundation of residential treatment. The milieu of the residential program was classically described by Bettelheim and Sylvester (1948), Noshpitz (1962, 1975), and Rinsley (1980a, 1980b), among others.

These authors defined the milieu as an integration of every facet of the children's lives in a comprehensive and coherent treatment program. In their ideal form, psychotherapy, family treatment, pharmacological interventions, educational and recreational programs, and specialized group and individual interventions (see following discussion) are woven together in a structure of care, validation, holding, support, and containment that encompasses the psychological, cognitive, social, and physical aspects of children's development and functioning.

This integration results from the joint effort of a team of professionals with distinct roles and areas of expertise. The team generally includes a child and adolescent psychiatrist, psychotherapist(s), a social worker, special education teachers, nurses, and child care workers. A team leader is responsible for articulating a diagnostic formulation, conceptualizing a treatment plan, and overseeing its implementation. The diagnostic formulation includes the following:

1. Cognitive–intellectual assessment (including psychoeducational assessment of developmental learning disorders).
2. Speech and hearing evaluation.
3. Physical and neurological examination (including diagnostic studies, EEG, and other studies as indicated).
4. Family history (including history of genetic loading for psychiatric disorders and response to medications).
5. Educational assessment and school history.
6. Substance abuse history and assessment (including evaluation of family and individual risk factors for substance abuse, and assessment of peer and family factors promoting or exacerbating substance abuse).
7. Psychosocial assessment (including assessment of risk and protective factors, and sources of support and stress).
8. Developmental assessment (including assessment of developmental achievements and failure to negotiate developmental tasks).
9. Family assessment (including evaluation of attachment patterns and family coping strategies, and assessment of interactive patterns that trigger coercive cycles).
10. Assessment of the child's relationship patterns and coping mechanisms (including specific experiences that precipitate inhibition of reflective function).

This formulation serves as the basis for the design of a specific milieu structure and treatment plan, which includes the following elements: (1) milieu treatment; (2) psychotherapy; (3) pharmacotherapy; (4) group treatment; (5) school and vocational programs; (6) recreational and life skills programs; (7) religious and spiritual activities; (8) substance abuse programs; and (9) eating disorders programs.

Milieu Treatment

The milieu consists of a way of structuring daily life defined by explicit rules and expectations that give predictability and consistency to interactions with peers and staff. The degree of supervision or autonomy that each youngster enjoys is based on the demonstrated capacity for adaptive functioning, particularly the ability to control behavior that is dangerous to self and/or others.

Psychotherapy

Youngsters in residential treatment become involved in integrated individual/family therapy treatment (outlined in Chapters 7, 8, and 9). The milieu's capacity to contain, regulate, and validate (see following discussion) creates a secure base for attachment and a "representational mismatch" (described in Chapter 7), which provides the necessary challenge to the youngsters' maladaptive inhibition of reflective function that is required to begin psychotherapy. Containment, regulation, and validation are also conditions that foster attachment and an inclination to conceive of treaters and other adults as a potential source of help and comfort—essential conditions for development of a working alliance.

Residential treatment requires particular attention to the caregivers' authority and executive position in the family. Focused residential treatment, in contrast to the open-ended variety, does not aim to take over parental functions but instead works to support the caregivers' competence and ability to set limits and offer support and validation to their children. A change in attitude and orientation toward families from the traditional psychoanalytic–developmental model of residential treatment is required to implement a focused approach of residential care.

The critical changes include (1) an appreciation of the children's problems within the context of their attachment, however disorganized, to their families; (2) a view of the parents as partners rather than as adversaries, or merely as a cause of, or contributor to, the children's dysfunction; (3) an emphasis on strength rather than an exclusive focus on psychopathology, which leads to the recognition and mobilization of the family's resources; (4) a focus on children and their families in the context of their culture, recognizing cultural differences related to areas such as discipline, rules, and expression of affect; and (5) a readiness to introduce and take advantage of resources and support systems in the neighborhood and community, such as churches, schools, job training programs, and self-help groups (Cafferty & Leichtman, 1999).

Thus, a focused residential treatment process with intensive family work pays particular attention to educating caregivers, whether through counseling, classes, support groups, or literature (Jenson & Whittaker, 1989), and to helping families, first, to clarify and articulate the necessary conditions that will allow children to return home and, second, to develop the skills and supports necessary to meet such conditions (Cafferty & Leichtman, 1999). Structured approaches to enhance the caregivers' parenting competence (described in Chapter 9), such as parent–child interaction therapy (Eyberg et al., 1995) or the Oregon social learning model (Patterson & Forgatch, 1995), are incorporated into the family treatment to further the caregivers' capacity to provide care, nurturance, protection, and containment of their youngsters.

When the primary goal of treatment is to help adolescents return to their families and community as rapidly as possible, treatment priorities change. Home visits and passes, for example, are not treated as rewards for good behavior but as essential opportunities to enhance the youngsters' and their caregivers' capacity to develop the necessary skills to interact with one another in a supportive and reflective fashion.

Pharmacotherapy

Children with severe personality disorders often require medication to target emerging symptoms or traits that impair their adjustment, particularly those that affect the exercise of reflective function. As I describe in Chapter 11, pharmacotherapy seeks to address the dysregulations of arousal, cognition, affect, and impulse that maintain, reinforce, and exacerbate these youngsters' maladjustment, promote the inhibition of reflective function, and evoke destructive responses from their environment.

Group Treatment

Group interventions encourage youngsters to discuss with peers and staff their problems and how they cope with them. Community meetings provide a forum to review the forms and range of interaction of the residential group members in relation to affect, support or disqualification of autonomy, interpersonal boundaries, communication, competition, collaboration, expression and resolution (or avoidance) of conflict, decision making, goal setting, distribution of power and authority, and any other significant aspect of social functioning that finds expression in the day-to-day life of the residential community. The group format also offers an opportunity for each youngster to define goals for treatment and the steps needed to return home. Peers and staff question what *prevents* youngsters from accomplishing the goals of treatment.

School and Vocational Programs

These programs seek to identify the specific cognitive, psychological, and interpersonal factors that interfere with the youngsters' capacity to learn and acquire the tools that will equip them to pursue a career. The purpose of the programs is to put the youngsters on track to utilize school or vocational training in the community. The programs are informed by a detailed understanding of the children's developmental learning disorders and attentional problems on the one hand, and of their deficits in learning skills and fund of knowledge on the other. This understanding is the basis for a remediation plan that can assist community schools in facilitating the youngsters' education after their discharge from the residential program. Helping them benefit from school and vocational training involves contending with their fear of failure and humiliation, their terror at exposing their vulnerability, and, in the case of predominantly antisocial–narcissistic youngsters, their difficulty acknowledging their ignorance or need for help.

Recreational and Life Skills Programs

An important component of residential treatment is a program designed to help youngsters with severe personality disorders develop adaptive recreational and life skills that can further their success in school and work. Recreational activities (e.g., participating in sports or crafts, attending theater or movies) help relieve these youngsters' isolation and sense of emptiness, and give them opportunities to share in more adaptive aspects of their peer culture. Adaptive functioning is also enhanced by specific life skills education in areas such as budgeting and money management, computer skills, cooking, and housekeeping, as well as education in issues such as anger management and conflict resolution. Recognizing and promoting youngsters' special interests and talents—musical, artistic, or athletic—can serve to arouse the strands of their own individuality, strands that these youngsters can use to weave a sense of self grounded in their own attributes.

Religious and Spiritual Activities

Youngsters with severe personality disorders are offered the opportunity to seek spiritual guidance and affiliation with their own faith and religious community. Such affiliation nurtures a sense of belonging, identity, meaning, and purpose that counters the pressures of their antisocial affiliations.

Substance Abuse Programs

Abuse of illegal drugs and alcohol is a major factor in maintaining, reinforcing, and exacerbating the maladjustment of many youngsters with severe personality disorders. A careful substance abuse assessment that involves taking a family history of addiction, a history of addictive behaviors—including addictive-like behaviors such as compulsive stealing, eating disorders, and sexual promiscuity—and a history of the youngsters' affiliation with substance-abusing peers is the basis for planning substance abuse interventions. Youngsters who do not exhibit significant substance abuse problems require only substance abuse education and the general components of residential treatment designed to help them cope more effectively with peer pressure to engage in substance misuse. For youngsters with substantial addictive problems, or for those at great risk for abusing drugs, a more targeted and comprehensive approach becomes necessary.

The substance abuse track of residential treatment aims to (1) break dependence on drugs as a primary coping strategy, mode of affiliation with peers, and source of comfort and identity; (2) prepare youngsters and their caregivers to utilize community-based substance abuse programs; and (3) develop a relapse prevention plan. These steps are implemented through chemical dependency counseling, which focuses on attitudes and behaviors disposing to drug abuse, on family and peer interactions that maintain and reinforce substance abuse, and on strategies for dealing with abuse-promoting attitudes and interactions. The relapse prevention plan involves self-study and assignments, including selected readings and the completion of a workbook that guides the youngsters in articulating a narrative of their history of substance abuse and its impact on themselves and their families. The plan also involves family and multifamily education designed to enable caregivers to interrupt family patterns of substance abuse more effectively. Finally, the plan includes orientation and links to community-based self-help substance abuse programs, such as 12-step programs. These programs are offered to youngsters and their families initially within the residential unit and then within the community.

Eating Disorders Programs

Eating problems are a significant element compounding the impairment in functioning of youngsters with severe personality disorders. The first step in the treatment of anorexia nervosa and bulimia nervosa is the correction of malnutrition. Correcting malnutrition is mandatory because starvation and the metabolic abnormalities associated with it can be life threatening. Malnutrition also seems to create a fight-or-flight state of impaired reflective functioning and a limited capacity for symbolic processing (Fahy & Russell, 1993). Treatment in a specialized eating disorders program capable of metabolic and cardiac monitoring and sophisticated refeeding is needed in life-threatening conditions.

For youngsters with eating disorders embedded in a severe personality disorder, residential treatment is often indicated as a step down from the inpatient crisis intervention (Fahy, Eisler, & Russell, 1993). Residential treatment with an eating disorder track allows youngsters to address the full extent of their personality and family problems, while focusing on a major aspect of their maladjustment.

The therapeutic focus on reflective function—as the mediating mechanism that allows the attainment of genuine autonomy, self-regulation, and healthy connections with others—addresses the central concerns of patients with eating disorders. Freeing their capacity for reflective function is reinforced by the specific elements of the eating disorder track that I will discuss. The residential staff manages the children's weight gain until their health is not in jeopardy. Serving meals family style, with a therapist present, is designed to help the caregivers of younger patients gain control of the children's eating using noncoercive means. The basic framework is that the caregivers' task is to return their children to physical health with a minimum of tension and upset. With older adolescents, the caregivers are asked to decide either to seek to gain control over their children's eating by noncoercive means, until the children have regained physical health, or to communicate consistently the attitude that the children's eating is not their concern; instead, the caregivers' goal is the children's overall health and their capacity to make their own choices (Russell, Treasure, & Eisler, 1998).

Specific components of the eating disorders program aim at interrupting the pattern of disturbed eating behavior and the coercive responses such behavior evokes from caregivers. The components of the eating disorders program include (1) psychoeducational techniques; (2) self-monitoring; (3) nutrition and exercise counseling; (4) cues and responses; (5) restructuring thoughts about body image; and (6) relapse prevention.

- *Psychoeducational techniques*. These techniques provide information about anorexia nervosa and bulimia nervosa, and the physical and psychosocial consequences of these disorders.
- *Self-monitoring*. Patients are taught to monitor their eating behavior, and the physical and emotional states associated with eating. This is an important step toward gaining self-control and discovering the connection between internal states and overt behavior (Agras, Schneider, Arnow, Raeburn, & Telch, 1989). A food diary can be a useful adjunct in this task.
- *Nutrition and exercise counseling*. Youngsters are instructed about the goal of developing healthy patterns of eating and exercise. Planning meals and exercise in advance avoids reactive bingeing, food restriction, or the compulsive overexercising triggered by internal or interpersonal cues that signal vulnerability.
- *Cues and responses*. Youngsters with severe personality disorders and, in particular, those who present with an eating disorder, need help to recognize the internal cues that trigger thoughts and behavior. The inhibition of reflective function generates inchoate internal states experienced as physical distress that can be relieved only by bingeing, vomit-

ing, or exercising. Bringing attention to the cues—social, situational, mental, and physiological—involved in the youngsters' eating behavior is a prelude to examining the consequences that result from it. As suggested earlier, the purpose of these discussions is to emphasize both the "helpful" aspects of the symptoms—relief of pain, stress, loneliness, and emptiness, and provision of a sense of control and power—and the longer-term maladaptive effects. Acknowledging how the eating disorders provide understandable benefits frees these youngsters to examine the price they pay for relying on such maladaptive behavior. When patients choose to give up their eating symptoms, they can be assisted to delay bingeing responses to internal or interpersonal cues and to develop alternative responses to such cues.

• *Restructuring thoughts about body image.* Cognitive-behavioral techniques are helpful in understanding and challenging the youngsters' nonreflective thoughts about weight and body image (Mitchell, Raymond, & Specker, 1993).

• *Relapse prevention.* A central goal of residential treatment is to help youngsters and their caregivers use community resources after discharge from the residential program and to develop plans to prevent relapse. Exposure to high-risk foods and situations while still in residential treatment offers the youngsters a chance to test the sturdiness of their newly acquired coping approach to trauma and parasuicidal behavior.

Maltreatment, particularly physical and/or sexual abuse, is an important antecedent of the severe personality disorders. The individual and family treatment described in Chapters 7, 8, and 9 is designed primarily to help youngsters overcome the pathological solutions they have developed for dealing with vulnerability and trauma. These interventions can be augmented in a residential setting with psychoeducational trauma groups that provide instruction on the effects of trauma and give youngsters opportunities to share traumatic experiences and how they have coped with them. Educational trauma groups help youngsters to create a narrative of their fragmented experience and to overcome feelings of isolation.

Several approaches can be helpful for one of the most notoriously resistant symptoms in youngsters with a history of physical and sexual abuse: persistent parasuicidal and self-mutilating behavior. Eye movement desensitization and reprocessing, or EMDR (Shapiro, 1995; Shapiro & Forrest, 1997), which seems to blend elements of cognitive-behavioral therapy with hypnotic suggestion, appears effective according to clinical accounts. But the questionable explanations about the neurophysiological basis of its effectiveness, coupled with an absence of empirical evidence of EMDR's effectiveness, make its use with youngsters with severe personality disorders somewhat controversial. Less controversial is the use of dialectical behavioral therapy (Linehan, 1993; Linehan, Armstrong, Suarez, Allmon, & Heard, 1991), which relies on a structured cognitive-behavioral approach. Originally designed to interrupt parasuicidal and self-destructive behavior but now expanded to address substance abuse, high-risk sexual practices, emotional lability, and other manifestations of borderline personality disorder, dialectical behavioral therapy emphasizes skills acquisition through the use of individual sessions, and by coaching *in vivo*, and by phone and skills training groups. The skills targeted by dialectical behavioral therapy—"mindfulness," distress tolerance, acceptance, emotional regulation, and interpersonal effectiveness—are very much in line with the focus on reflective function proposed in this book.

But perhaps more than the availability of a comprehensive array of treatment components, what best defines a residential model for youngsters is the conceptual and practical integration of every facet of treatment. A focus is provided by the conceptual framework that defines the severe personality disorders in terms of selective inhibition of reflective function in response to internal and interpersonal cues. The team shares a coherent formulation of the treatment plan and its goals. This integration of views is a powerful rejoinder to the youngsters'—and their families'—fragmented experience. The coherent treatment formulation helps the youngsters and their caregivers build their own coherent narrative of their experience.

Coherence, however, will be routinely tested by the currents of feeling and the fight-or-flight responses that these youngsters and their caregivers evoke in others, including the treaters. Countertransference reactions are powerfully amplified in a residential program as each staff member's responses resonate with everyone else's reactions. Thus, the range of typical responses experienced by clinicians in the individual and family treatment of youngsters with severe personality disorders, described in Chapter 8, can easily reach the boiling point in the hothouse environment of the residential unit.

Youngsters with severe personality disorders, with their uncanny ability to detect the specific vulnerabilities of each staff member, "select" individuals to play particular roles in their coercive, unreflective dramas. Some staff members find themselves enraged and exasperated, wishing that the patients would run away, disappear, or succeed in killing themselves. At times, these countertransference reactions become so compelling that certain staff members in fact conspire, in subtle or not-so-subtle ways, to foster the patients' self-destructiveness. In turn, these feelings evoke staff members' guilt and contrition and, at times, the need to make amends to the patients by showing them exaggerated devotion and concern.

Sometimes the patients' rejection and mistreatment by some staff members elicits other staff members' rescue fantasies. Open battles among the staff members, threatening to bring the treatment to a standstill, attest to the power of coercive patterns of relatedness to trigger unreflectiveness in an entire group. Not infrequently, factions develop within the staff, with some members experiencing great sympathy, concern, and compassion for the plight of a maltreated and misunderstood patient. This faction generally experiences other staff members as unempathetic or unable to connect with the troubled, frightened child. The second group, however, believes that the patient is a cunning manipulator who has seduced staff members into indulging his or her personal whims and colluding with efforts to sabotage treatment.

Treatment failures—and outright therapeutic catastrophes—result from staff entanglements in coercive, unreflective patterns of experience and relationship. Staff members can be seduced by some youngsters into blurring professional boundaries. At times, self-disclosure and special treatment deteriorate into sexual relationships. Some staff members rationalize their transgression on the basis of the special needs of children whose experience of trauma and extraordinary suffering requires exceptional measures to rekindle hope and even prevent suicide.

Bright, aggressive youngsters can intimidate staff with their short fuses, explosive rage, and ruthless ability to zero in on others' vulnerable spots. Staff helplessness in the face of such intimidation leads to a failure to confront patient misbehavior and, at times, encourages these youngsters' sense of entitlement and antisocial behavior.

As pointed out in Chapter 8, such countertransference reactions can also offer a unique window into the patient's inner world, in particular, into specific patterns of fractionation of reflective and nonreflective modes of functioning. Gaining perspective on this information requires all team members to systematically examine their own emotional reactions to the patients, the caregivers, and the rest of the team. Ongoing communication and the routine discussion of internal experience and interpersonal problems among staff members and between patients and staff—as opposed to discussions driven by a breakdown of the treatment—offer the only protection against the potentially destructive impact of staff countertransference. The maturity and cohesiveness of the team, and the strength and clarity of the team leader, are tested time and time again by the forces of coerciveness and unreflectiveness, threatening the team with paralysis or fragmentation, dissent or aimlessness, or the perilous enactment of interpersonal scenarios generated by the patients' desperate efforts to cope and survive.

The Course of Residential Treatment

An essential feature of a focused residential program is the capacity of the team to provide a conceptually coherent formulation of the treatment goals and an emotionally consistent and integrated response to patients and their caregivers that can withstand the pulls of coercion and unreflectiveness. Such coherence and consistency are first and foremost designed to create the conditions in which secure attachments can flourish. The basic premise of this approach, of course, is that only in the context of secure attachments can youngsters and families in treatment disinhibit reflective function when buffeted by the pressures of stress and vulnerability. Disinhibition enables them to disengage from coercive patterns of interaction.

Several features of the residential milieu serve to provide a "secure base" (Bowlby, 1969) for attachment and reflective function, and can be grouped into a holding and containing environment, an attuned environment, an involved and interactive environment, or a facilitating environment.

• *A holding environment* (Winnicott, 1965). This feature of the milieu refers to the capacity of the residential program to offer consistency, structure, predictability, and responsiveness to stress, loss of control, and psychological or physiological dysregulation. At its most basic level, "holding" refers to the capacity of the milieu to provide reliable and effective care, nurturance, support, and limits. Holding involves protecting children from their own rage, impulsivity, and self-destructiveness, as well as from disorganizing or overwhelming environmental stimulation. An important aspect of the holding is the structure of the milieu, which is the organization of daily activities and the regularity of relationships with staff members. Such regularity includes predictable arrivals and departures, and an expected range of responses to the patients, including predictable—noncoercive—consequences for maladaptive or destructive behavior.

• *An attuned environment.* This aspect of the milieu entails staff members' capacity to respond to each youngster as a unique, intentional being. Attunement involves the staff's ability to recognize, respect, and respond to the entire range of children's internal states, without failing to confront and contain their maladaptive defensive measures.

• *An involved, interactive environment* (Gunderson, 2000). Involvement refers to staff activities designed to foster the youngsters' active attention and interaction with their social environment. Opportunities to give and receive feedback from staff members and peers, and to participate in group activities, are aspects of involvement built into the interactive milieu.

• *A facilitating environment* (Winnicott, 1965). This aspect of the milieu refers to the staff's capacity to recognize children's potential for development and to encourage and support them in achieving greater mastery and competence. The staff responds to the children on the basis of not only their current level of functioning but also the level of developmental attainment they are ready to achieve. As Friedman (1982) pointed out, staff members treat patients not only as the persons they are but also as the persons they are about to become.

In the traditional psychodynamic–developmental long-term residential model, treatment was conceptualized as a series of stages. Masterson (1972) and Rinsley (1980a, 1980b), for example, defined three distinct stages in the residential treatment of youngsters with severe personality disorders: (1) a resistance (testing) stage, (2) an introjective (working-through) stage, and (3) a resolution (separation) stage. The basic premise underlying this conceptualization is that after these youngsters' resistance to engagement in treatment is overcome, the residential milieu allows them to internalize the holding, attuning, interactive, and facilitating features of the environment, and enables them to achieve greater autonomy and self-regulation.

In the model of short-term, focused residential treatment I present here, on the other hand, the goal of treatment is to create the conditions that will permit youngsters to become engaged in treatment after discharge from the residential program. Such conditions involve (1) developing a working alliance with the youngsters; (2) promoting the caregivers' ability to provide an environment supportive of secure attachments that can lead to an interruption of coercive cycles of interaction; and (3) identifying the therapeutic elements and relationships that will provide the continuity of treatment necessary to enhance reflective function, foster self-regulation, and increase awareness of others' mental states.

Not long after they enter a residential program, children with severe personality disorders busily endeavor to shape the milieu to fit the fragmentation of their internal world. Such attempts may be subtle or blatant. Jay's (Chapter 6) first 3 weeks in the residential program were a therapeutic honeymoon. He behaved like a perfect gentleman, a model of civility and propriety. Elliot (Chapter 6), an extremely bright and verbal boy, could espouse with great poise and clarity the issues underlying his narcissistic problems. Pseudocompliance and pseudoinsight are frequent maneuvers employed by narcissistic children in their effort to secure a sense of control. Seductive efforts to sexualize the relationship with staff, become good "buddies" with the treaters, or turn into the staff's designated assistants render the staff ineffective and reinforce the youngsters' illusory omnipotence.

In contrast, borderline and antisocial–narcissistic youngsters may be more openly defiant, assaultive, threatening, contemptuous, or bent on avoiding or defeating treatment by running away or instigating chaos in the residential program. Mike, for example, an 8-year-old who had already accumulated a rather impressive record of assaultive incidents, greeted his doctor with the announcement that he would be the one to decide on the details of his daily routine. He warned that any effort to impinge on his privileges would have the direst consequences. With his exceptional sensitivity to everyone's vulnerable spots, Mike also ruthlessly poured salt on other people's wounds. Like a puppeteer pulling the strings, he sat back and grinned smugly while other children became anxious or aggressive, as his perfectly targeted zingers never failed to wreak havoc in the group.

Borderline children will typically seek to turn staff members into transitional objects, invested with regulating functions that in the children's fantasy are completely under their control. Pam, an opinionated and spirited 10-year-old girl, rapidly developed an intense attachment with one female child care worker, Mrs. H. When Ms. H had the audacity to go on vacation, in spite of Pam's desperate pleas that she remain with her, the child exploded with rage. At night she was awakened by terrifying dreams of monsters coming to torment and murder her. Most distressing was that no amount of reassurance seemed to convince her that the monsters were only a nightmare rather than a real threat.

Pam's solution to the breakdown of her illusory control over Mrs. H, and the associated threat of a breakdown in her grip on reality, was to falsify reality further. Smiling impishly the next morning, she proclaimed that she did not have to miss Mrs. H anymore. All she had to do was turn on the television and Mrs. H would appear and comfort her. She then proceeded excitedly to turn on the television, claiming against all evidence that Mrs. H was at her beck and call.

Mary offers another instance of a borderline child's reliance on people as regulating objects. This 12-year-old girl's history was replete with abandonment, neglect, and aborted adoptions. Shortly after her admission to the residential program, Mary declared her joy at having found in Mrs. C, a child care worker, the perfect person to love and to be loved by. In lengthy letters to Mrs. C, Mary extolled the virtues of their unique relationship. In reality, however, Mary seemed to go out of her way to avoid having much contact with Mrs. C, as if she feared that a real interaction would disrupt the ideal relatedness she had constructed.

As swiftly and arbitrarily as Mary's and Mrs. C's ideal love came to life, it also fell apart. Without apparent provocation, Mary attacked Mrs. C. For days following this incident, Mary cried bitter tears of anguish, mourning the loss of her perfect love. She resumed her epistolary communication with Mrs. C, this time begging for forgiveness and an opportunity to rebuild their shattered relationship, without which she could not imagine living. Again, Mary rebuffed Mrs. C's attempts to examine with her what had happened between them. The girl's elaborate choreography seemed designed to ensure the enactment of an unreflective script in which she alternatively created, then destroyed, and finally resurrected an ideal relationship. She was thus fully in control, but only as long as she could prevent reality, in the form of genuine exchanges with other people's internal states, from disturbing her illusionary scenarios.

These examples illustrate the challenge of striking a balance between holding, containment, and limit setting on the one hand, and validation and promotion of self-expression on the other. Mike, for example, received the consistent message that everyone on staff recognized that he had far more confidence in his ability to trick or set up other people than in his capacity to trust or get help from anyone. Such recognition, however, did not preclude clear limits and consequences for provocative and manipulative behavior. In a similar fashion, staff members were careful *not* to respond to Mary's letters, while Mrs. C insisted on face-to-face meetings.

Violent, assaultive youngsters present a special challenge. Optimally containing their assaultiveness requires that they be restrained before they can attack anyone. Staff members in residential programs capable of treating impulsively violent youngsters must be skilled at identifying the cues that signal a violent assault—at times, cues as subtle as the trembling of an upper lip or the flaring of the nostrils—and they must be able to intervene effectively to prevent the violent outburst. Such containment must be provided as a response to these youngsters' need for safety and reassurance in the face of their own impulsivity rather than as a countertransferential reaction to the youngsters' unreflective behavior. Staff members are vulnerable to feeling compelled to retaliate sadistically to the violence of these youngsters, a response that reinforces the power the youngsters experience when they can evoke unreflective reactions from others. Unreflective responses on the part of staff members can also reinforce the sexualization of the physical restraining of defiant and provocative youngsters. Thus, violent youngsters and staff members can become trapped in sadomasochistic patterns of interaction that reek of unreflective hostility and disguised sexual excitement.

A reflective response of containment and attunement requires staff members who can dispassionately restrain youngsters physically in an emergency. (Optimally, restraint is applied with medications, as described in Chapter 11.) Restraining conveys the following messages: (1) The milieu is designed to ensure the physical well-being and safety of the youngsters and all others, including staff members; (2) the milieu is capable of preventing the youngsters from harming themselves or others; and (3) restraining occurs without sadism or satisfaction, in a matter-of-fact, almost mechanical fashion, communicating that human connection occurs under the aegis of attachment and reflective function, and not as a disguised by-product of coercive interaction.

Recognizing, respecting, and responding to the mental states of youngsters with severe personality disorders can be challenging for the staff of the residential program. While giving Mike a time-out when other children acted up after his provocation, child care staff members also commented, in group sessions and in informal contacts, how hard it seemed for him to stop pushing people's buttons and just relax and be himself.

After 6 weeks of confrontation, Mike's affect and demeanor seemed to change. He appeared sad and worried, and gave hints of how exquisitely sensitive he was to humiliation and burdened by the threat of being found inadequate. Reluctantly, he acknowledged that his bravado and provocativeness in school were meant to cover the void in his fund of knowledge and learning skills. He believed he possessed the potential of a genius (although his IQ tests placed him only in the above-average range), yet he experienced a painful discrepancy between his real achievements and the brilliance he felt compelled to achieve. Nothing short of utter embarrassment and permanent banishment to prison or a mental hospital would be the consequence of failure to live up to his genius potential. When he was able to admit these feelings, he began individual psychotherapy.

As these examples illustrate, a crucial task of the milieu is to convey to youngsters in residential treatment the message that signals of distress—however disguised by the inhibition of reflective function and the activation of coercive, unreflective modes of functioning—will not drive the caregivers away, turn them into unreflective monsters, or hinder their ability to provide a holding, attuning, and facilitating environment. The end of residential treatment is signaled by indications that the patients have developed some degree of conviction that they can derive help from collaborating with the treaters and are able to share some aspects of their experience. Discharge from the residential program is indicated when individual and family treatment is established and a plan is in place to address continuity of educational, pharmacological, and other treatment components, including substance abuse and eating disorders treatment, if needed. The plan must also include caregiver support and contingencies in case of crisis.

To achieve these goals, staff members, from the outset, must focus on preparing youngsters and caregivers to deal with the challenges of being together. In contrast to the traditional residential treatment model, frequent passes and home visits are necessary to build opportunities to practice new ways of coping and relating. Therefore, home visits are not "granted" as a reward for good behavior in the unit but instead are prescribed as part of the treatment program. Reversing the traditional sequence, unit status is earned by successfully completing tasks assigned on family visits; visits are not earned for achieving a high status in the unit.

Home visits and family sessions also serve to develop relapse prevention and crisis plans, based on "mapping" the pitfalls and land mines that youngsters and their families are likely to encounter. As soon as youngsters show evidence of a working alliance, the residential staff begins to work on a relapse prevention plan. Youngsters work on identifying the problems that led to their admission, and for several weeks they are helped to produce a detailed description of each problem. The description includes (1) manifestations of the problem in the past; (2) thoughts, feelings, and actions that indicate an imminent recurrence; (3) thoughts, feelings, and actions that may trigger a recurrence; (4) steps to take in order to gain control of the problem before it gets out of hand; and (5) ways to ask and receive help from others (Leichtman & Leichtman, 1999).

A subsequent task consists of articulating detailed rules to deal with problems and the consequences the youngsters should expect to face when the problems arise. Generally, after a discharge date has been set, youngsters and their caregivers prepare a crisis plan that includes information on how to recognize the cues that signal an imminent crisis, steps for family members to give feedback when youngsters are doing well and when problems emerge, and steps to take when the problems have reached crisis proportions. Youngsters and caregivers also spell out the steps they will take to prevent a crisis from escalating. For purposes of illustration, I now describe in some detail the residential treatment of a borderline child.

Larry was 6 years old when he was admitted to the Menninger residential program. His mother's pregnancy with Larry was difficult. She felt nauseated and sick, and during the seventh month required an emergency cesarean section because of fetal distress. Unable to breathe independently, Larry needed resuscitation and the assistance of a respirator. He weighed only 3 pounds at birth and had difficulty tolerating formula. To compound the family strain, his mother suffered postpartum complications that required a hysterectomy. She also developed a severe postpartum depression.

When Larry was 8 months old, his parents became alarmed when he developed severe neurological symptoms, including listlessness and lethargy. These symptoms turned out to be secondary to a communicating hydrocephalus, which was treated with a ventriculoperitoneal shunt that drained the fluid from his brain to his abdomen. A few months later, when Larry again became lethargic and started vomiting, doctors attributed this to a malfunction of the shunt.

From that time on, the family became organized around the parents' belief that the risk of shunt malfunction would hang like a sword over their child's head for the rest of his life. If that dreaded crisis arrived, they believed that only immediate attention would save Larry from death or brain damage. More and more, the idea that Larry was on the brink of death held the family in a tight grip. His mother hovered anxiously over him, seeking to divine the slightest indication of increased intracranial pressure. The shunt ensnarled mother and child in a suffocating noose. Larry soon learned the enormous power of his physical symptoms and complaints. Before long, his complaints of headache and nausea frequently precipitated frantic trips to the emergency room.

When Larry was 3 years old, his father, an engineer with an oil company, was assigned to an overseas post. After several months, his wife joined him, leaving Larry in the care of her parents. This separation marked another crisis for Larry's family. While Larry's mother was overseas, her brother died in a car accident. She herself developed urological problems and was hospitalized for several weeks. At that point, Larry's behavior got out of control. He became more aggressive and oppositional, and threw furious temper tantrums when anyone attempted to set limits on him. He also tried to hurt himself by trying to pull his toenails out, banging his head against the wall, and trying to jump out of the car. He slept fitfully, awoke often, and was tormented by nightmares. When awake, he could not find much peace either, since he was haunted by the fear of being bitten in the neck by Dracula or of being stabbed in the head. In spite of outpatient treatment and several brief hospitalizations, these problems only worsened as the boy grew older.

Larry was a small, straggly-haired, waif-like child at the time of admission. He appeared much younger than his stated age of 6, but the sad expression on his face made him look older and betrayed the pain behind his frantic activity. He was indeed a small engine of destruction and could hardly sit still for more than a few seconds.

The residential program provided Larry with a clear, reliable daily routine. He was given the consistent message that the program was designed to help him learn to feel safe. After a careful physical and neurological examination revealed no abnormalities, both Larry and his parents were repeatedly told that he was physically healthy, not defective, and not in danger of imminent death. His physical complaints were treated expeditiously and matter-of-factly, without providing Larry undue gratification. The boy was repeatedly told that he gave the impression that it was hard for him to ask people for help unless his body was hurting.

Larry met diagnostic criteria for attention-deficit/hyperactivity disorder and was thus prescribed methylphenidate, which not only helped to improve his attention span and decrease his overactivity but also enhanced his ability to grasp social cues (to be discussed in Chapter 11). After 4 weeks on the stimulant regimen, Larry had improved but was still struggling with impulsivity and overactivity, as well as significant sleep problems. Thus, clonidine was added to his medication regimen.

Larry's school program was focused initially on helping him tolerate the stress of learning, then on strengthening cognitive weaknesses and assisting the development of better learning skills. At the same time, a structure was set up to provide him with clear and firm consequences for impulsive and aggressive behavior. At first, containing his aggression literally required physically holding him. While being held, he always complied with staff comments about his difficulty in communicating thoughts and feelings in words. By the fourth week of treatment, staff members shared with Larry their conviction that he had grown enough to begin taking over the containment of his destructive behavior. From then on, the staff reminded Larry when his aggressive or destructive behavior required containment. Instead of physically restraining him, however, staff members asked him to go to his room for a 15-minute time-out. The duration of the time-out was signaled by the bell on a timer. The timer eventually became a transitional object for Larry and seemingly helped him curb his impulsivity.

By the fourth month in the residential program, Larry's behavior had noticeably improved. The first signs were a lessening of somatic complaints and improved sleep, which seemed to benefit from the combination of clonidine, structure, and the boy's growing capacity to experience others as soothing and comforting. In the family process, Larry's parents focused first on acquiring the "skills" of remaining calm and clear when the boy was anxious and in need of comfort, or impulsive and destructive and in need of limits and consequences. Home visits were scheduled to assist the parents in practicing to help Larry sleep through the night, which initially required a routine of a warm bath, a glass of milk, and a bedtime story. Four months into the family process, Larry began individual psychotherapy.

The combination of an individualized school program, psychotherapy (individual and family), a medication regimen, and milieu treatment appeared to help Larry develop a measure of security in his attachments and allowed him to sustain reflective function even in times of stress. With enthusiasm, he discovered the pleasures of learning, making sense of things, and using a growing capacity to understand the human world to anticipate, plan, and resolve problems. Eight months after admission, Larry was discharged from the residential program to continue in a treatment program along the lines I describe in the next section. Larry's somatic complaints were identified as a cue to his parents and to the treatment team brought into individual and family therapy, as well as to the wraparound team (see later description), so that they could assist him in figuring out ways to ask for help with words.

Setting a discharge date a few weeks in advance provides children with an essential opportunity to test their (and their caregivers') readiness to pursue treatment without the support of the milieu. The reality of the discharge confronts youngsters with the loss of perhaps their first human context with holding, attainment, involvement, and facilitation. Some reactivation of old symptoms can be expected, yet a facilitating stance on the staff's part necessitates a relaxation of supervision, expanded privileges, and increased responsibility for the youngsters, even in the presence of symptomatic regression.

As suggested in the section on individual psychotherapy in Chapter 9, facilitating comments may provide a much-needed boost to the therapeutic process. Pointing out, for example, the courage needed to go forward in an adaptive direction aligns staff members with the children's proximal area of development. Friedman (1982, cited in Stern, 1985) suggested treating patients as though they are roughly the persons they are about to become: "The patient will explore being treated that way, and fill in the personal details" (p. 43). Seeing in the minds of the treaters a conviction about his potential to grow up as a healthy boy seemed in fact to help Larry advance in the direction of his own growth.

To summarize:

1. Residential treatment is conceptualized as a focused, relatively short-term immersion in the total therapeutic environment indicated for certain youngsters with severe personality disorders, for whom a less intense and restrictive approach is likely to be counterproductive or inadequate.
2. Residential treatment aims to interrupt coercive patterns of family interaction and establish the conditions in the youngsters and the family that would permit secure attachments and the exercise of reflective function.
3. The essence of the residential program is the integration of the goals of treatment, and the therapeutic modalities designed to achieve those goals, in a coherent formulation shared by all those involved in the treatment, including the caregivers.
4. Planning for discharge begins at the time of admission, as staff members seek to identify the treatment modalities and social supports needed to return youngsters to the community, while maintaining continuity of planning and relationships. Development of relapse prevention and crisis plans are crucial aspects of the treatment process.

WRAPAROUND AND COMMUNITY-BASED SERVICES

Following discharge from a residential program, youngsters with severe personality disorders require an array of services and programs to maintain their gains and to support the continuation of treatment into the middle and termination phases described in Chapter 9. Outcome studies clearly point out that although behavior and adjustment seem improved at the end of most youngsters' residential treatment, in the absence of a transition to effective community-based services, gains are frequently lost (Curry, 1991).

The principles that govern the transition from residential to community-based programs are essentially the same as those that guide the design of a community-based program for youngsters with severe personality disorders who do *not* require a phase of residential care:

• *Empowering the caregivers as full partners in treatment.* Treatment success depends to a large degree on the caregivers' capacity to experience a sense of ownership and control over the treatment. They must also be able to use the process to gain competence in interrupting coercive cycles and in functioning in a reflective mode, as well as in becoming more generally effective at parenting their children. Such greater competence includes the ability to access supports for themselves and their families.

• *Building on the strengths and resources of the caregivers, their families, and the community.* Success in treatment depends heavily on how much the process helps youngsters and caregivers recognize, mobilize, and build on their strengths, resources, supports, and adaptive coping capacities.

• *Designing the treatment program within the specific family and community cultural and economic context.* Financial resources, educational background, and the cultural, religious, and value systems of the family and the community in which youngsters' lives are embedded are crucial determinants of the resources available for treatment. Also critical are the particular rules and expectations that "make sense" to youngsters and families trying to stop coercive cycles and develop the capacity to create a base for secure attachments and reflective function. Although the literature emphasizes sensitivity to the specific challenges and features of families from minority or low-income groups, families of wealth and privilege offer a no less significant test of the treaters' ability to retain a reflective perspective. The ordinary fabric of the day-to-day life of families of wealth generates feelings of envy and accusations of entitlement, narcissism, and child-spoiling parental behavior.

• *Normalizing the caregivers' support system by drawing on community resources.* The principle of normalization involves identifying current or potential natural supports in the community, such as friends, neighbors, clergy, schoolteachers, extended family, and community self-help groups.

Providing Child- and Family-Centered Treatment: The Wraparound Model

The focus principles just described call for an integration of services and resources. Efforts to provide such integration led to the development of the continuum of services. The concept of a "continuum of care" (Axelson, 1997; Behar, 1990; England & Cole, 1992; Tuma, 1989) was first designed as a step-down from inpatient or residential services. The continuum consists of an array of services that extend from the most restrictive inpatient setting to the least restrictive outpatient interventions. The continuum was meant to provide a more gradual transition from the controlled structure of the hospital or the residential treatment program at one end of the continuum, to outpatient services at the other end of the spectrum. A full spectrum of services (see Table 10.1)

TABLE 10.1. Continuum of Services

Hospitalization

Residential treatment

  Specialized residential center
  Group home
  Professional parenting/specialized foster home
  Supervised independent living

Day treatment

  High management—full day
  Moderate management—full day
  Moderate management—half day
  Therapeutic vocational placement
  Therapeutic preschool

Evening treatment

  After school or work

Therapeutic camping

  Weekend, summer

Outpatient

  Individual treatment (office or home)
  Family treatment (office or home)
  In-school support
  24-hour emergency services—crisis intervention
  Intensive outpatient

Wraparound services

  Family preservation services
  In-home crisis stabilization
  Natural supports

thus included a number of midrange services, including group homes, specialized foster care, day treatment, school-based services, vocational placements, after-school or after-work evening treatment, weekend or summer therapeutic camping, emergency services, and in-home crisis stabilization and family preservation services.

The view of the continuum as a series of categorical services that youngsters traverse in one direction—from more to less restrictive settings—has several significant shortcomings. First, the continuum of services, as it exists in most communities, is mired in logistical and planning problems. Some services are publicly funded, while others access third-party and private reimbursement. The diversity of criteria for admission and funding streams, the vagaries of state legislative policies, and the parochial biases and interests of each agency's staff hinder the possibility of coordinating services and achieving a smooth integration of the planning and implementation of the treatment along the various components of the continuum (Stroul & Friedman, 1988).

Second, youngsters with severe personality disorders and their families live chaotic lives marked by crisis resulting from developmental, interpersonal, and social pressures. Thus, they rarely sail in a smooth and orderly fashion from one end of the continuum to the other. Instead, individual youngsters and their families typically need to go in and out of various parts of the continuum of services, and they need to access various combinations of services at any given time. For example, during the middle phase of psychotherapy, a suicidal crisis can develop from a confrontation with previously dissociated experiences. The severity of the life-threatening risk may require a brief hospitalization followed by a specific crisis plan. Such a plan can resolve the crisis in a few days or weeks, enabling the youngster and family to resume individual and family psychotherapy augmented by pharmacotherapy and in-school support.

A way of addressing these limitations is the creation of flexible teams that "wrap" services around the children and their families. Wraparound is an approach to planning and providing individualized, integrated treatment for youngsters with complex problems. Wraparound is remarkably well suited to provide community-based treatment for youngsters with severe personality disorders. The essence of wraparound lies in the process of bringing together patients, families, natural supports (e.g., teachers, coaches, extended family, clergy, neighbors), and mental health professionals to work as a team. This team endeavors to develop a community-based plan specifically designed to address the needs of particular youngsters and their families.

The process of developing a team begins by asking the caregivers to identify those persons who can help them think about how to meet their needs. Caregivers need support and help in building their skill and comfort in providing a secure environment for themselves and their families. They also need specific assistance to enable them to support their child's treatment.

Caregivers are encouraged to develop a support system that draws as much as possible on "normal" community supports, such as friends, coworkers, extended family, and clergy. Professionals include therapists, case managers, and agency representatives, such as school personnel, probation officers, and managed care reviewers. A typical team consists of 8 to 10 people (Adkins, Safier, & Parker, 1998).

A paid team coordinator facilitates the decision-making process, keeps meetings on task, and oversees the implementation of the wraparound plan. The team coordinator promotes a culture that protects the team's reflective function by attending to the feedback, needs, and concerns of all team members, and by helping them articulate their points of view. The team coordinator ensures communication and coordination among all team members and keeps the caregivers at the center of the decision-making process.

An essential factor in the implementation of wraparound programs is access to funding. A collaborative relationship with third-party payers can result in the flexible use of funds to cover nontraditional services in lieu of inpatient or residential treatment. Managed care reviewers participate as members of the wraparound team and are actively involved in ensuring that the wraparound plan is cost-effective.

For example, Adkins and colleagues (1998) reported the case of Sally, a 16-year-old borderline girl, who had been repeatedly hospitalized for suicide attempts and suicidal ideation. The individual psychotherapist discovered that Sally became suicidal when she was left alone at home, Monday through Thursday, between 3:00 and 6:00 P.M. The wraparound team developed a plan to provide Sally with attendant care for those 12 hours. During the next 3 years, Sally neither attempted suicide nor required hospitalization.

Payers are often convinced by experiences with cases such as Sally's of the benefits of their active participation in treatment planning and use of financial resources in flexible ways. Even more convincing is the cost-effectiveness of recruiting normal community supports into the process.

The benefits of promoting the use of normal supports goes, of course, beyond the obvious cost advantage of utilizing free, or relatively free, services. Incorporating normal community resources goes a long way toward decreasing stigma and countering the marginalization of youngsters and families whose dysfunction has cut them off from normal sources of help and support. By intertwining the lives of these youngsters and their families with the broader community, wraparound programs provide them with opportunities to develop adaptive models of coping and communication, and sturdier sources of support that will stay in place after the engagement with professional staff has come to an end.

As Leichtman and Leichtman (1999) point out, optimally, community resources and activities are integrated into the treatment of youngsters in a residential program every bit as much as they are in the treatment of youngsters living at home. For both groups, community activities expose youngsters to normal social demands. Thus, participation in these activities offers the wraparound team a chance to dissect the specific pressures that bring about inhibition of reflective function and trigger unreflective and coercive modes of functioning. Leichtman and Leichtman describe how participation in community activities becomes a critical aspect of the middle and final stages of residential treatment, serving to facilitate the transition back to the community, and providing the basis for postdischarge planning.

Perhaps the most important area of community involvement for children and adolescents is school. School is obviously the crucial center of children and adolescents' learning of social and academic skills. It is also the hub of their social life and, particularly for older children and adolescents, a significant source of their sense of identity.

Leichtman and Leichtman (1999) describe the transition from the residential program's school to a school program in the community. During the first few weeks of treatment, youngsters in residential treatment typically require an educational program embedded in the residential unit. This program serves to assess the specific educational interventions needed to remediate learning disabilities and overcome chronic academic problems that include long-standing academic failure, conflicts with authority, association with antisocial peers, and poorly developed academic skills.

By the middle phase of treatment, as a working alliance and attachment to the treaters become evident, youngsters in residential treatment often begin to take some classes at a community school and, as their discharge date looms, most youngsters attend school full-time and are encouraged to participate in after-school activities, such as plays, sports events, and school dances. During the latter stages of residential treatment, the wraparound team begins to plan for the continuation of treatment after discharge from the residential program. This team includes a school representative that brings to the community school the academic approaches that support the youngsters' success in school. The school representative and other members of the wraparound team consult with teachers and other school personnel to help them appreciate the nature of the youngsters' problems and how best to deal with them. At the same time, the school representative brings feedback to the wraparound team about problems and successes the youngsters encounter as they seek to redress years of school failure and frustration.

For youngsters in residential treatment, religious activities are another avenue for involvement in the community. Religious interests are explored as part of the diagnostic assessment. By the middle stage of residential treatment, youngsters attend youth groups and other religious programs (Leichtman & Leichtman, 1999). The wraparound team for these youngsters, as well as for those living at home, typically includes a rabbi, a minister, or another religious representative.

Another crucial bridge to youngsters' adaptive functioning in the community is the development of vocational interests and work skills that are in line with their talents. Leichtman and Leichtman (1999) describe a community-based workshop designed to help adolescents identify their vocational interests, write résumés, obtain letters of reference, apply for jobs, and interview with employers. An interesting opportunity to practice reflective function occurs in a series of exercises designed to help youngsters appreciate what interests the employers who are hiring.

Obtaining a part-time job provides a substantial boost to the self-esteem of adolescents with severe personality disorders. Work provides a structured activity that limits contact with antisocial peers and introduces these youngsters to money management and budgeting skills. Working as volunteers in community services (e.g., soup kitchens, delivering meals to the elderly) offers antisocial youngsters an opportunity for restitution. Leichtman and Leichtman (1999), for example, describe a youngster whom they required to calculate how much his penchant for stealing car stereos had cost others and then make restitution through community service. Although this youngster's residential milieu structure was highly restrictive, he still spent 4 hours per day, with limited supervision, remodeling homes for homeless families. In this particular aspect of treatment, this youngster never sought to cheat or to manipulate the rules, and when he completed residential treatment, he reported that it had given him the greatest pride and sense of accomplishment he had ever experienced.

Other community-based programs help youngsters improve relationships, learn or develop skills, and pursue recreational interests. One interesting example is a program combining martial arts and meditation. The "gentle warrior" model offered as part of the Peaceful Schools program (Twemlow et al., 2001), developed by the Child and Family Center at Menninger, stresses meditation, control over emotions and impulsivity, and mindfulness of martial arts, as well as the security and gentleness that come from genuine strength.

Community-Based Treatment of Substance Abuse Problems

Misuse of illicit drugs is often the Achilles' heel of the treatment of youngsters with severe personality disorders. Relapse into substance abuse hovers like a dark cloud over the most thoughtfully constructed treatment plan, threatening to sap the commitment of the youngsters and their families. Peers, often youngsters who themselves suffer from severe personality disorders, pressure the patients to reconnect with them by consuming drugs. The pull of drugs is powerful. They offer momentary relief from stress and a "rush" that obliterates, at least for an instant, dreadful feelings of inner deadness. But they also resonate with a family theme, since the abuse of drugs is not infrequently implanted in the very fabric of the family's genetics and history. Drugs thus have the "smell" of home and are at times subtly or blatantly encouraged by caregivers. The combination of substance abuse and a severe personality disorder is a common indication for residential treatment, which integrates the components previously described, including milieu therapy, pharmacotherapy, individual and family therapy, and educational programs, with specialized approaches that specifically address substance abuse problems (Cooperman & Frances, 1989; Rounds-Bryant, Kristiansen, & Hubbard, 1999).

Specialized substance abuse interventions are the responsibility of a chemical dependency counselor, who develops individualized plans for all youngsters. These plans, as described earlier, include individual counseling, chemical dependency groups, and workbook assignments (Jaffe, 1990). Emphasis is placed on relapse prevention, including after-care plans. These plans typically include random urinalysis and participation in Alcoholics Anonymous (AA) or Narcotics Anonymous (NA) groups in the community.

Youngsters in a residential program are gradually introduced to community self-help programs (Leichtman & Leichtman, 1999). First, they become involved in 12-step programs without leaving the unit, where staff members provide information about the philosophy and expectations of NA/AA groups. Then, as they show evidence of engaging in a working alliance with the treatment team (typically after 4 to 8 months of residential treatment), youngsters begin to participate in community-based NA/AA groups. As discharge approaches, sponsors are recruited to help the youngsters attend community meetings after discharge. Sponsors and NA/AA groups thus become important components of the structure of support and holding that can allow youngsters with severe personality disorders to persist in their journey to healthier development and improved adjustment.

11

Pharmacological Treatment

In clinical practice, the treatment of most youngsters with severe personality disorders includes medications, typically in combination with some form of psychosocial treatment or case management. Such practice is based largely on the clinical impression that medications improve outcome and give despairing clinicians something to offer to patients and families faced with the constraints of limited reimbursement for more time-consuming interventions.

A growing literature documents the effectiveness of pharmacological agents in the treatment of adults with personality disorders (Coccaro & Kavoussi, 1997; Coccaro et al., 1989; Kapfhammer & Hippius, 1998; Soloff, 1998). Very limited empirical evidence, however, supports the use of pharmacological interventions with children and adolescents. Also lacking are studies that compare psychotherapy alone, pharmacotherapy alone, and a combination of psychotherapy and pharmacotherapy.

In this chapter, I discuss a clinical rationale for the use of pharmacotherapy as a component of an integrated treatment plan for youngsters with severe personality disorders. This rationale, given the limitations in empirical research just mentioned, is based to a significant degree on the models derived from clinical studies and research with adult patients (Cloninger, Svrakic, & Przybeck, 1993; Gabbard, 2000; Gunderson & Links, 1995; Soloff, 1998). It is also grounded in clinical experience with these youngsters and in studies that document the effectiveness of pharmacotherapy in a range of related or comorbid child and adolescent problems.

At the heart of this treatment model is the evidence presented in Chapters 4, 5, and 6, which suggests that neurobiological vulnerabilities, mediated by variations in neurotransmitter activity, are crucial factors in generating, maintaining, reinforcing, and exacerbating these youngsters' maladaptive patterns of coping, relating, and experiencing. These vulnerabilities, as described earlier, stem from a genetic disposition and/or the biological alterations brought about by disadvantage, trauma, or maltreatment. More specifically, the dysregulations of arousal, cognition, affect, and impulse that underlie the severe personality disorders promote the selective inhibition of reflective function in at least four ways.

1. They generate in the youngsters a heightened need for attuned responses to restore psychophysiological regulation. (Arguably, these dysregulations also signal a heightened innate capacity in these youngsters for reading caregivers' violent or rejecting internal states.)
2. The dysregulations evoke distress, frustration, and inhibition of reflective function in the caregivers (and the fight-or-flight response that gives rise to their need to flee or to destroy the children who "provoke" such a response). Caregivers are thus less likely to provide the caregiving responses that trigger the phenotypic expression of reflective function.
3. They increase the intensity of distress, anxiety, or hyperarousal that leads to fight-or-flight reactions of sufficient intensity to block the exercise of reflective function.
4. They decrease the availability of symbolic capacities, energy level, or concentration necessary for reflective function. These dysregulations are ultimately dependent on specific neurotransmitter and neurophysiological activation (Soloff, 1998).

The role of pharmacotherapy in the treatment of youngsters with severe personality disorders is to target the symptoms associated with such dysregulation and the traits of vulnerability that compromise healthy adjustment and development, particularly the exercise of reflective function. Pharmacotherapy targets both the symptoms that emerge during episodes of acute psychosociobiological decompensation and the trait vulnerabilities that represent an enduring diathesis to dysfunction. By influencing the neurobiological underpinnings of arousal, cognition, affect, and impulse, pharmacotherapy can create more optimal conditions for psychotherapy and family treatment. When youngsters are not buffeted by subjective distress, anxiety, or hyperarousal, or when their depressed energy level and reduced capacity for concentration have improved, they can more readily engage in reflective function. Likewise, the collaborative work between treater and caregiver that results in the prescription and administration of effective medication places the adults in a position of helping the patient to gain control and self-regulation. Thus, caregivers promote the development of secure attachment by their ability to respond effectively to their children's distress. In summary, although medications do not change personality or, by themselves, alter children's developmental trajectory, they act synergistically with individual and family treatment to promote new experiences and learning, and to facilitate the creation of a different interpersonal context.

As described in Chapter 4, no one-to-one congruity has been identified at this point between specific neurobiological vulnerabilities and types of personality disorder. In particular, at the borderline end of the cluster, youngsters present various combinations of vulnerability and corresponding Axis I disorders, such as depression, anxiety disorders, substance abuse, ADHD, eating disorders, and mood disorders. In addition, they manifest varying degrees of explosiveness, impulsive aggression, and self-destructiveness. Thus, rather than presenting a set protocol of pharmacological intervention, it is more practical, given the current level of knowledge, to target, as Soloff (1998) proposes, personality dimensions such as affective dysregulation and impulsive–behavioral dysregulation. These dimensions can be assessed for all children in the cluster of severe personality disorders, although they are much more prominent at the borderline end of the cluster. Currently, no pharmacological strategy exists to address the predatory–ruthless dimension that predominates at the antisocial–narcissistic end of the cluster.

I thus follow Soloff's dimensional approach to define treatment algorithms based on different levels of support from research and clinical experience. In particular, they reflect the overlap between personality dimensions and Axis I conditions for which well-established medication algorithms have been developed. The dimension of affective dysregulation overlaps with the Axis I conditions of bipolar disorder, intermittent explosive disorder, and depression. The dimension of impulsive-behavioral dysregulation overlaps with Axis I ADHD. These algorithms follow the rules proposed by Soloff (1998): (1) preference for medications for which efficacy is most strongly supported by empirical evidence; (2) preference for safer medication, with less risk for overdose, abuse, or noncompliance; and (3) preference for fast-acting drugs whenever the clinical need warrants a rapid response.

PHARMACOLOGICAL TREATMENT OF AFFECTIVE DYSREGULATION, BIPOLAR DISORDER, INTERMITTENT EXPLOSIVE AGGRESSION, AND DEPRESSION

Affective dysregulation is a major component of the problems of youngsters with severe personality disorders, particularly those at the borderline end of the cluster. Affective dysregulation includes a range of symptoms, such as mood lability; intermittent, explosive anger; depressive "crashes"; and temper outbursts.

Some of these youngsters meet the criteria for juvenile-onset bipolar disorder, including the hallmark feature of a manic episode. These children are candidates for the algorithm developed for childhood bipolar disorder (see Figure 11.1, see also Davanzo & McCracken, 2000). Some youngsters display distinct periods of abnormality and persistently elevated, explosive, or irritable mood that do not meet criteria for bipolar disorder but, clinically, these children are also considered for treatment with mood stabilizers (Lewinsohn, Klein, & Seeley, 1995). Thus, they are included in the same algorithm. Other youngsters display prominent features of anxiety, labile mood, and heightened sensitivity to slights, rejection, frustration, or abandonment. Frequently, they meet DSM-IV diagnostic criteria for depression but lack the clear-cut features of bipolar disorder or intermittent explosive aggression. These youngsters are included in the algorithm for affective dysregulation–depression *without* bipolar disorder–intermittent explosive aggression (see Figure 11.2 on page 280).

The Bipolar Disorder–Intermittent Explosive Aggression Algorithm

This algorithm, illustrated in Figure 11.1, applies to youngsters with severe personality disorders who also are likely to have an underlying bipolar disorder that both exacerbates and is exacerbated by these chil-

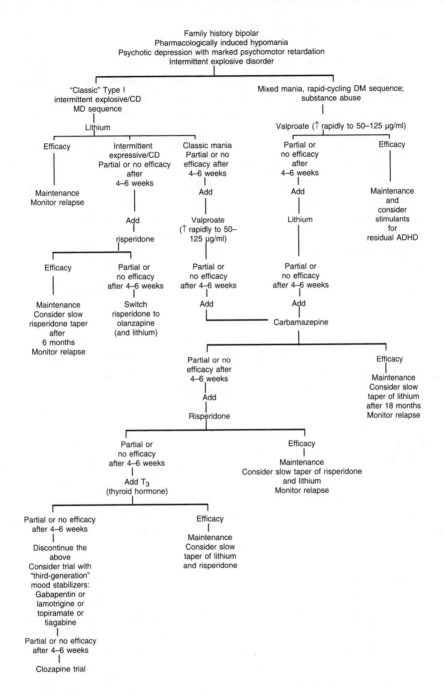

FIGURE 11.1. Algorithm for bipolar disorder–intermittent explosive aggression (Davanzo & McCracken, 2000). CD, conduct disorder; DM, depression–mania; MD, mania–depression.

dren's experience and interpersonal context. Predictors of bipolarity are (1) a history of bipolar disorder in a first-degree relative; (2) a switch to hypomania after the administration of antidepressants; (3) episodes of exacerbation of disruptive behavior, moodiness, low frustration tolerance, and explosive anger, followed by guilt, depression, and difficulty sleeping at night; and (4) depression with marked psychomotor retardation, neurovegetative symptoms, and delusions.

The case of Travis, discussed in Chapter 4, illustrates a youngster for whom the bipolar disorder–intermittent explosive aggressive algorithm applies. Travis's father, paternal uncle, and paternal grandfather all suffered from bipolar disorder. Mood lability, irritability, and intermittent storms of rage and aggression were the most striking features of this boy's clinical picture when he was first seen at age 7.

A trial of lithium is the first step for children with the classical presentation of bipolar disorder, that is, those who present a clear-cut family history of a mood disorder and/or an identifiable manic episode. Lithium is also the initial pharmacological treatment for those who present with intermittent episodes of explosive violence. Open-label studies (Carlson, Rapport, Pataki, & Kelly, 1992; Hsu, 1986) as well as double-blind, placebo-controlled studies of adolescent mania (Geller, Cooper, Sun, et al., 1998; Geller, Cooper, Zimerman, et al., 1998) suggest that lithium is effective in juvenile mania, even though it is less effective than in adult bipolar disorder. Differences in effectiveness are particularly evident in early-onset bipolar disorder. Strober and colleagues (1988) reported that adolescents with prepubertal onset responded more poorly to lithium (33% response), compared to adolescents with later onset (66% response). Lithium was also the first medication shown to be effective in the treatment of impulsive aggression (Sheard, 1975; Sheard, Marini, Bridges, & Wagner, 1976). More recent studies support the use of lithium for the treatment of explosive anger (Campbell et al., 1995; Fava, 1997).

Starting children on lithium using the mg/kg body weight/day dosage method has been discouraged because of the high serum levels attained with this approach (Fetner & Geller, 1992). Davanzo and McCracken (2000) recommend a lithium titration schedule of a starting daily dose of 300 mg for children who weigh less than 25 kg (target dose: 600 mg); 600 mg for children who weigh between 25 kg and 40 kg (target dose: between 750 and 900 mg); and 900 mg for youngsters who weigh over 40 kg (target dose: 1,200 mg/day). These authors suggest titrating the dose every 3–5 days until the desired serum level of 1.0–1.2 mEq/liter is reached.

The Cooper nomogram has been reported to show good predictive value for serum lithium in children (Geller & Fetner, 1989). It permits the adjustment of the dosage based on the 24-hour serum levels drawn after a single 600-mg dose. This method results in a more rapid attainment of a therapeutic blood concentration, which may be associated with better remission of manic episodes (Goldberg, Garno, Leon, Kocsis, & Portera, 1998). A more recent application of this approach, however, suggested possible toxicity and the potential for overestimating the dose needed to produce therapeutic blood levels (Davanzo & McCracken, 2000).

Lithium, however, has several disadvantages and limitations:

1. The need for gradual dosing because of possible toxicity, which impedes rapid loading and creates a narrow therapeutic index.
2. Serious side effects, including diarrhea, tremor, hypothyroidism (found in roughly 5–10% of patients, particularly women; Lenox, Manji, McElroy, Keck, & Dubovsky, 1995), and cognitive dulling (which may be a source of poor medication compliance).
3. A capacity to induce birth defects, which, although perhaps occurring less frequently than previously thought (Altshuler et al., 1996), is a particularly serious concern with adolescent girls with severe personality disorders—who often engage in poorly protected and otherwise self-destructive sexual relationships.
4. The need for thyroid, renal, and serum level monitoring.
5. The likelihood that monotherapy with lithium will not succeed in sustaining mood stability.

In addition to these disadvantages, lithium is only of limited effectiveness in the treatment of mixed manic and depressive states, rapid-cycling bipolar disorder, and comorbid substance abuse, all of which are particularly common conditions in children and adolescents with severe personality disorders.

Because of such limitations, clinicians have actively looked for alternative medications. The anticonvulsants have become an increasingly important alternative in the acute and prophylactic treatment of bipolar disorder and affective aggression. Divalproex sodium is currently the first indication for children and adolescents presenting with mixed mania, rapid-cycling bipolar disorder, or a mood disorder combined with substance abuse (Calabrese, Rapport, Kimmel, Reese, & Woyshville, 1993; McElroy, Keck, Pope, & Hudson, 1992; Post, Ketter, Denicoff, et al., 1996; Post, Ketter, Pazzaglia, et al., 1996; Post, Kramlinger, Altshuler, Ketter, & Denicoff, 1990). It was the medication selected for Travis, who tolerated it well and responded with a significant reduction in affective storms and impulsive aggression.

Case studies (Papatheodorou, Kutcher, Katic, & Szalai, 1995) suggest that divalproex sodium may be both effective and well tolerated in adolescents with bipolar disorder (Kastner & Friedman, 1992) and in youngsters with affective aggression and behavioral dyscontrol (Donovan et al., 1997). These studies suggest that anticonvulsants such as divalproex sodium seem to reduce not only angry outbursts but also irritability and increase the capacity to reflect before acting, an effect that made it possible for Travis to begin psychotherapy.

Davanzo and McCracken (2000) recommended a starting dose of divalproex sodium of 250 mg/day in divided doses for children who weigh less than 25 kg (target dose: 500 mg); 375 mg for youngsters who weigh between 25 kg and 40 kg (target dose: 750 mg); and 500 mg for children who weigh over 40 kg (target dose: over 1,000 mg as needed to achieve the desired serum level of 50–125 mg/ml) (see Table 11.1). Davanzo and McCracken report that the best clinical results, particularly in acute mania, are obtained when the optimal serum level is attained rapidly.

The use of divalproex sodium addresses a major limitation of lithium, namely, the chance of relapse. Davanzo and McCracken (2000) report recent studies showing that the probability of relapse by the third year is considerably reduced with divalproex sodium, compared to lithium (20% vs. 50%). Use of divalproex sodium, however, requires moni-

TABLE 11.1. Recommended Dosage Schedule for Divalproex Sodium

Body weight	Initial dose	Target dose	Target serum level
< 25 kg	250 mg	500 mg	50–125 mg/ml
25–40 kg	375 mg	750 mg	50–125 mg/ml
> 40 kg	500 mg	1,000 mg	50–125 mg/ml

toring of liver enzymes. Common side effects include transient gastro-intestinal symptoms, rash, appetite increase or anorexia, hair loss, and lower prothrombin time and platelet counts. A particular concern with girls is the potential for the occurrence of polycystic ovaries (Isojarvi, Laatikainen, Pakarinen, Juntunen, & Myllyla, 1993), which requires monitoring of early signs of menstrual irregularities or hirsutism.

In the event of efficacy with either lithium or divalproex sodium, the medication should be maintained for at least 18 months after the first manic episode before considering gradual discontinuation (Kowatch et al., 2000). Abrupt discontinuation of lithium increases the rate of relapse at least threefold (Strober, Morrell, Lampert, & Burroughs, 1990).

One of the atypical antipsychotics may be added when youngsters with intermittent explosive aggression receiving lithium show only partial or no response, or when the clinical need is urgent. These medications have antipsychotic effects with few or no side effects (particularly in regard to movement disorders), and they have demonstrated therapeutic effects on a broad range of symptoms, including depression (Tollefson, Sanger, Lu, & Thieme, 1998), cognitive symptoms (Hagger et al., 1993), and mania (Tohen et al., 1999). A number of other studies of patients with borderline personality disorder treated with atypical antipsychotics (e.g., Frankenburg & Zanarini, 1993; Schulz, Camlin, Berry, & Jesberger, 1999) suggest that the atypical antipsychotics may be safe and well tolerated by patients with severe personality disorders. These medications also appear safe in combination with other medications. Their usefulness extends beyond reducing psychotic symptoms in these patients. Atypical antipsychotics may be especially helpful for intermittently explosive patients and for those showing symptoms of refractory depression (see subsequent discussion).

Given the absence of controlled research with children and adolescents, the use of atypical antipsychotics, although widespread, must be regarded as unsupported by empirical evidence. Pam, whose case is described in Chapter 10, illustrates this sequence. Lithium was first prescribed to help modulate her irritability, mood swings, and fits of rage and impulsive aggression. After 4 weeks, she showed partial improvement but remained vulnerable to affective storms, during which her reality contact was impaired. The addition of risperidone greatly reduced her intermittent explosiveness and also seemed to strengthen her capacity to avoid lapses in reality testing.

Risperidone should be considered the first choice among the atypical antipsychotics given its relatively benign profile of adverse effects and the extent of available clinical experience with children and adolescents (Grcevich, Findling, Rowane, Friedman, & Schulz, 1996). Daily dosages range from 2 mg to 10 mg (mean: 6 mg). The main adverse effects include mild sedation and extrapyramidal symptoms, but reports of liver enzyme abnormalities point to the need for careful monitoring of liver function (Kumra, 2000).

For children with a severe personality disorder comorbid with a "classic" bipolar disorder who fail to respond to lithium, the next step is to add divalproex sodium. In a controlled study, Findling and Calabrese (2000) found evidence of the safety and efficacy of a combination of mood stabilizers. These results are consistent with studies of adults showing that a combination of mood stabilizers is more effective than monotherapy in preventing relapse (Davanzo & McCracken, 2000). Accordingly, lithium should be added to the treatment of children with mixed mania, rapid-cycling bipolar disorder, or bipolar disorder comorbid with substance abuse, who respond partially or fail to respond to divalproex sodium.

To summarize the algorithm so far: Youngsters with intermittent explosive "affective" aggression should first be treated with lithium. If they are not responsive, risperidone should be added to their treatment. Children with "classic" mania should first be treated with lithium and, if not responsive, have divalproex sodium added. For youngsters with mixed mania, rapid-cycling bipolar disorder, or bipolar disorder comorbid with substance abuse, the first choice is divalproex sodium. If they fail to respond to this medication, lithium should be added to their treatment.

If there has been only partial or no response after 4–6 weeks of lithium and risperidone treatment for controlling intermittent explosive aggression, risperidone can be replaced with olanzapine. Olanzapine has been well tolerated by children with schizophrenia (Kumra et al., 1998). The most commonly reported adverse effects are relatively minor, including increased appetite, constipation, nausea and vomiting, headache, somnolence, difficulty concentrating, nervousness, and transient increases in liver enzymes. The incidence of minor adverse effects is comparable to that found with use of clozapine but without the potentially fatal blood dyscrasias associated with clozapine. No studies have been conducted with children or adolescents with severe personality disorders, but open-label studies of adults with borderline personality disorder are promising. If a youngster fails to respond to olanzapine plus lithium after 4–6 weeks, the algorithm outlined for rapid-cycling and mixed states, that is, a combination of lithium and valproex sodium, should be considered as a next step.

The addition of carbamazepine is the next choice for youngsters with a classic bipolar disorder, a mixed state, or a rapid-cycling condition—as well as for those with intermittent explosive aggression—who have failed to respond to the combination of lithium and divalproex sodium. Travis exemplifies an instance of a youngster whose signs of a mixed, rapid-cycling mood disorder and explosive, impulsive aggression improved only partially with the combination of lithium and divalproex sodium. The addition of carbamazepine had a marked effect in decreasing his temper outbursts and explosive aggression.

Carbamazepine is effective for acute and prophylactic treatment of mania and depression in adults with bipolar disorder (Post, Ketter, Denicoff, et al., 1996; Post, Ketter, Pazzaglia, et al., 1996). Although no controlled studies on children and adolescents have been published, several studies have documented the effectiveness of carbamazepine in decreasing temper outbursts and explosive aggression (Cueva et al., 1996; Kafantaris et al., 1992). The initial dose for children who weigh less than 25 kg is 100 mg/day, which can be increased every 5–7 days by 100–200 mg, until the target dose of 400 mg and the desired serum level of 4–14 mg/ml are achieved. The initial dose for children weighing 25–40 kg is 200 mg, titrated every 5–7 days, until the target dose of 800 mg/day and the desired serum level of 4–14 mg/ml are reached. Children who weigh over 40 kg should start with a dose of 400 mg, until a target dose of 1,200 mg/day and the desired serum level of 4–14 mg/ml are reached (see Table 11.2). The use of carbamazepine requires careful monitoring of blood, platelet, and reticulocyte counts. This medication interacts with multiple drugs and has potentially serious adverse effects in children, including

TABLE 11.2. Recommended Dosage Schedule for Carbamazepine

Body weight	Initial dose	Target dose	Target serum level
< 25 kg	100 mg	400 mg	4–14 mg/ml
25–40 kg	200 mg	800 mg	4–14 mg/ml
> 40 kg	400 mg	1,200 mg	4–14 mg/ml

rashes, leukopenia, and, more rarely, aplastic anemia and thrombocytopenia.

In case of failure to respond to the combination of the first- and second-line mood stabilizers, children and adolescents with severe personality disorders and intermittent explosive aggression may be candidates for discontinuation of divalproex sodium and carbamazepine in favor of a trial with one of the new anticonvulsants that have emerged as a potential third generation of mood stabilizers. Four new anticonvulsants have been approved for the treatment of epilepsy: lamotrigine, gabapentin, topiramate, and tiagabine. Lamotrigine and gabapentin have shown efficacy in the treatment of adults with refractory bipolar depression and rapid-cycling mood disorder (Ghaemi, 2000; Kusumakar & Yatham, 1997). Case studies suggest a robust response to lamotrigine in adults with borderline personality (Pinto & Akiskal, 1998). Clinical experience with children and adolescents has fueled a surge of interest in the use of the new anticonvulsants, particularly lamotrigine and gabapentin, for the treatment of not only refractory bipolar and rapid-cycling depression but also the broader range of affective aggression and behavioral dyscontrol. In the absence of controlled studies on safety and efficacy, the use of these agents requires extreme care. Of particularly serious concern is the high prevalence of skin rash in children receiving lamotrigine, particularly given a number of reports of Steven Johnson syndrome, a potentially lethal condition (Davanzo & McCracken, 2000). The risk of such reactions may be at least partially related to higher dosage and concomitant use of divalproex sodium.

The Affective Dysregulation–Depression Algorithm

For those youngsters—typically, children at the borderline end of the clusters—who present prominent features of affective dysregulation and depression *without* the characteristics of a bipolar disorder or intermittent explosive aggression, the first line of treatment is the selective serotonin reuptake inhibitors (SSRIs). These medications appear to be both safe and effective (Emslie et al., 1997; March et al., 1998; Strober et al., 1999).

Research with adult patients with borderline personality disorder supports the use of SSRI antidepressants to reduce their depressive mood, dysregulated anger, hypersensitivity to rejection, mood lability, impulsive behavior, and self-mutilation (Markovitz, 1995; Salzman et al., 1995; Soloff, 1998). These clinical findings are consistent with the evidence discussed in Chapter 4 regarding the significantly higher vulnerability of rhesus monkeys who carry the short allele of the serotonin transporter (5-HTT) gene to be affected by maternal deprivation. To briefly recapitulate, these genetically vulnerable monkeys, *if* they are also deprived of maternal caregiving, grow up with features highly congruent with the dimensions of affective dysregulation and impulsive behavioral dyscontrol discussed in this and the next section. These monkeys grow up to be socially anxious, emotionally labile, impulsive, and fearful (Higley, King, et al., 1996; Suomi, 1997). They consume large amounts of alcohol (Higley et al., 1991) and develop tolerance to it more rapidly. These behavioral abnormalities correlate with lower concentrations of the serotonin metabolite 5-hydroxyindoleacetic acid (5-HIAA) in the cerebrospinal fluid (Heinz, Higley, et al., 1998; Heinz, Ragan, et al., 1998; Higley, Suomi, et al., 1996), pointing to decreased serotonergic turnover.

The relationship between affective dysregulation and impulsive aggression—including violent suicide attempts—and low levels of the central nervous system's serotonin is also well established in humans (Brown, Pulido, Grota, & Niles, 1984; Heinz, Higley, et al., 1998; Heinz, Ragan, et al., 1998; Lesch et al., 1996). Direct measures of brain serotonergic activity support the proposed central role of serotonin in aggression and behavioral dyscontrol. Postmortem analyses of the brains of suicide victims demonstrate that these individuals carry a reduced number of serotonin transporters, compared to autopsy specimens obtained from individuals who have not committed suicide (Stanley & Mann, 1983). A compensatory increase in the number of serotonin 5-HT$_2$ postsynaptic receptor sites is noted in the frontal cortex samples obtained from individuals who committed suicide (Stanley & Mann, 1983).

Arguably, reduced production or release of serotonin in violent or suicidal individuals could account for the decreased number of serotonin transports and the increased number of postsynaptic receptors. Coccaro and colleagues (1989) reported that similar decreases in serotonergic neurotransmission were associated with a history of suicide attempts and impulsive aggressive behavior among patients with personality disorders, but only with suicide attempts and no impulsive aggression in patients with a mood disorder.

Recent functional brain imaging studies have also demonstrated serotonergic abnormalities related to aggressive behavior. Siever and colleagues (1999) used positron emission tomography (PET) scanning to compare glucose utilization in the brains of impulsive–aggressive patients with personality disorders and of normal controls after a challenge with fenfluramine. The personality disorder patients showed significantly less response to fenfluramine, again pointing to decreased serotonin turnover.

This body of evidence points to a dysfunction in the serotonergic system in individuals with affective dysregulation, impulsivity, and impulsive aggression, whether directed outward or toward the self, and also provides a rationale for the use of SSRIs in the treatment of this behavioral dimension in individuals with severe personality disorder. The overlap between the dimensions of affective dysregulation and impulsivity–behavioral dyscontrol is paralleled by the overlap between the two pharmacological algorithms, both of which start with an SSRI. The dimension of affective dysregulation, however, typically includes manifestations of dysthymia or major depressive disorder, according to DSM-IV (American Psychiatric Association, 1994). Recent studies, as mentioned earlier, point out that SSRIs are equally effective in the treatment of childhood and adult depression.

In an effort to integrate the clinical and research evidence currently available for the treatment of depression in children and adolescents, the Texas Children's Medication Algorithm Project (Hughes et al., 1999) has endeavored to create a consensus algorithm for the medication treatment of childhood major depressive disorder. This algorithm, illustrated in Figure 11.2, resulted from a conference attended by national experts in child and adolescent mood disorders who reviewed current research on childhood depression. It represents state-of-the-art medication treatment for youngsters with major depressive disorder, with or without a severe personality disorder.

The algorithm begins with one of the SSRIs, which are deemed first-line treatment because of supporting efficacy data for fluoxetine in children and adolescents (Emslie et al., 1997), paroxetine in adolescents (Keller et al., 1998), and open trials of sertraline (Ambrosini et al., 1999) and fluoxetine (Strober et al., 1999), as well as clinical experience. Fluvoxamine has shown safety and efficacy in the treatment of children and adolescents with obsessive–compulsive disorder (Apter et al., 1994; Grados & Riddle, 1999; Riddle et al., 2001) and is being investigated for the treatment of major depression and anxiety disorder (Martin, Kaufman, & Charney, 2000).

SSRIs are not only effective but also appear significantly safer than the tricyclics. The tricyclics have not been shown to be effective in child and adolescent depression. In addition, they carry a high risk of toxicity, including lethality in overdose (Birmaher, Ryan, Williamson, Brent, & Kaufman, 1996). In contrast, the adverse effects of SSRIs tend to be mild and transient, including nausea (Leonard, March, Rickler, & Allen, 1997), insomnia (Apter et al., 1996), and behavioral activation shading into agitation, hypomania, and full-blown mania (Grados & Riddle, 1999; Peet, 1994). Children who develop a manic or hypomanic response to SSRIs are candidates for the bipolar disorder algorithm previously described.

One important advantage of SSRIs is that they appear relatively safe in overdose (Grados & Riddle, 1999) and seem to have little effect on cardiac conduction (Leonard et al., 1997). Of course, these features are of great importance when medicating youngsters with high potential for suicide and self-destructive behavior.

Because there are no data available to predict which SSRI will work better with a particular child, the decision to choose one of the currently available SSRIs is generally related to the clinician's experience, drug interactions, pharmacokinetic profiles, and cost. The dose of SSRIs must be individualized, taking into account adverse effects and efficacy. The following are suggested initial and target doses: sertraline, 25 mg, with a target dose of 50 mg (young children may respond better to an initial dose of 12.5 mg); fluoxetine, 5 mg, with a target dose of 20 mg; fluvoxamine, 50 mg, with a target dose of 200 mg; and paroxetine, 10 mg, with a target dose of 20 mg (Kutcher, 1998).

A trial of SSRIs should be continued for 8–12 weeks (Emslie, Mayes, & Hughes, 2000). In patients who fail to respond to an initial adequate trial with an SSRI, the Texas algorithm project and clinical experience suggest switching to a different SSRI (Emslie et al., 2000). An augmentation strategy is indicated after unsuccessful trials with two different SSRIs on the basis of data derived from studies with adults and clinical experience (Hughes et al., 1999). This approach is particularly appropriate in case of a partial response to SSRIs (Ryan, Meyer, Dachille, Mazzie, & Puig-Antich, 1988; Strober, Freeman, Rigali, Schmidt, & Diamond, 1992). The current consensus (Hughes et al., 1999) is to recommend lithium as the first choice as an agent to potentiate the effects of the first-line medications. If anxiety is a prominent symptom, however, buspirone can also be considered (Emslie, Walkup, Pliszka, & Ernst,

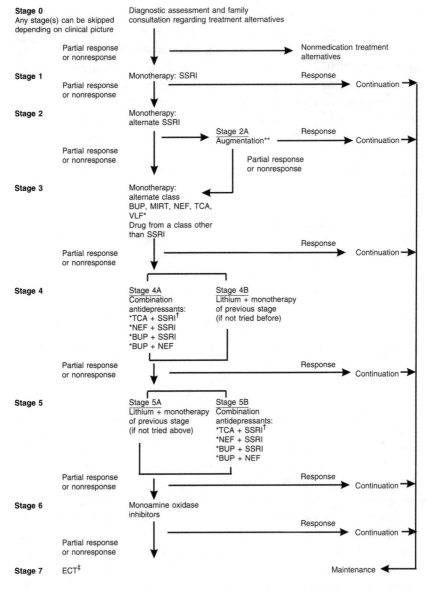

Stage 0
Any stage(s) can be skipped depending on clinical picture

Diagnostic assessment and family consultation regarding treatment alternatives

Partial response or nonresponse → Nonmedication treatment alternatives

Stage 1
Partial response or nonresponse

Monotherapy: SSRI

Response → Continuation →

Stage 2
Monotherapy: alternate SSRI

Stage 2A Augmentation** Response → Continuation →

Partial response or nonresponse

Partial response or nonresponse

Stage 3
Monotherapy: alternate class BUP, MIRT, NEF, TCA, VLF* Drug from a class other than SSRI

Partial response or nonresponse

Response → Continuation →

Stage 4
Stage 4A Combination antidepressants: *TCA + SSRI† *NEF + SSRI *BUP + SSRI *BUP + NEF

Stage 4B Lithium + monotherapy of previous stage (if not tried before)

Partial response or nonresponse

Response → Continuation →

Stage 5
Stage 5A Lithium + monotherapy of previous stage (if not tried above)

Stage 5B Combination antidepressants: *TCA + SSRI† *NEF + SSRI *BUP + SSRI *BUP + NEF

Partial response or nonresponse

Response → Continuation →

Stage 6
Monoamine oxidase inhibitors

Response → Continuation →

Partial response or nonresponse

Stage 7 ECT‡

Maintenance ←

*Consider TCA/VLF.   **Lithium + buspirone.   †Most studied combination in adults.   ‡ECT not allowed in Texas.

FIGURE 11.2. Texas Children's Medication Algorithm for affective dysregulation–depression (Hughes et al., 1999). BUP, bupropion; MIRT, mirtazapine; NEF, nefazodone; TCS, tricyclic antidepressant; VLF, venlafaxine.

1999). Buspirone may offer some benefit against anxiety and enhance the efficacy of SSRIs, without the risk of abuse and the potential to precipitate behavioral dyscontrol associated with other antianxiety medications (Gardner & Cowdry, 1985).

In case of partial or no response, several strategies can be pursued, depending on the clinical picture. These strategies are not supported by data and are largely based on clinical experience. If impulsive anger and explosiveness are prominent, the algorithm for intermittent explosive aggression (see Figure 11.1) can be followed, beginning with the addition of risperidone. If mood symptoms such as mood lability, irritability, and depressive crashing predominate, clinicians can follow the algorithm for mixed or rapid-cycling bipolar disorder (see Figure 11.1), beginning with the addition of divalproex sodium. On the other hand, if depressive symptoms predominate, clinical experience suggests following the next steps of the Texas algorithm, which recommends discontinuing the SSRI and switching to an alternative antidepressant, such as venlafaxine, nefazodone, bupropion, or mirtazapine (Emslie et al., 2000; Hughes et al., 1999). In cases of children with major depression who continue to show only a partial or no response, the Texas algorithm (Hughes et al., 1999) recommends a combination of the alternative antidepressant with either lithium or an SSRI. Finally, after lack of response or intolerance to the combination of lithium and an antidepressant or SSRI and alternative antidepressant, Emslie and colleagues (1999) and the Texas algorithm project recommend a trial with monoamine oxidase inhibitors (MAOIs).

Controlled studies of adults with personality disorders document the effectiveness of MAOIs, particularly in reducing behavioral impulsivity, mood lability, sensitivity to rejection, and intense anger (Cowdry & Gardner, 1988; Liebowitz et al., 1988). MAOIs, however, have serious limitations, including potentially fatal hypertensive crises due to drug–drug and drug–diet interactions. There is also a lack of data demonstrating their efficacy in treating children and adolescents. The potential of dietary indiscretions resulting in a life-threatening crisis is a particular problem, given these youngsters' impulsivity, suicidality, and proneness to substance abuse. MAOIs should thus be considered only when other medications and forms of treatment have been ineffective, when the benefits warrant the risks, and when there is an adequate capacity to monitor the youngsters' compliance with dietary restrictions.

The introduction of selective and reversible MAOIs such as moclobemide and brofaromine has greatly increased interest in these agents and may offer safer alternatives for the treatment of affective dysregulation in children and adolescents. Other promising pharmacological approaches loom on the horizon. Of particular interest are corticotropin-releasing hormone Type I receptor antagonists, which may not only serve as novel antidepressants but also be particularly effective in correcting the hypothalamic–pituitary–adrenocortical (HPA) axis dysregulation, described in Chapter 4, that is present in affectively dysregulated and maltreated individuals (Holsboer, 1999; Kaufman et al., 1997).

The final step in the Texas Children's Medication Algorithm is electroconvulsive therapy (ECT), which is reserved for refractory youngsters whose symptoms have not improved and/or who suffer intolerable side effects but continue to experience serious and debilitating depression. This last-resort treatment is supported by good efficacy studies in adults (Fink, 1989; Prudic et al., 1996) and by open trials and clinical experience in children and adolescents (Cohen, Flament, Taieb, Thompson, & Basquin, 2000; Cohen, Taieb, et al., 2000; Duffett, Hill, & Lelliott, 1999).

Jay, described in Chapter 6, an example of a youngster with prominent borderline features who also demonstrates the signs of gender-identity confusion and depression, serves to illustrate the intertwining of psychotherapy and pharmacotherapy. When Jay entered treatment at age 6, he was started on an SSRI. He struggled with taking the medication because he feared it would poison him, control him, and reveal to everyone that he was defective. After 4 weeks, however, he was sleeping better. His appetite remained poor and he was still irritable. When lithium was added as an augmentation agent, marked improvement was subsequently noted in the boy's irritability.

At that point, Jay began individual psychotherapy. In therapy, he developed a repetitive play centering on Cinderella, Snow White, and Sleeping Beauty. Jay invariably played the role of the heroine, the beautiful yet tormented princess. Concerns about separation and loss slowly crept into the sessions. Jay initiated hide-and-seek games or pretended to be lost, challenging his therapist to find him. Increasingly, he became preoccupied with food and nurturance. He spoke of the medication as food that he pretended to share with his therapist. As he pretended to feed himself and the therapist with the "pills that helped him sleep," he also inquired about getting pregnant and pretended that his stuffed animals were pregnant.

Talking about pills that helped him sleep brought up the theme of Sleeping Beauty. The therapist helped Jay link the Sleeping Beauty fantasy both to his worries and fears of being left alone and to his resultant feeling of loneliness. Over several weeks, the therapist was able to show Jay how he became bossy and demanding when he thought he was going to be alone. Jay spontaneously linked these feelings to the memory of his dead mother. Without much assistance, he added a new element to the story themes of Snow White and Sleeping Beauty: If Snow White died but came back to life and Sleeping Beauty was not really dead but only sleeping, then perhaps his mother could also be brought to life. He would not have to feel little or helpless if he could become the mother—Sleeping Beauty, waiting to be awakened from her 100-year sleep. Perhaps his father would not have become depressed and left him if he could offer himself to his dad as a lovely princess to replace his dead mother.

At this point, 6 months after Jay's admission to the residential program, his father and stepmother decided to separate. Jay's father was also about to undergo surgery to repair an inguinal hernia. Jay became concerned that his father would again become depressed and unavailable, and he also worried intensely that his father might die during the surgery.

Jay became anxious, demanding, and provocative. Because of his readily apparent, intense anxiety, buspirone was added to the medication regimen. In the therapy sessions, Jay demanded absolute control over the therapist and their joint activities. He instructed the therapist to play a pregnant woman who was giving birth to twins, a boy and a girl. Jay played the role of a nurse or an obstetrician who removed the babies from the "mother" and then thwarted her efforts to hold them, care for them, and take them home. Instead, the babies were sent away to have surgery to remove their genitals or to amputate a limb. But the babies were kidnapped before the surgery. Jay then instructed the therapist to attempt to rescue the babies but made certain that the therapist's efforts would fail.

Jay responded to the therapist's comments about his anger and worry about possible abandonment with a request that the therapist feed a doll with a toy bottle. Jay then pretended to urinate on the therapist. "Squirt, squirt, pee on you!" yelled the boy, in a challenging display of anger that barely concealed his fear of retaliation. "It's okay to do that," responded the therapist. "Babies get very upset when they are left without someone to help them get food and to understand how they feel." With obvious relief and a mixture of glee and fury, Jay pretended to urinate and vomit on the therapist. Then the therapist commented: "The baby is angry at mom for leaving and angry at the babies who get food from their moms." Jay immediately shifted to become the baby himself and asked to be fed. He seemed to relax when the therapist offered him a cup of hot cocoa. Two months later, Jay was ready to continue treatment on an outpatient basis.

Algorithms for the Treatment of Impulsivity, Behavioral Dyscontrol, and Attention-Deficit/Hyperactivity Disorder

Impulsivity and behavioral dyscontrol plague these children's lives and strain their families' resources. In children who are made vulnerable by a proneness to hyperarousal, inattentiveness, or physiological hyper-reactivity, which are typically potentiated by maltreatment and trauma, they represent a prominent expression of the absence of the modulating influence afforded by reflective function.

The most dramatic manifestations of impulsivity and behavioral disinhibition in youngsters with personality disorders are also the clearest indications for pharmacotherapy: suicide attempts; parasuicidal behavior, including recurrent self-mutilation; or assaultiveness resulting from affective, impulsive aggression (Vitiello & Stoff, 1997). Reckless behavior, binge eating, sexual promiscuity, and abuse of drugs are also manifestations of impulsivity and disinhibition targeted by pharmacotherapy. These algorithms overlap with those presented for affective dysregulation because they likely share common aspects of underlying neurophysiological vulnerability reflected in the extensive comorbidity of Axis I disorders such as ADHD, anxiety disorders, mood disorders, and depression.

Controlled studies of adults with severe personality disorders suggest that SSRIs are the first choice for treatment of impulsivity and behavioral dyscontrol (Coccaro & Kavoussi, 1997; Salzman et al., 1995). There are no comparable studies of children and adolescents to support this recommendation.

A number of youngsters with severe personality disorders meet DSM-IV diagnostic criteria for ADHD. For these youngsters, a treatment algorithm such as that delineated in the Texas Children's Medication Algorithm Project (Pliszka et al., 2000a, 2000b) and the Multimodal

Treatment Study of Children with Attention-Deficit/Hyperactivity Disorder (MTA Cooperative Group, 1999a, 1999b; Swanson et al., 2001) offers a systematic approach to integrate available research information and expert clinical experience (see Figure 11.3).

The first line of treatment in the algorithm is a stimulant such as methylphenidate (MPH). Psychostimulants have consistently shown robust efficacy in more than 100 randomized controlled trials with children and adolescents with ADHD (Greenhill, Halperin, & Abikoff, 1999; Pliszka et al., 2000a, 2000b).

The effects of stimulants in the brain are complex. Preclinical studies have shown that the stimulants block the reuptake of dopamine (DA) and norepinephrine (NE) into the presynaptic neuron (Volkow et al., 1998) and the release of these neurotransmitters into the extraneuronal space (Spencer, Biederman, & Wilens, 2000). Alteration in dopaminergic and noradrenergic function appears necessary for clinical efficacy of the stimulants in the treatment of ADHD.

The stimulants bind to the DA transporter protein, with resultant inhibition of the DA reuptake presynaptically. A proposed model to explain the effects of stimulants in ADHD includes the inhibitory influence of frontal cortical activity, predominantly noradrenergic, acting on lower striatal structures related to direct DA agonists. In contrast, effects on serotonin metabolism seem only minimally related to the stimulant's clinical efficacy.

This model is consistent with the hypothesis discussed in Chapter 4 that the core deficit in ADHD is the impairment in the executive and gating functions of the prefrontal cortex, such as working memory (verbal and nonverbal) and affect regulation (Heilman et al., 1991; Pliszka et al., 1996). The disruption in the development of reflective function fits with this model.

The A_1A_2 allele (previously described in Chapter 4) may be a marker for low dopamine transporter binding, which may be related to the dysfunctions in executive function just described. This marker of low dopaminergic turnover, as pointed out, has been shown to be elevated in a number of problems that overlap significantly with severe personality disorders: alcoholism, gambling, substance abuse, and eating disorders. This marker is also seen in traumatized individuals who develop borderline personality disorder.

A more specific association with ADHD has been claimed for the DR D_4 receptor III exon polymorphism (LaHoste et al., 1996; Swanson

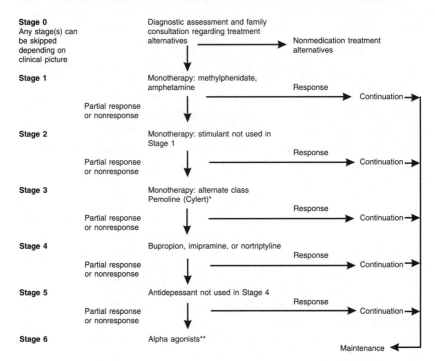

Stage 0
Any stage(s) can be skipped depending on clinical picture

Diagnostic assessment and family consultation regarding treatment alternatives → Nonmedication treatment alternatives

Stage 1
Monotherapy: methylphenidate, amphetamine
Response → Continuation →

Partial response or nonresponse

Stage 2
Monotherapy: stimulant not used in Stage 1
Response → Continuation →

Partial response or nonresponse

Stage 3
Monotherapy: alternate class Pemoline (Cylert)*
Response → Continuation →

Partial response or nonresponse

Stage 4
Bupropion, imipramine, or nortriptyline
Response → Continuation →

Partial response or nonresponse

Stage 5
Antidepessant not used in Stage 4
Response → Continuation →

Partial response or nonresponse

Stage 6
Alpha agonists**

Maintenance ←

*Plus liver function monitoring and substance abuse history.   **Cardiovascular side effects.

FIGURE 11.3. Texas Children's Medication Algorithm for ADHD (Pliszka et al., 2000b).

et al., 1998). This research supports choosing a stimulant as a first step in the treatment of ADHD with behavioral dyscontrol. There are no clinical predictors of which stimulant will produce the best results. MPH is preferred because it enjoys the largest clinical experience and number of citations in the literature. A large number of controlled studies document the efficacy of stimulants, particularly MPH, on the core features of ADHD (motor overactivity, impulsivity, and inattention) as well as on cognition, social function, and aggression (Spencer et al., 2000). Controlled studies also demonstrate continued effectiveness throughout adolescence and into adulthood (Spencer et al., 1996).

Stimulants have a striking impact on social skills and emotional functioning. They appear to "normalize" the understanding of peer communications, self-perception, and the ability to grasp social cues; that is, stimulants appear to facilitate the development of reflective function in youngsters who are otherwise compromised in this ability. Children with ADHD who are treated with stimulants show improved modulation of communication and an enhanced capacity to modulate their affect and behavior (Whalen, Henker, & Granger, 1990). These cognitive and behavioral changes, in turn, have a clear and well-documented positive impact in the children's environment (Cunningham, Siegel, & Offord, 1991; Whalen & Henker, 1992). Parents, teachers, siblings, and peers are more positive and less critical and rejecting of children with ADHD who have been so treated. These studies lend support to the concept of transactional processes in which the children's dysfunction shapes and reinforces family dysfunction, which in turn is shaped and reinforced by the family's responses.

A large number of controlled studies document the reduction in aggression and conduct disorder symptoms in children receiving stimulants (e.g., Amery, Minichiello, & Brown, 1984; Barkley, 1997a, 1997b; Barkley, McMurray, Edelbrock, & Robbins, 1989; Gadow, Nolan, Sverd, Sprafkin, & Paolicelli, 1990; Hinshaw, Heller, & McHale, 1992). In these and other studies, stimulants are shown to be effective in decreasing physical and verbal aggression both at home and in school, and also to have a positive effect on some covert antisocial behavior such as stealing and vandalism (but not on cheating).

The NIMH multisite, multimodal treatment study of children with ADHD (1992–1997) generated an MTA Psychopharmacology Treatment Manual (Arnold et al., 1997; MTA Cooperative Group, 1999a, 1999b) that provides guidelines for the length of washout period from previous medications, choice of the order in which drugs should be tried, ranges of starting doses and administration schedule, choice of rating forms, and target symptoms and algorithms for changing doses and drugs. The MTA's titration trial is quite complex and may not be suitable for ordinary office practice (Greenhill, 1998). Greenhill recommends dividing the dose into three parts, with the last one—a 4:00 P.M. dose— "sculpted" to equal at least half the noon and morning doses. The starting dose is 15 mg of MPH in three equal amounts. For smaller children (weighing less than 25 kg), the MTA protocol limits the highest dose of MPH to 15 mg/dose on a 15 mg—15 mg—5 mg schedule. Larger children (weighing over 25 kg) receive a maximum of 20 mg—20 mg—10 mg, for a total of 50 mg/day. The medication is increased every 3–4 days until children respond—or adverse effects prevent any further increases (Greenhill et al., 2001).

Common adverse effects of MPH tend to be mild, of short duration, or responsive to timing or dosage adjustments. They include appetite suppression and sleep disturbance, stomachache, headache, and dizziness. Sleep problems usually respond to lowering the late afternoon dose or to adding clonidine (Prince, Wilens, Biederman, Spencer, & Wozniak, 1996). Mild increases in blood pressure and heart rate have been described (Brown, Wynne, & Slimmer, 1984), but the significance of this report is unclear. Long-standing concerns about growth deficits in children receiving stimulants mandate that these youngsters' growth progression be monitored. Current evidence suggests that drug holidays are not needed in the absence of documented growth deficits (Spencer et al., 2000).

Stimulants are not associated with increased rates, severity, or persistence of tic disorder (Gadow, Sverd, Sprafkin, Nolan, & Ezor, 1995). Nonetheless, a longitudinal study of children with Tourette's syndrome and ADHD reports that 30% of the patients discontinued stimulant treatment because of a worsening of tics, which was attributed to the medication (Castellanos et al., 1997). Prudent practice warrants a careful weighing of risks and benefits, and a thorough discussion with the patient and family before prescribing stimulants to children with ADHD and tics, or a family history of tics.

Although stimulants can be abused—a particular concern with impulsive youngsters with personality disorder—current evidence indicates that treatment with stimulants actually reduces substantially the risk that children with ADHD will abuse drugs (Biederman, Wilens, Mick, Spencer, & Faraone, 1999). This evidence notwithstanding, adolescents with ADHD and severe personality disorder who are receiving stimulants require education and monitoring.

If a 2- to 4-week trial with MPH fails to produce results, current evidence suggests a trial with a different stimulant. The MTA study and the Texas Children's Algorithm for ADHD recommend switching first to dextroamphetamine, followed by a switch to pemoline, if necessary. This sequence is based on experience, preference for short-acting agents over longer acting ones, and a number of studies of safety and effectiveness (Safer, Zito, & Fine, 1996) rather than on evidence of superiority of one agent over another. Pemoline is associated with liver failure (Pliszka et al., 2000a, 2000b) and thus requires twice-monthly monitoring of liver function. Because of the risks and inconvenience, pemoline is recommended only for children with ADHD who fail to respond to trials of MPH and amphetamine.

If trials with stimulants are ineffective, a number of alternatives are available. Controlled studies demonstrate the effectiveness of tricyclic antidepressants with ADHD (e.g., Biederman, Baldessarini, Wright, Keenan, & Farone, 1993; Biederman, Baldessarini, Wright, Knee, & Harmatz, 1989). The secondary amines, desipramine and nortriptyline, are more selective for noradrenergic function and have fewer adverse effects. A large, controlled trial with desipramine reported that 68% of clinically referred children with ADHD were considered improved or very much improved (Biederman et al., 1989). Many of these children had previously failed to respond to stimulants. Studies of nortriptyline and desipramine have consistently shown a robust, positive response not only of ADHD symptoms but also of comorbid depression and anxiety (Biederman, Faraone, et al., 1993; Wilens & Biederman, 1993). These agents also appear effective in ADHD with comorbid tic symptoms (Spencer, Biederman, Kerman, Steingard, & Wilens, 1993; Spencer, Biederman, Wilens, Steingard, & Geist, 1993). Desipramine and nortriptyline are thus reasonable alternatives for children with a severe personality disorder and ADHD who fail to respond to stimulants, particularly if they also present symptoms of depression, anxiety, or tics.

The use of these drugs, however, has been limited by reports of sudden unexplained deaths in four children with ADHD treated with desipramine. The current view is that most of these deaths were due to preexisting cardiac conditions, such as hypertrophic cardiomyopathy. Biederman, Thisted, Greenhill, and Ryan (1995) estimate that the risk of sudden death associated with desipramine use in children may not be much greater than the baseline risk of sudden death in this age group. However, the panel of experts who developed the Texas Children's Medication Algorithm excluded desipramine because of the risk of sudden death (Pliszka et al., 2000a, 2000b). Prudent practice dictates careful cardiovascular assessment, including electrocardiogram and perhaps a consultation with a pediatric cardiologist as part of the evaluation of the risks and benefits of utilizing these drugs.

Other nontricyclic antidepressants appear promising and are perhaps safer alternatives for youngsters who do not respond to stimulants, and who have comorbid symptoms of depression, anxiety, or tics. In controlled studies, bupropion has been shown to be effective, safe, and well tolerated by children and adolescents with ADHD (Casat, Pleasants, & Van Wyck Fleet, 1987; Conners et al., 1996). Barrickman and colleagues (1995) reported that bupropion is equivalent to MPH in the treatment of children with ADHD. The slightly increased risk for bupropion-induced seizures has been linked to high doses, a previous history of seizures, and eating disorders (Spencer et al., 2000). Bupropion may be a particularly appropriate choice for children with affective dysregulation and ADHD. Other antidepressants also appear to be effective. Studies of venlafaxine in children with ADHD show promising results (Spencer et al., 2000). Encouraging findings have also been reported with tomoxetine (Spencer et al., 2000), a highly specific noradrenergic agent, in terms of both safety and effectiveness.

The final step in the ADHD algorithm is the addition of clonidine or other alpha noradrenergic agonists. Use of clonidine and guanfacine, noradrenergic agonists that have been widely used with children with ADHD and tics, is partially supported by a number of studies (Horrigan & Barnhill, 1995; Hunt, Minderaa, & Cohen, 1985; Steingard, Biederman, Spencer, Wilens, & Gonzalez, 1993; van der Meere, Gunning, & Stemerdink, 1999). These agents have also been used for the treatment of disruptive behavior and affective aggression (Hunt, 1987). Reports of deaths of children receiving clonidine plus other medications have raised concerns about its cardiovascular safety, particularly in combination with MPH. Many clinicians will therefore now use clonidine only when other drugs have failed.

The case of Larry, presented in Chapter 10, represents an example of the use of the ADHD algorithm. Larry, a distractible, impulsive, overactive child, responded favorably to MPH. However, he continued to have sleep problems and to display impulsive aggression, so clonidine was added to his regimen. The close monitoring available in a residential program allowed the use of the combination with a reasonable sense of safety.

Many youngsters with severe personality disorders show marked impulsivity and behavioral dyscontrol without meeting diagnostic criteria for ADHD, or, alternatively, they meet the criteria but respond only partially to the ADHD algorithm. For these youngsters, the first choice is SSRI antidepressants. The effects of SSRI antidepressants on impulsivity and behavioral dyscontrol appear to be independent of the effects on depression (Soloff, 1998). These effects are documented in controlled studies of adults with severe personality disorders (Coccaro & Kavoussi, 1997; Kavoussi, Liu, & Coccaro, 1994; Markovitz, 1995; Salzman et al., 1995) and seem to appear earlier than the effects on depression (Soloff, 1998).

Other agents should be considered for particular types of impulsive behavior. Clinically, clonidine appears to work most effectively with motorically impulsive and affectively aggressive children. Both the tablet and the transdermal preparation are equally effective. The oral preparation has the disadvantage of requiring multiple doses, while the transdermal form is not tolerated by some children. A low dose (0.5–1.5 mg) of clonidine can help overaroused children such as Larry, who have difficulty falling asleep at night (Prince et al., 1996).

In the event of partial response to SSRI antidepressants, or when there is an urgent clinical need (e.g., dangerous destructive or self-destructive behavior), low-dose antipsychotics are indicated. These medications have demonstrated effectiveness in reducing impulsivity and behavioral dyscontrol in patients with severe personality disorders (Soloff, 1998). Low-dose neuroleptics, such as haloperidol (2–5 mg intramuscularly, if needed), can provide rapid control over escalating impulsive aggression or self-destructiveness. Because of the risk of extrapyramidal symptoms and tardive dyskinesia, many child and adolescent clinicians now prefer atypical neuroleptics as first-line agents.

A specific form of behavioral dyscontrol, bulimia nervosa, typically develops in older adolescents and young adults. It is frequently associated with severe personality disorder, mainly borderline personality. The disordered and impulsive binge eating, followed by vomiting and purging, that is characteristic of bulimia nervosa responds to SSRI antidepressants (Fairburn, 1995, 1997; Fichter et al., 1991). The high comorbidity of bulimia nervosa with mood disorders provided the stimulus to use these agents in individuals with bulimia nervosa. Yet improvements in out-of-control eating, vomiting, and purging with antidepressants are observed equally in depressed or nondepressed individuals with bulimia nervosa.

Despite significant symptomatic improvement, patients with bulimia nervosa rarely reach complete remission with medication alone. Nearly half the patients just on medication will relapse after 3–4 months (Casper, 2000). Case reports and controlled studies show that various forms of psychotherapy—group, cognitive-behavioral, and family—can be as effective as, or more effective than, medication (Carter & Fairburn, 1998; Mitchell et al., 1993). These and other studies suggest that long-term improvement requires psychological and family interventions.

If there is no response with an SSRI antidepressant, a trial with a second SSRI or an alternative antidepressant, such as venlafaxine, may be considered. This "salvage" strategy (Soloff, 1998) is based solely on clinical experience. A second alternative, better supported by controlled studies, is the addition of lithium, which arguably can augment the effects of the SSRI antidepressant on impulsivity and behavioral dyscontrol (Sheard, 1975). When impulsivity and dyscontrol persist after a 4- to 6-week trial with these medications, the clinician should consider following the algorithm for bipolar disorder, which calls for the addition of divalproex sodium and, in case of no response or partial response, the subsequent addition of carbamazepine (as previously described). This proposed sequence is largely supported by clinical experience and some preliminary reports in adults (Hollander, 1999). Finally, a trial with clozapine should be considered as a last resort.

One group of borderline youngsters presents a particular treatment challenge: those who recurrently engage in self-injurious behavior. Their internal experience is a build-up of tension, an inchoate dysphoria that can be relieved only by self-cutting. The self-destructive act is generally not painful and serves to terminate the state of dysphoria (Roth et al., 1996). The first step in the pharmacological treatment of these youngsters is SSRIs. When self-mutilation and related parasuicidal behavior fail to respond to SSRI antidepressants, an alternative to the addition of mood stabilizers is a trial with naltrexone, a long-acting opiate antagonist that can block the "reward" of enhanced exogenous and endogenous opioids triggered by self-destructive behavior.

Roth and colleagues (1996) reported on an open-label trial of 50 mg/day naltrexone for seven women with borderline personality disorder and self-mutilating behavior. In this trial, six of the seven patients completely eliminated their self-injurious behavior within 10 weeks. The evidence supporting the use of naltrexone for self-mutilation is limited. Nonetheless, it is compelling to consider that a neurochemical abnormality underlying self-mutilating behavior in patients with severe personality disorders creates a need for supernormal levels of endorphins to deal with stress (Roth et al., 1996). By blocking endorphin receptors, naltrexone prevents the analgesia that often accompanies self-mutilation and the relief of dysphoria that follows.

An additional compelling argument for the use of naltrexone is its well-demonstrated effectiveness in helping patients to avoid relapsing into alcohol abuse. Youngsters with a severe personality disorder and self-mutilation also frequently present with substance abuse, perhaps reflecting their limited capacity to manage stress without hypernormal levels of endorphins, which are stimulated by alcohol (Volpicelli, Davis, & Olgin, 1986). In clinical practice, the association of self-mutilation and substance abuse in youngsters with severe personality disorders makes naltrexone a logical choice for patients with this combination of problems (Links, Heslegrave, & Villella, 1998).

Naltrexone is one of the most promising agents in the treatment of substance abuse, whether or not it is associated with self-mutilation. Volpicelli, Volpicelli, and O'Brien (1995), in a controlled study of 70 patients addicted to alcohol, demonstrated that naltrexone significantly reduced relapse rates and the number of drinks per day. O'Malley and colleagues (1992) obtained similar results with a group of alcohol-dependent individuals. Despite these favorable results and FDA approval for its use to prevent relapse, naltrexone is not widely used in clinical practice.

Newer opiate antagonists may offer additional options for addressing this crucial aspect of the dysfunction of youngsters with personality disorders. Among the most promising agents, nalmefene has been successful in small, controlled studies with alcohol-dependent individuals (Mason et al., 1994), and calcium acetylhomotaurinate has shown considerable effectiveness in both animal studies and in controlled studies with human subjects (Lhuintre et al., 1985; Sass, Soyka, Mann, & Zieglgansberger, 1996).

PRACTICAL CONSIDERATIONS

One important practical consideration is the decision about whether one clinician will be responsible for both medication management and psychosocial treatment, or if these roles will be divided among two or more clinicians. Gabbard (2000) discusses the relative advantages and complications of what he calls the "one-person" versus the "two-person" model. As Gabbard points out, psychiatrists have particular advantages in integrating the biological, psychological, and social aspects of the treatment of severe personality disorders. For child and adolescent psychiatrists who are both trained and able to work in pharmacological and psychosocial modalities, the "one-person model" offers definite advantages.

One advantage is that the fragmentation and splitting that can be expected in the treatment of youngsters with severe personality disorders may be decreased when a single clinician is involved in all aspects of the treatment. A particular problem that is perhaps better addressed by a single clinician is the high rate of treatment dropout. More than 50% of patients with borderline personality disorder interrupt treatment before it is completed (Links, Steiner, Boiago, & Irwin, 1990). Although there are no empirical data about dropout rates in the treatment of children and adolescents with severe personality disorders, there is considerable face validity to support the notion that such rates run very high. A single clinician may decrease dropout by integrating every aspect of treatment, by minimizing chances of things "falling into the cracks," and by assuring that each modality potentiates the others and strengthens the overall treatment alliance with the youngsters and their families.

An example of how one modality reinforces the others is when clinicians take advantage of the frequent idealization of the medication often observed early in treatment, as was the case with Larry and Jay. The medication can become imbued with soothing and comforting properties that can serve as an alternative to more maladaptive ways of responding to stress. Eventually, medication may serve as a substitute for the therapist at times of separation or frustration. The magical expectation placed on the medication almost inevitably leads to bitter disappointment and often to an urgent demand for a new magic pill. The single therapist/pharmacologist is optimally positioned to find the right balance between allowing patients to benefit from the "magic" of the idealized medication while helping them to regain reflective function when disappointment and frustration ensue.

Gabbard (2000) points out that when physicians are both conducting psychotherapy and managing medications, they must shift back and forth between an empathic–subjective approach and a more objective–descriptive stance. Going back and forth between these two levels implicitly emphasizes a basic premise of symbolic–reflective functioning: the multiplicity of meanings and roles that are part of human relationships and the flexibility needed to respond appropriately. Along these lines, when acting in a "therapist" mode, the clinician may encourage the patient to talk and reflect on the meaning of a particular exchange. On the other hand, in a "medication management" mode, the clinician may give information about adverse effects and instruct patients about expected therapeutic results.

In practice, however, the roles of therapist and medication manager are often divided. Many child and adolescent psychiatrists are not adequately skilled as psychotherapists or, if they have devoted themselves primarily to psychosocial interventions, they are insufficiently experienced in the use of the latest medications. Obviously, in cases where the primary clinician is not a physician, a referral to a child and adolescent psychiatrist is mandatory. Managed care providers often require this arrangement by stipulating that psychotherapy must be conducted by a less expensive, nonmedical clinician.

Such a division of labor offers some advantages (Waldinger & Frank, 1989a, 1989b). Clinicians can consult with one another, which is often helpful to lessen the impact of nonreflective, coercive exchanges with the youngsters and their caregivers. The very intensity of these exchanges can be diluted by having two treaters, which can facilitate the rescue of reflective function from the throes of unreflective, coercive modes of operation that are mobilized by vulnerability and stress. Observing clinicians who can integrate their perspectives while retaining their individuality offer patients and caregivers a model of how it is possible to bring coherence to their internal fragmentation and to connect with others, resolve differences, and share a common direction without sacrificing one's distinctive voice and identity.

At the same time, the two-person model is also fraught with potential pitfalls. First, as Gabbard (2000) argues, it is a setup for problems involving splitting. In a pointed clinical vignette, Gabbard illustrates how the two-clinician model can become an arena where the patient— or the caregiver, in the case of children and adolescents—pits one treater against the other, undermining their effectiveness and derailing a treatment process that challenges the patient's internal and interpersonal adjustment.

Splitting is bound to be exacerbated by the difficulties that busy clinicians have in finding the time to communicate, share their individual perspectives, integrate their views with other clinicians, and coordinate their actions in a coherent plan. Finding the time to communicate and consult is made more problematic by the fact that these efforts are not generally reimbursed by third-party payers.

YOGI, COMMISSAR, AND ALCHEMIST

The usefulness of medication as an integral component of the treatment of youngsters with severe personality disorders reflects the complex interaction among genetic predisposition, neurobiological vulnerability, and environmental forces, mediated by processing mechanisms such as reflective function. Treatment marshals these same sets of factors to create the conditions in which youngsters and their families can set in motion the representational and regulating processes that can alter or moderate both environmental and genetic effects. When impulsive youngsters with ADHD receive MPH, for example, functional magnetic resonance imaging (MRI) studies show an admittedly preliminary finding of improved frontostriatal function and response inhibition (Vaidya et al., 1998). Children's improvement, in turn, changes the quality of caregivers' and peers' responses, and reduces the risk of substance abuse (Buhrmester, Whalen, Henker, MacDonald, & Hinshaw, 1992; Cunningham et al., 1991; Whalen & Henker, 1992). These children and their caregivers are in a better position to develop the reflective capacities that, in turn, will further modify the environment and perhaps the triggering of the very genes underlying a disposition to develop severe personality disorders. Indeed, this biopsychosocial model of treatment calls for an integration of the perspectives of the neurobiological–genetic pharmacologist, the environmental–contextual family systems therapist, and the intrapsychic psychotherapist. Yogis, commissars, and alchemists come together to generate the optimal therapeutic outcome.

As youngsters acquire the interpersonal and mental mechanisms for holding on to other people's attention and for getting across something about their internal status, their automatic propensity to inhibit reflective function and to move into a fight-or-flight mode of unreflectiveness and coercion begins to lessen. As it does, they slowly make the momentous discovery that their experience is not only distinctly their own but also part of what can be shared with other human beings.

References

Adelson, J., & Doehrman, M. J. (1980). The psychodynamic approach to adolescence. In J. Adelson (Ed.), *Handbook of adolescent psychology* (pp. 99–116). New York: Wiley.

Adkins, S. L., Safier, E. J., & Parker, N. N. (1998). Evolution of wraparound services at the Menninger Clinic. *Bulletin of the Menninger Clinic, 62,* 243–255.

Adler, G. (1985). *Borderline psychopathology and its treatment.* New York: Aronson.

Agras, W. S., Schneider, J. A., Arnow, B., Raeburn, S., & Telch, C. F. (1989). Cognitive-behavioral and response–prevention treatments for bulimia nervosa. *Journal of Consulting and Clinical Psychology, 57,* 215–221.

Aichhorn, A. (1935). *Wayward youth.* New York: Viking Press.

Ainsworth, M. D. S., & Bell, S. M. (1974). Mother–infant interaction and the development of competence. In J. Bruner & K. Connolly (Eds.), *The growth of competence* (pp. 97–118). New York: Academic Press.

Ainsworth, M. D. S., Bell, S. M. V., & Stayton, D. J. (1971). Individual differences in Strange-Situation behaviour of one-year-olds. In H. R. Schaffer (Ed.), *The origins of human social relations* (pp. 17–57). New York: Academic Press.

Ainsworth, M. D. S., Blehar, M. C., Waters, E., & Wall, S. (1978). *Patterns of attachment: A psychological study of the Strange Situation.* Hillsdale, NJ: Erlbaum.

Akhtar, S. (1992). *Broken structures: Severe personality disorders and their treatment.* Northvale, NJ: Aronson.

Akiskal, H. S. (1981). Subaffective disorders: Dysthymic, cyclothymic and bipolar II disorders in the "borderline" realm. *Psychiatric Clinics of North America, 4,* 25–46.

Allen, J. G. (2001). *Traumatic relationships and serious mental disorders.* Chichester, UK: Wiley.

Allen, J. G., Gabbard, G. O., Newsom, G., & Coyne, L. (1990). Detecting patterns of change in patients' collaboration within individual psychotherapy sessions. *Psychotherapy: Theory, Research, Practice, Training, 27,* 522–530.

Altshuler, L. L., Cohen, L., Szuba, M. P., Burt, V. K., Gitlin, M., & Mintz, J. (1996).

Pharmacologic management of psychiatric illness during pregnancy: Dilemmas and guidelines. *American Journal of Psychiatry, 153,* 592–606.

Alvarez, A. (1992). *Live company: Psychoanalytic psychotherapy with autistic, borderline, deprived, and abused children.* New York: Routledge.

Ambrosini, P. J., Wagner, K. D., Biederman, J., Glick, I., Tan, C., Elia, J., Hebeler, J. R., Rabinovich, H., Lock, J., & Geller, D. (1999). Multicenter open-label sertraline study in adolescent outpatients with major depression. *Journal of the American Academy of Child and Adolescent Psychiatry, 38,* 566–572.

American Psychiatric Association. (1980). *Diagnostic and statistical manual of mental disorders* (3rd ed.). Washington, DC: Author.

American Psychiatric Association. (1987). *Diagnostic and statistical manual of mental disorders* (3rd ed., rev.). Washington, DC: Author.

American Psychiatric Association. (1994). *Diagnostic and statistical manual of mental disorders* (4th ed.). Washington, DC: Author.

Amery, B., Minichiello, M. D., & Brown, G. L. (1984). Aggression in hyperactive boys: Response to d-amphetamine. *Journal of the American Academy of Child Psychiatry, 23,* 291–294.

Anan, R. M., & Barnett, D. (1999). Perceived social support mediates between prior attachment and subsequent adjustment: A study of urban African-American children. *Developmental Psychology, 35,* 1210–1222.

Andrulonis, P. A. (1991). Disruptive behavior disorders in boys and the borderline personality disorder in men. *Annals of Clinical Psychiatry, 3,* 23–26.

Anthony, E. J. (1982). Normal adolescent development from a cognitive viewpoint. *Journal of the American Academy of Child Psychiatry, 21,* 318–327.

Apter, A., Fallon, T. J., Jr., King, R. A., Ratzoni, G., Zohar, A. H., Binder, M., Weizman, A., Leckman, J. F., Pauls, D. L., Kron, S., & Cohen, D. J. (1996). Obsessive–compulsive characteristics: From symptoms to syndrome. *Journal of the American Academy of Child and Adolescent Psychiatry, 35,* 907–912.

Apter, A., Ratzoni, G., King, R. A., Weizman, A., Iancu, I., Binder, M., & Riddle, M. A. (1994). Fluvoxamine open-label treatment of adolescent inpatients with obsessive–compulsive disorder or depression. *Journal of the American Academy of Child and Adolescent Psychiatry, 33,* 342–348.

Arendt, H. (1994). *Eichmann in Jerusalem: A report on the banality of evil.* New York: Peter Smith.

Arnold, L. E., Abikoff, H. B., Cantwell, D. P., Conners, C. K., Elliott, G., Greenhill, L. L., Hechtman, L., Hinshaw, S. P., Hoza, B., Jensen, P. S., Kraemer, H. C., March, J. S., Newcorn, J. H., Pelham, W. E., Richters, J. E., Schiller, E., Severe, J. B., Swanson, J. M., Vereen, D., & Wells, K. C. (1997). National Institute of Mental Health Collaborative Multimodal Treatment Study of Children with ADHD (the MTA): Design challenges and choices. *Archives of General Psychiatry, 54,* 865–870.

Astington, J. W., & Jenkins, J. M. (1995). Theory of mind development and social understanding. *Cognition and Emotion, 9,* 151–165.

Axelson, A. A. (1997). Alternative treatment services for children and adolescents. In R. K. Schreter, S. S. Sharfstein, & C. A. Schreter (Eds.), *Managing care, not dollars: The continuum of mental health services* (pp. 151–176). Washington, DC: American Psychiatric Press.

Baden, A. D., & Howe, G. W. (1992). Mothers' attributions and expectancies regarding their conduct-disordered children. *Journal of Abnormal Child Psychology, 20,* 467–485.

Bahrick, L. R., & Watson, J. S. (1985). Detection of intermodal proprioceptive–visual contingency as a potential basis of self-perception in infancy. *Developmental Psychology, 21,* 963–973.

Baldwin, A. L., Baldwin, C., & Cole, R. E. (1990). Stress-resistant families and stress-resistant children. In J. E. Rolf, A. S. Masten, D. Cicchetti, K. H. Nuechterlein, & S. Weintraub (Eds.), *Risk and protective factors in the development of psychopathology* (pp. 257–280). New York: Cambridge University Press.

Bank, L., Marlowe, J. H., Reid, J. B., Patterson, G. R., & Weinrott, M. R. (1991). A comparative evaluation of parent-training interventions for families of chronic delinquents. *Journal of Abnormal Child Psychology, 19,* 15–33.

Barkley, R. A. (1997a). Behavioral inhibition, sustained attention, and executive functions: Constructing a unifying theory of ADHD. *Psychological Bulletin, 121,* 65–94.

Barkley, R. A. (1997b). *ADHD and the nature of self-control.* New York: Guilford Press.

Barkley, R. A., McMurray, M. B., Edelbrock, C. S., & Robbins, K. (1989). The response of aggressive and nonaggressive ADHD children to two doses of methylphenidate. *Journal of the American Academy of Child and Adolescent Psychiatry, 28,* 873–881.

Baron-Cohen, S. (1994). How to build a baby that can read minds: Cognitive mechanisms in mind reading. *Cahiers de Psychologie Cognitive [Current Psychology of Cognition], 13,* 513–552.

Baron-Cohen, S., & Swettenham, J. (1996). The relationship between SAM and ToMM: Two hypotheses. In P. Carruthers & P. K. Smith (Eds.), *Theories of theories of mind* (pp. 158–168). Cambridge, MA: Cambridge University Press.

Baron-Cohen, S., Tooby, J., & Cosmides, L. (1995). *Mindblindness: An essay on autism and theory of mind.* Cambridge, MA: Bradford, MIT Press.

Barrickman, L. L., Perry, P. J., Allen, A. J., Kuperman, S., Arndt, S. V., Herrmann, K. J., & Schumacher, E. (1995). Bupropion versus methylphenidate in the treatment of attention-deficit hyperactivity disorder. *Journal of the American Academy of Child and Adolescent Psychiatry, 34,* 649–657.

Barrnett, R. J., Docherty, J. P., & Frommelt, G. M. (1991). A review of child psychotherapy research since 1963. *Journal of the American Academy of Child and Adolescent Psychiatry 30,* 1–14.

Bateman, A., & Fonagy, P. (1999). Effectiveness of partial hospitalization in the treatment of borderline personality disorder: A randomized controlled trial. *American Journal of Psychiatry, 156,* 1563–1569.

Bateman, A. W. (1998). Thick- and thin-skinned organisations and enactment in borderline and narcissistic disorders. *International Journal of Psycho-Analysis, 79,* 13–25.

Battagliola, M. (1994, June). Breaking with tradition. *Business and Health, 12*(6), 53–54, 56.

Beebe, B., Jaffe, J., & Lachmann, F. M. (1992). A dyadic systems view of communication. In N. J. Skolnick & S. C. Warshaw (Eds.), *Relational perspectives in psychoanalysis* (pp. 61–81). Hillsdale, NJ: Analytic Press.

Beebe, B., & Lachmann, F. M. (1988). The contribution of mother–infant mutual influence to the origins of self- and object representations. *Psychoanalytic Psychology, 5,* 305–337.

Beeghly, M., & Cicchetti, D. (1994). Child maltreatment, attachment, and the self system: Emergence of an internal state lexicon in toddlers at high social risk. *Development and Psychopathology, 6,* 5–30.

Behar, L. (1990). Financing mental health services for children and adolescents. *Bulletin of the Menninger Clinic, 54,* 127–139.

Bemporad, J. R., Smith, H. F., Hanson, G., & Cicchetti, D. (1982). Borderline syndromes in childhood: Criteria for diagnosis. *American Journal of Psychiatry, 139,* 596–602.

Beren, P. (1992). Narcissistic disorders. *Psychoanalytic Study of the Child, 47,* 265–278.

Berman, S. M., & Noble, E. P. (1997). The D_2 dopamine receptor (DRD_2) gene and family stress: Interactive effects on cognitive functions in children. *Behavior Genetics, 27,* 33–43.

Bettelheim, B., & Sylvester, E. (1948). A therapeutic milieu. *American Journal of Orthopsychiatry, 18,* 191–206.

Biederman, J., Baldessarini, R. J., Wright, V., Keenan, K., & Faraone, S. (1993). A double-blind placebo controlled study of desipramine in the treatment of ADD: III. Lack of impact of comorbidity and family history factors on clinical response. *Journal of the American Academy of Child and Adolescent Psychiatry, 32,* 199–204.

Biederman, J., Baldessarini, R. J., Wright, V., Knee, D., & Harmatz, J. S. (1989). A double-blind placebo controlled study of desipramine in the treatment of ADD: I. Efficacy. *Journal of the American Academy of Child and Adolescent Psychiatry, 28,* 777–784.

Biederman, J., Faraone, S. V., Spencer, T., Wilens, T., Norman, D., Lapey, K. A., Mick, E., Lehman, B. K., & Doyle, A. (1993). Patterns of psychiatric comorbidity, cognition, and psychosocial functioning in adults with attention deficit hyperactivity disorder. *American Journal of Psychiatry, 150,* 1792–1798.

Biederman, J., Rosenbaum, J. F., Hirshfeld, D. R., Faraone, S. V., Bolduc, E. A., Gersten, M., Meminger, S. R., Kagan, J., Snidman, N., & Reznick, J. S. (1990). Psychiatric correlates of behavioral inhibition in young children of parents with and without psychiatric disorders. *Archives of General Psychiatry, 47,* 21–26.

Biederman, J., Thisted, R. A., Greenhill, L. L., & Ryan, N. D. (1995). Estimation of the association between desipramine and the risk for sudden death in 5- to 14-year-old children. *Journal of Clinical Psychiatry, 56,* 87–93.

Biederman, J., Wilens, T., Mick, E., Spencer, T., Faraone, S. V. (1999). Pharmacotherapy of attention-deficit/hyperactivity disorder reduces risk for substance use disorder [Editorial]. *Pediatrics, 104,* 20.

Bierman, K. L. (1989). Improving the peer relationships of rejected children. In B. B. Lahey & A. E. Kazdin (Eds.), *Advances in clinical child psychology* (Vol. 12, pp. 53–84). New York: Plenum Press.

Bigelow, A. E. (1998). Infants' sensitivity to familiar imperfect contingencies in social interaction. *Infant Behavior and Development, 21,* 149–161.

Bion, W. R. (1959). Attacks on linking. *International Journal of Psycho-Analysis, 40,* 308–315.

Bion, W. R. (1962). *Learning from experience.* New York: Basic Books.

Birmaher, B., Ryan, N. D., Williamson, D. E., Brent, D. A., & Kaufman, J. (1996). Childhood and adolescent depression: A review of the past 10 years. Part II. *Journal of the American Academy of Child and Adolescent Psychiatry, 35,* 1575–1583.

Bleiberg, E. (1984). Narcissistic disorders in children: A developmental approach to diagnosis. *Bulletin of the Menninger Clinic, 48,* 501–517.

Bleiberg, E. (1988). Developmental pathogenesis of narcissistic disorders in children. *Bulletin of the Menninger Clinic, 52,* 3–15.

Bleiberg, E. (1994). Normal and pathological narcissism in adolescence. *American Journal of Psychotherapy, 48,* 30–51.

Block, J. H., & Block, J. (1980). The role of ego-control and ego-resiliency in the organization of behavior. In W. A. Collins (Ed.), *Development of cognition, affect, and social relations: The Minnesota Symposia on Child Psychology* (Vol. 13, pp. 39–101). Hillsdale, NJ: Erlbaum.

Blos, P. (1967). The second individuation process of adolescence. *Psychoanalytic Study of the Child, 22,* 162–186.

Blum, K., Braverman, E. R., Wood, R. C., Gill, J., Li, C., Chen, T. J., Taub, M., Montgomery, A. R., Sheridan, P. J., & Cull, J. G. (1996). Increased prevalence of the Taq I A$_1$ allele of the dopamine receptor gene (DRD$_2$) in obesity with comorbid substance use disorder: A preliminary report. *Pharmacogenetics, 6,* 297–305.

Booth, C. L., Rubin, K. H., & Rose-Krasnor, L. (1998). Perceptions of emotional support from mother and friend in middle childhood: Links with social–emotional adaptation and preschool attachment security. *Child Development, 69,* 427–442.

Bower, G. H., & Sievers, H. (1998). Cognitive impact of traumatic events. *Development and Psychopathology, 10,* 625–654.

Bowlby, J. (1951). *Maternal care and mental health* (WHO Monograph Series, No. 2). Geneva: World Health Organization.

Bowlby, J. (1969). *Attachment and loss: Vol. 1. Attachment.* New York: Basic Books.

Bowlby, J. (1973). *Attachment and loss: Vol. 2. Separation: Anxiety and anger.* New York: Basic Books.

Bowlby, J. (1980). *Attachment and loss: Vol. 3. Loss: Sadness and depression.* New York: Basic Books.

Branscomb, L. (1991). Dissociation in combat-related post-traumatic stress disorder. *Dissociation, 4,* 13–20.

Braun, B. G., & Sacks, R. G. (1985). The development of multiple personality disorder: Predisposing, precipitating, and perpetuating factors. In R. P. Kluft (Ed.),

Childhood antecedents of multiple personality (pp. 38–65). Washington, DC: American Psychiatric Press.

Brazelton, T. B., Koslowski, B., & Main, M. (1974). The origins of reciprocity: The early mother–infant interaction. In M. Lewis & L. A. Rosenblum (Eds.), *The effect of the infant on its caregiver* (pp. 49–76). New York: Wiley.

Bremner, J. D., & Narayan, M. (1998). The effects of stress on memory and the hippocampus throughout the life cycle: Implications for childhood development and aging. *Development and Psychopathology, 10,* 871–885.

Bremner, J. D., Randall, P., Vermetten, E., Staib, L., Bronen, R. A., Mazure, C., Capelli, S., McCarthy, G., Innis, R. B., & Charney, D. S. (1997). Magnetic resonance imaging–based measurement of hippocampal volume in posttraumatic stress disorder related to childhood physical and sexual abuse: A preliminary report. *Biological Psychiatry, 41,* 23–32.

Brennan, P. A., Mednick, S. A., & Jacobsen, B. (1996). Assessing the role of genetics in crime using adoption cohorts. In G. R. Bock & J. A. Goode (Eds.), *Genetics of criminal and antisocial behaviour* (CIBA Foundation Symposium 194, pp. 115–128). Chichester, UK: Wiley.

Bretherton, I. (1991). Pouring new wine into old bottles: The social self as internal working model. In M. R. Gunnar & L. A. Sroufe (Eds.), *Self processes and development: The Minnesota Symposia on Child Psychology* (Vol. 23, pp. 1–41). Hillsdale, NJ: Erlbaum.

Bretherton, I., Bates, E., Benigni, L., Camaioni, L., & Volterra, V. (1979). Relationships between cognition, communication, and quality of attachment. In E. Bates (with L. Benigni, I. Bretherton, L. Camaioni, & V. Volterra, Eds.), *The emergence of symbols: Cognition and communication in infancy* (pp. 223–269). New York: Academic Press.

Breuer, J., & Freud, S. (1955). Studies on hysteria. In J. Strachey (Ed. & Trans.), *The standard edition of the complete psychological works of Sigmund Freud* (Vol. II, pp. 1–311). London: Hogarth Press. (Original work published 1893–1895)

Briere, J., & Runtz, M. (1988). Symptomatology associated with childhood sexual victimization in a nonclinical adult sample. *Child Abuse and Neglect, 12,* 51–59.

Brinich, P. M. (1980). Some potential effects of adoption on self and object representations. *Psychoanalytic Study of the Child, 35,* 107–133.

Britton, R. (1989). The missing link: Parental sexuality in the Oedipus complex. In R. Britton, M. Feldman, & E. O'Shaughnessy, *The Oedipus complex today: Clinical implications* (J. Steiner, Ed.; pp. 83–102). London: Karnac Books.

Britton, R. (1992). The Oedipus situation and the depressive position. In R. Anderson (Ed.), *Clinical lectures on Klein and Bion* (pp. 34–45). New York: Tavistock/Routledge.

Brown, G. M., Pulido, O., Grota, L. J., & Niles, L. P. (1984). N-acetylserotonin in the central nervous system. *Progress in Neuro-Psychopharmacology and Biological Psychiatry, 8,* 475–480.

Brown, R. T., Wynne, M. E., & Slimmer, L. W. (1984). Attention deficit disorder and the effect of methylphenidate on attention, behavioral, and cardiovascular functioning. *Journal of Clinical Psychiatry, 45,* 473–476.

Bruner, J. S. (1990). *Acts of meaning: Four lectures on mind and culture.* Cambridge, MA: Harvard University Press.

Bruner, J. S. (with Watson, R.). (1983). *Child's talk: Learning to use language.* Oxford, UK: Oxford University Press.

Buhrmester, D., Whalen, C. K., Henker, B., MacDonald, V., & Hinshaw, S. P. (1992). Prosocial behavior in hyperactive boys: Effects of stimulant medication and comparison with normal boys. *Journal of Abnormal Child Psychology, 20,* 103–121.

Cafferty, H., & Leichtman, M. (1999). Facilitating the transition from residential treatment into the community: II. Changing social work roles. In C. Waller (Ed.), *Contributions to residential treatment 1999* (pp. 88–97). Washington, DC: American Association of Children's Residential Centers.

Cain, A. C. (1964). On the meaning of "playing crazy" in borderline children. *Psychiatry, 27,* 278–289.

Calabrese, J. R., Rapport, D. J., Kimmel, S. E., Reese, B., & Woyshville, M. J. (1993). Rapid cycling bipolar disorder and its treatment with valproate. *Canadian Journal of Psychiatry, 38*(Suppl. 2), S57–S61.

Campbell, M., Adams, P. B., Small, A. M., Kafantaris, V., Silva, R. R., Shell, J., Perry, R., & Overall, J. E. (1995). Lithium in hospitalized aggressive children with conduct disorder: A double-blind and placebo-controlled study. *Journal of the American Academy of Child and Adolescent Psychiatry, 34,* 445–453.

Campos, J. J., & Stenberg, C. (1981). Perception, appraisal, and emotion: The onset of social referencing. In M. E. Lamb & L. A. Sherrod (Eds.), *Infant social cognition: Empirical and theoretical considerations* (pp. 273–314). Hillsdale, NJ: Erlbaum.

Cantwell, D. P. (1981). Hyperactivity and antisocial behavior revisited: A critical review of the literature. In D. O. Lewis (Ed.), *Vulnerabilities to delinquency* (pp. 21–38). New York: SP Medical & Scientific Books.

Carlson, E. A., & Sroufe, L. A. (1995). Contribution of attachment theory to developmental psychopathology. In D. Cicchetti & D. J. Cohen (Eds.), *Developmental psychopathology* (pp. 581–617). New York: Wiley.

Carlson, G. A., Rapport, M. D., Pataki, C. S., & Kelly, K. L. (1992). Lithium in hospitalized children at 4 and 8 weeks: Mood, behavior and cognitive effects. *Journal of Child Psychology and Psychiatry and Allied Disciplines, 33,* 411–425.

Carpy, D. V. (1989). Tolerating the countertransference: A mutative process. *International Journal of Psycho-Analysis, 70,* 287–294.

Carter, J. C., & Fairburn, C. G. (1998). Cognitive-behavioral self-help for binge eating disorder: A controlled effectiveness study. *Journal of Consulting and Clinical Psychology, 66,* 616–623.

Casat, C. D., Pleasants, D. Z., & Van Wyck Fleet, J. (1987). A double-blind trial of bupropion in children with attention deficit disorder. *Psychopharmacology Bulletin, 23,* 120–122.

Casper, R. C. (2000). Update on the treatment of eating disorders. *Psychiatric Clinics of North America: Annual of Drug Therapy, 1,* 219–234.

Castellanos, F. X., Giedd, J. N., Elia, J., Marsh, W. L., Ritchie, G. F., Hamburger, S. D., & Rapoport, J. L. (1997). Controlled stimulant treatment of ADHD and comorbid Tourette's syndrome: Effects of stimulant and dose. *Journal of the American Academy of Child and Adolescent Psychiatry, 36,* 589–596.

Chethik, M., & Fast, I. (1970). A function of fantasy in the borderline child. *American Journal of Orthopsychiatry, 40,* 756–765.

Christiansen, K. O. (1977). A review of studies of criminality among twins. In S. A. Mednick & K. O. Christiansen (Eds.), *Biosocial bases of criminal behavior* (pp. 89–108). New York: Gardner Press.

Chu, J. A. (1998). *Rebuilding shattered lives: The responsible treatment of complex post-traumatic and dissociative disorders.* New York: Wiley.

Chu, J. A., & Dill, D. L. (1990). Dissociative symptoms in relation to childhood physical and sexual abuse. *American Journal of Psychiatry, 147,* 887–892.

Cicchetti, D., & Cohen, D. (Eds.). (1995). *Developmental psychopathology.* New York: Wiley.

Cicchetti, D., & Rogosch, F. A. (1997). The role of self-organization in the promotion of resilience in maltreated children. *Development and Psychopathology, 9,* 797–815.

Cicchetti, D., & Toth, S. L. (1995). A developmental psychopathology perspective on child abuse and neglect. *Journal of the American Academy of Child and Adolescent Psychiatry, 34,* 541–565.

Cicchetti, D., & Tucker, D. (1994). Development and self-regulatory structures of the mind. *Development and Psychopathology, 6,* 533–549.

Clarkin, J. F., Yeomans, F. E., & Kernberg, O. F. (1999). *Psychotherapy for borderline personality.* New York: Wiley.

Cleckley, H. M. (1941). *The mask of sanity: An attempt to clarify some issues about the so-called psychopathic personality.* St. Louis, MO: Mosby.

Clifford, P. L. (1999). The FACE Recording and Measurement System: A scientific approach to person-based information. *Bulletin of the Menninger Clinic, 63,* 305–331.

Cloninger, C. R., Svrakic, D. M., & Przybeck, T. R. (1993). A psychobiological model of temperament and character. *Archives of General Psychiatry, 50,* 975–990.

Cloward, R. A., & Ohlin, L. E. (1960). *Delinquency and opportunity: A theory of delinquent gangs.* Chicago: Free Press.

Coates, S. W., & Wolfe, S. (1995). Gender identity disorder in boys: The interface of constitution and early experience. *Psychoanalytic Inquiry, 15,* 6–38.

Coccaro, E. F., & Kavoussi, R. J. (1997). Fluoxetine and impulsive–aggressive behavior in personality-disordered subjects. *Archives of General Psychiatry, 54,* 1081–1088.

Coccaro, E. F., Siever, L. J., Klar, H. M., Maurer, G., Cochrane, K., Cooper, T. B., Mohs, R. C., & Davis, K. L. (1989). Serotonergic studies in patients with affective and personality disorders: Correlates with suicidal and impulsive aggressive behavior. *Archives of General Psychiatry, 46,* 587–599.

Cohen, D., Flament, M., Taieb, O., Thompson, C., & Basquin, M. (2000). Electroconvulsive therapy in adolescence. *European Child and Adolescent Psychiatry, 9,* 1–6.

Cohen, D., Taieb, O., Flament, M., Benoit, N., Chevret, S., Corcos, M., Fossati, P.,

Jeammet, P., Allilaire, J. F., & Basquin, M. (2000). Absence of cognitive impairment at long-term follow-up in adolescents treated with ECT for severe mood disorder. *American Journal of Psychiatry, 157,* 460–462.

Cohen, Y. (1991). Grandiosity in children with narcissistic and borderline disorders: A comparative analysis. *Psychoanalytic Study of the Child, 46,* 307–324.

Coie, J. D., & Dodge, K. A. (1998). Aggression and antisocial behavior. In W. Damon & N. Eisenberg (Eds.), *Handbook of child psychology: Social, emotional, and personality development* (Vol. 3, 5th ed., pp. 779–862). New York: Wiley.

Colombo, J., Mitchell, D. W., Coldren, J. T., & Atwater, J. D. (1990). Discrimination learning during the first year: Stimulus and positional cues. *Journal of Experimental Psychology: Learning, Memory, and Cognition, 16,* 98–109.

Combrinck-Graham, L. (1990). Developments in family systems theory and research. *Journal of the American Academy of Child and Adolescent Psychiatry, 29,* 501–512.

Comer, J. P. (1988). *Maggie's American dream: The life and times of a black family.* New York: New American Library.

Comings, D. E., Muhleman, D., & Gysin, R. (1996). Dopamine D_2 receptor (DRD_2) gene and susceptibility to posttraumatic stress disorder: A study and replication. *Biological Psychiatry, 40,* 368–372.

Conners, C. K., Casat, C. D., Gualtieri, C. T., Weller, E., Reader, M., Reiss, A., Weller, R. A., Khayrallah, M., & Ascher, J. (1996). Bupropion hydrochloride in attention deficit disorder with hyperactivity. *Journal of the American Academy of Child and Adolescent Psychiatry, 35,* 1314–1321.

Coons, P. M., Bowman, E. S., & Milstein, V. (1988). Multiple personality disorder: A clinical investigation of 50 cases. *Journal of Nervous and Mental Disease, 176,* 519–527.

Cooperman, S., & Frances, R. J. (1989). Adolescent alcohol and substance abuse. In R. D. Lyman, S. Prentice-Dunn, & S. Gabel (Eds.), *Residential and inpatient treatment of children and adolescents* (pp. 341–360). New York: Plenum Press.

Cowdry, R. W., & Gardner, D. L. (1988). Pharmacotherapy of borderline personality disorder: Alprazolam, carbamazepine, trifluoperazine, and tranylcypromine. *Archives of General Psychiatry, 45,* 111–119.

Crits-Cristoph, P., Luborsky, L., Dahl, L., Popp, C., Mellon, J., & Mark, D. (1988). Clinicians can agree in assessing relationship patterns in psychotherapy: The Conflictual Relationship Theme method. *Archives of General Psychiatry, 45,* 1001–1004.

Crittenden, P. M. (1994). Peering into the black box: An exploratory treatise on the development of self in young children. In D. Cicchetti & S. L. Toth (Eds.), *Disorders and dysfunctions of the self: Rochester Symposium on Developmental Psychopathology* (Vol. 5, pp. 79–148). Rochester, NY: University of Rochester Press.

Cueva, J. E., Overall, J. E., Small, A. M., Armenteros, J. L., Perry, R., & Campbell, M. (1996). Carbamazepine in aggressive children with conduct disorder: A double-blind and placebo-controlled study. *Journal of the American Academy of Child and Adolescent Psychiatry, 35,* 480–490.

Cunningham, C. E., Siegel, L. S., & Offord, D. R. (1991). A dose–response analysis of the effects of methylphenidate on the peer interactions and simulated class-room performance of ADD children with and without conduct problems. *Journal of Child Psychology and Psychiatry and Allied Disciplines, 32,* 439–452.

Curry, J. F. (1991). Outcome research on residential treatment: Implications and suggested directions. *American Journal of Orthopsychiatry, 61,* 348–357.

Damasio, A. R. (1989). Time-locked multiregional retroactivation: A systems-level proposal for the neural substrate of recall and recognition. *Cognition, 33,* 25–62.

Damasio, A. R. (1998). Emotion in the perspective of an integrated nervous system. *Brain Research Reviews, 26,* 83–86.

Davanzo, P. A., & McCracken, J. T. (2000). Mood stabilizers in the treatment of juvenile bipolar disorder: Advances and controversies. *Child and Adolescent Psychiatric Clinics of North America, 9,* 159–182.

Davis, M. (1992). The role of the amygdala in fear and anxiety. *Annual Review of Neuroscience, 15,* 353–375.

Dell, P. F., & Eisenhower, J. W. (1990). Adolescent multiple personality disorder: A preliminary study of eleven cases. *Journal of the American Academy of Child and Adolescent Psychiatry, 29,* 359–366.

Dennett, D. C. (1987). *The intentional stance.* Cambridge, MA: MIT Press.

Devinsky, O., Morrell, M. J., & Vogt, B. A. (1995). Contributions of anterior cingulate cortex to behaviour. *Brain, 118,* 279–306.

Diamond, G. S., & Liddle, H. A. (1999). Transforming negative parent–adolescent interactions: From impasse to dialogue. *Family Process, 38,* 5–26.

Dishion, T. J., Andrews, D. W., & Crosby, L. (1995). Antisocial boys and their friends in early adolescence: Relationship characteristics, quality, and interactional process. *Child Development, 66,* 139–151.

Dodd, B. (1979). Lip reading in infants: Attention to speech presented in- and out-of-synchrony. *Cognitive Psychology, 11,* 478–484.

Dodge, K. A. (1991). The structure and function of reactive and proactive aggression. In D. J. Pepler & K. H. Rubin (Eds.), *The development and treatment of childhood aggression* (pp. 201–218). Hillsdale, NJ: Erlbaum.

Donovan, S. J., Susser, E. S., Nunes, E. V., Stewart, J. W., Quitkin, F. M., & Klein, D. F. (1997). Divalproex treatment of disruptive adolescents: A report of 10 cases. *Journal of Clinical Psychiatry, 58,* 12–15.

Duffett, R., Hill, P., & Lelliott, P. (1999). Use of electroconvulsive therapy in young people. *British Journal of Psychiatry, 175,* 228–230.

Edelman, G. M. (1987). *Neural Darwinism: The theory of neuronal group selection.* New York: Basic Books.

Edelman, G. M. (1992). *Bright air, brilliant fire: On the matter of the mind.* New York: Basic Books.

Egan, J., & Kernberg, P. F. (1984). Pathological narcissism in childhood. *Journal of the American Psychoanalytic Association, 32,* 39–62.

Ekstein, R., & Wallerstein, J. (1954). Observations on the psychology of borderline and psychotic children. *Psychoanalytic Study of the Child, 9,* 344–372.

Elicker, J., Englund, M., & Sroufe, L. A. (1992). Predicting peer competence and peer relationships in childhood from early parent–child relationships. In R. D.

Parke & G. W. Ladd (Eds.), *Family–peer relationships: Modes of linkage* (pp. 77–106). Hillsdale, NJ: Erlbaum.

Elman, J. L., Bates, A. E., Johnson, M. H., Karmiloff-Smith, A., Parisi, D., & Plunkett, K. (1996). *Rethinking innateness: A connectionist perspective on development.* Cambridge, MA: MIT Press.

Emch, M. (1944). On the "need to know" as related to identification and acting out. *International Journal of Psycho-Analysis, 25,* 13–19.

Emde, R. N. (1983). The prerepresentational self and its affective core. *Psychoanalytic Study of the Child, 38,* 165–192.

Emde, R. N. (1988). Development terminable and interminable: I. Innate and motivational factors from infancy. *International Journal of Psycho-Analysis, 69,* 23–42.

Emde, R. N. (1989). The infant's relationship experience: Developmental and affective aspects. In A. J. Sameroff & R. N. Emde (Eds.), *Relationship disturbances in early childhood: A developmental approach* (pp. 31–51). New York: Basic Books.

Emslie, G. J., Mayes, T. L., & Hughes, C. W. (2000). Special article: Updates in the pharmacologic treatment of childhood depression. *Psychiatric Clinics of North America: Annual of Drug Therapy, 23,* 811–836.

Emslie, G. J., Rush, A. J., Weinberg, W. A., Kowatch, R. A., Hughes, C. W., Carmody, T., & Rintelmann, J. (1997). A double-blind, randomized, placebo-controlled trial of fluoxetine in children and adolescents with depression. *Archives of General Psychiatry, 54,* 1031–1037.

Emslie, G. J., Walkup, J. T., Pliszka, S. R., & Ernst, M. (1999). Nontricyclic antidepressants: Current trends in children and adolescents. *Journal of the American Academy of Child and Adolescent Psychiatry, 38,* 517–528.

England, M. J., & Cole, R. (1992). Building systems of care for youth with serious mental illness. *Hospital and Community Psychiatry, 43,* 630–633.

England, M. J., & Goff, V. V. (1993). Health reform and organized systems of care. *New Directions for Mental Health Services, 59,* 5–12.

Erikson, E. H. (1950). *Childhood and society.* New York: Norton.

Erikson, E. H. (1959). Identity and the life cycle: Selected papers. *Psychological Issues, 1,* 1–171.

Erikson, E. H. (1968). *Identity, youth, and crisis.* New York: Norton.

Eyberg, S. M., Boggs, S. R., & Algina, J. (1995). Parent–child interaction therapy: A psychosocial model for the treatment of young children with conduct problem behavior and their families. *Psychopharmacology Bulletin, 31,* 83–91.

Fahy, T. A., Eisler, I., & Russell, G. F. (1993). Personality disorder and treatment response in bulimia nervosa. *British Journal of Psychiatry, 162,* 765–770.

Fahy, T. A., & Russell, G. F. (1993). Outcome and prognostic variables in bulimia nervosa. *International Journal of Eating Disorders, 14,* 135–145.

Fairbairn, W. R. D. (1954). *An object-relations theory of the personality.* New York: Basic Books. (Original work published 1952)

Fairburn, C. G. (1997). Bulimia outcome. *American Journal of Psychiatry, 154,* 1791–1792.

Fairburn, C. G., Norman, P. A., Welch, S. L., O'Connor, M. E., Doll, H. A., & Peveler, R. C. (1995). A prospective study of outcome in bulimia nervosa and the long-term effects of three psychological treatments. *Archives of General Psychiatry, 52,* 304–312.

Famularo, R., Kinscherff, R., & Fenton, T. (1991). Posttraumatic stress disorder among children clinically diagnosed as borderline personality disorder. *Journal of Nervous and Mental Disease, 179,* 428–431.

Farrington, D. P. (1983). Offending from 10 to 25 years of age. In K. T. Van Dusen & S. A. Mednick (Eds.), *Prospective studies of crime and delinquency* (pp. 17–37). Boston: Kluwer–Nijhoff.

Farrington, D. P., Loeber, R., & van Kammen, W. B. (1990). Long-term criminal outcomes of hyperactivity–impulsivity–attention deficit and conduct problems in childhood. In L. N. Robins & M. Rutter (Eds.), *Straight and devious pathways from childhood to adulthood* (pp. 62–81). New York: Cambridge University Press.

Fava, M. (1997). Psychopharmacologic treatment of pathologic aggression. *Psychiatric Clinics of North America, 20,* 427–451.

Fergusson, D. M., & Horwood, L. J. (1999). Prospective childhood predictors of deviant peer affiliations in adolescence. *Journal of Child Psychology and Psychiatry and Allied Disciplines, 40,* 581–592.

Fetner, H. H., & Geller, B. (1992). Lithium and tricyclic antidepressants. *Psychiatric Clinics of North America, 15,* 223–224.

Fichter, M. M., Leibl, K., Rief, W., Brunner, E., Schmidt-Auberger, S., & Engel, R. R. (1991). Fluoxetine versus placebo: A double-blind study with bulimic inpatients undergoing intensive psychotherapy. *Pharmacopsychiatry, 24,* 1–7.

Field, T., Healy, B., Goldstein, S., Perry, S., Bendell, D., Schanberg, S., Zimmerman, E. A., & Kuhn, C. (1988). Infants of depressed mothers show "depressed" behavior even with nondepressed adults. *Child Development, 59,* 1569–1579.

Findling, R. L., & Calabrese, J. R. (2000). Rapid-cycling bipolar disorder in children. *American Journal of Psychiatry, 157,* 1526–1527.

Fink, M. (1989). The efficacy of electroconvulsive therapy in therapy-resistant psychotic patients. *Journal of Clinical Psychopharmacology, 9,* 231–232.

Fischer, K. W., Kenny, S. L., & Pipp, S. L. (1990). How cognitive processes and environmental conditions organize discontinuities in the development of abstractions. In C. N. Alexander & E. J. Langer (Eds.), *Higher stages of human development: Perspectives on adult growth* (pp. 162–187). New York: Oxford University Press.

Fletcher, A. C., Darling, N., & Steinberg, L. (1995). Parental monitoring and peer influences on adolescent substance use. In J. McCord (Ed.), *Coercion and punishment in long-term perspectives* (pp. 259–271). New York: Cambridge University Press.

Fonagy, P. (1999a). Process and outcome in mental health care delivery: A model approach to treatment evaluation. *Bulletin of the Menninger Clinic, 63,* 288–304.

Fonagy, P. (1999b). Male perpetrators of violence against women: An attachment theory perspective. *Journal of Applied Psychoanalytic Studies, 1,* 7–27.

Fonagy, P. (2000a, January). *The development of psychopathology from infancy to adulthood: The mysterious unfolding of disturbance in time.* Paper presented at the World Association of Infant Mental Health Congress, Montreal, Canada.

Fonagy, P. (2000b). The treatment of disturbance of conduct. In P. Fonagy, M. Target, D. Cottrell, J. Phillips, & Z. Kurtz (Eds.), *A review of the outcomes of all treatments of psychiatric disorder in childhood* (pp. 135–206). London: National Health Service Executive.

Fonagy, P., Steele, H., & Steele, M. (1991). Maternal representations of attachment during pregnancy predict the organization of infant–mother attachment at one year of age. *Child Development, 62,* 891–905.

Fonagy, P., Steele, M., Steele, H., Higgitt, A., & Target, M. (1994). The Emanuel Miller Memorial Lecture 1992: The theory and practice of resilience. *Journal of Child Psychology and Psychiatry and Allied Disciplines, 35,* 231–257.

Fonagy, P., Steele, M., Steele, H., Leigh, T., Kennedy, R., Mattoon, G., & Target, M. (1995). Attachment, the reflective self, and borderline states: The predictive specificity of the Adult Attachment Interview and pathological emotional development. In S. Goldberg, R. Muir, & J. Kerr (Eds.), *Attachment theory: Social, developmental, and clinical perspectives* (pp. 233–278). Hillsdale, NJ: Analytic Press.

Fonagy, P., Steele, M., Steele, H., Moran, G. S., & Higgitt, A. C. (1991). The capacity for understanding mental states: The reflective self in parent and child and its significance for security of attachment. *Infant Mental Health Journal, 12,* 201–218.

Fonagy, P., & Target, M. (1995). Understanding the violent patient: The use of the body and the role of the father. *International Journal of Psycho-Analysis, 76,* 487–501.

Fonagy, P., & Target, M. (1996). Predictors of outcome in child psychoanalysis: A retrospective study of 763 cases at the Anna Freud Centre. *Journal of the American Psychoanalytic Association, 44,* 27–77.

Fonagy, P., & Target, M. (1997). Attachment and reflective function: Their role in self-organization. *Development and Psychopathology, 9,* 679–700.

Fonagy, P., & Target, M. (2000). Playing with reality III: The persistence of dual psychic reality in borderline patients. *International Journal of Psycho-Analysis, 81,* 853–873.

Fonagy, P., Target, M., & Gergely, G. (2000). Attachment and borderline personality disorder: A theory and some evidence. *Psychiatric Clinics of North America, 23,* 103–122.

Fonagy, P., Target, M., Steele, M., Steele, H., Leigh, T., Levinson, A., & Kennedy, R. (1997). Morality, disruptive behavior, borderline personality disorder, crime, and their relationship to security of attachment. In L. Atkinson & K. J. Zucker (Eds.), *Attachment and psychopathology* (pp. 223–274). New York: Guilford Press.

Forehand, R., & Long, N. (1988). Outpatient treatment of the acting out child: Procedures, long-term follow-up data, and clinical problems. *Advances in Behaviour Research and Therapy, 10,* 129–177.

Forehand, R., Sturgis, E. T., McMahon, R. J., Aguar, D., Green, K., Wells, K., & Breiner, J. (1979). Parent behavioral training to modify child noncompliance: Treatment generalization across time and from home to school. *Behavior Modification, 3,* 3–25.

Fraiberg, S., Adelson, E., & Shapiro, V. (1975). Ghosts in the nursery: A psychoanalytic approach to the problems of impaired infant–mother relationships. *Journal of the American Academy of Child Psychiatry, 14*, 387–421.

Frankenburg, F. R., & Zanarini, M. C. (1993). Clozapine treatment of borderline patients: A preliminary study. *Comprehensive Psychiatry, 34*, 402–405.

Freud, A. (1958). Adolescence. *Psychoanalytic Study of the Child, 13*, 255–278.

Freud, A. (1960). Discussion of Dr. John Bowlby's paper on "Grief and mourning in infancy." *Psychoanalytic Study of the Child, 15*, 32–62.

Freud, A. (1966). The ego and the mechanisms of defense. In C. Baines (Trans.), *The writings of Anna Freud: The ego and the mechanisms of defense* (Vol. 2, rev. ed., pp. 3–191). New York: International Universities Press. (Original work published 1936)

Freud, S. (1953). The interpretation of dreams. In J. Strachey (Ed. & Trans.), *The standard edition of the complete psychological works of Sigmund Freud* (Vol. 5, pp. 339–622). London: Hogarth Press. (Original work published 1900)

Freud, S. (1955). "A child is being beaten": A contribution to the study of the origin of sexual perversions. In J. Strachey (Ed. & Trans.), *The standard edition of the complete psychological works of Sigmund Freud* (Vol. 17, pp. 175–204). London: Hogarth Press. (Original work published 1919)

Freud, S. (1958). Remembering, repeating and working-through. In J. Strachey (Ed. & Trans.), *The standard edition of the complete psychological works of Sigmund Freud* (Vol. 12, pp. 145–156). London: Hogarth Press. (Original work published 1914)

Freud, S. (1959). Inhibitions, symptoms and anxiety. In J. Strachey (Ed. & Trans.), *The standard edition of the complete psychological works of Sigmund Freud* (Vol. 20, pp. 75–175). London: Hogarth Press. (Original work published 1926)

Freud, S. (1962). The aetiology of hysteria. In J. Strachey (Ed. & Trans.), *The standard edition of the complete psychological works of Sigmund Freud* (Vol. 3, pp. 187–221). London: Hogarth Press. (Original work published 1896)

Freud, S. (1963). On narcissism: An introduction. In J. Strachey (Ed. & Trans.), *The standard edition of the complete psychological works of Sigmund Freud* (Vol. 14, pp. 67–102). London: Hogarth Press. (Original work published 1914)

Freud, S. (1966). Project for a scientific psychology. In J. Strachey (Ed. & Trans.), *The standard edition of the complete psychological works of Sigmund Freud* (Vol. 1, pp. 281–397). London: Hogarth Press. (Original work published 1950)

Freyd, J. J. (1996). *Betrayal trauma: The logic of forgetting childhood abuse.* Cambridge, MA: Harvard University Press.

Friedman, L. (1982). The humanistic trend in recent psychoanalytic theory. *Psychoanalytic Quarterly, 51*, 353–371.

Frijling-Schreuder, E. C. (1969). Borderline states in children. *Psychoanalytic Study of the Child, 24*, 307–327.

Furman, E. (1974). *A child's parent dies: Studies in childhood bereavement.* New Haven, CT: Yale University Press.

Gabbard, G. O. (1989). Two subtypes of narcissistic personality disorder. *Bulletin of the Menninger Clinic, 53*, 527–532.

Gabbard, G. O. (1994). *Psychodynamic psychiatry in clinical practice: The DSM-IV edition* (2nd ed.). Washington, DC: American Psychiatric Press.

Gabbard, G. O. (1995). Countertransference: The emerging common ground. *International Journal of Psycho-Analysis, 76,* 475–485.

Gabbard, G. O. (2000). Combining medication with psychotherapy in the treatment of personality disorders. In J. G. Gunderson & G. O. Gabbard (Eds.), *Psychotherapy for personality disorders* (pp. 65–93). Washington, DC: American Psychiatric Press.

Gabbard, G. O., & Wilkinson, S. M. (1994). *Management of countertransference with borderline patients.* Washington, DC: American Psychiatric Press.

Gadow, K. D., Nolan, E. E., Sverd, J., Sprafkin, J., & Paolicelli, L. (1990). Methylphenidate in aggressive–hyperactive boys: I. Effects on peer aggression in public school settings. *Journal of the American Academy of Child and Adolescent Psychiatry, 29,* 710–718.

Gadow, K. D., Sverd, J., Sprafkin, J., Nolan, E. E., & Ezor, S. N. (1995). Efficacy of methylphenidate for attention-deficit hyperactivity disorder in children with tic disorder. *Archives of General Psychiatry, 52,* 444–455.

Gardner, D. L., & Cowdry, R. W. (1985). Alprazolam-induced dyscontrol in borderline personality disorder. *American Journal of Psychiatry, 142,* 98–100.

Geleerd, E. R. (1958). Borderline states in childhood and adolescence. *Psychoanalytic Study of the Child, 13,* 279–295.

Geller, B., Cooper, T. B., Sun, K., Zimerman, B., Frazier, J., Williams, M., & Heath J. (1998). Double-blind and placebo-controlled study of lithium for adolescent bipolar disorders with secondary substance dependency. *Journal of the American Academy of Child and Adolescent Psychiatry, 37,* 171–178.

Geller, B., Cooper, T. B., Zimerman, B., Frazier, J., Williams, M., Heath, J., & Warner, K. (1998). Lithium for prepubertal depressed children with family history predictors of future bipolarity: A double-blind, placebo-controlled study. *Journal of Affective Disorders, 51,* 165–175.

Geller, B., & Fetner, H. H. (1989). Children's 24–hour serum lithium level after a single dose predicts initial dose and steady-state plasma level [Letter to the editor]. *Journal of Clinical Psychopharmacology, 9,* 155.

George, C., Kaplan, N., & Main, M. (1985). *The Adult Attachment Interview.* Unpublished manuscript, Department of Psychology, University of California, Berkeley.

Gergely, G. (1995, March). *The role of parental mirroring of affects in early psychic structuration.* Paper presented at the International Psychoanalytic Association's 5th Conference on Psychoanalytic Research: "Advances in our Understanding of Affects: Clinical Implications," London.

Gergely, G., Magyar, J., & Balazs, A. (1999, June). *Childhood autism as "blindness" to less-than-perfect contingencies.* Poster session presented at the biennial conference of the International Society for Research in Childhood and Adolescent Psychopathology (ISRCAP), Barcelona, Spain.

Gergely, G., & Watson, J. S. (1996). The social biofeedback theory of parental affect-mirroring: The development of emotional self-awareness and self-control in infancy. *International Journal of Psycho-Analysis, 77,* 1181–1212.

Gergely, G., & Watson, J. S. (1999). Early socio-emotional development: Contingency perception and the social-biofeedback model. In P. Rochat (Ed.), *Early social cognition: Understanding others in the first months of life* (pp. 101–136). Hillsdale, NJ: Erlbaum.

Gershberg, F. B., & Shimamura, A. P. (1995). Impaired use of organizational strategies in free recall following frontal lobe damage. *Neuropsychologia, 13,* 1305–1333.

Gerstley, L., McLellan, A. T., Alterman, A. I., Woody, G. E., Luborsky, L., & Prout, M. (1989). Ability to form an alliance with the therapist: A possible marker of prognosis for patients with antisocial personality disorder. *American Journal of Psychiatry, 146,* 508–512.

Ghaemi, S. N. (2000). New treatments for bipolar disorder: The role of atypical neuroleptic agents. *Journal of Clinical Psychiatry, 61*(14, Suppl.), 33–42.

Gladwell, M. (1998). Do parents matter? *The New Yorker, 74*(24), 54–64.

Glover, A. J. J. (1992). Identification of violent incarcerates using the Test of Criminal Thinking and the revised Psychopathy Checklist (Doctoral dissertation, University of Toronto, 1992). *Dissertation Abstracts International, 53*(12A), 4253.

Goel, V., Grafman, J., Sadato, N., & Hallett, M. (1991). Modeling other minds. *Neuroreport: An International Journal for the Rapid Communication of Research in Neuroscience, 6,* 1741–1746.

Goenjian, A. K., Yehuda, R., Pynoos, R. S., Steinberg, A. M., Tashjian, M., Yang, R. K., Najarian, L. M., & Fairbanks, L. A. (1996). Basal cortisol, dexamethasone suppression of cortisol, and MHPG among adolescents after the 1988 earthquake in Armenia. *American Journal of Psychiatry, 153,* 929–934.

Goldberg, J. F., Garno, J. L., Leon, A. C., Kocsis, J. H., & Portera, L. (1998). Rapid titration of mood stabilizers predicts remission from mixed or pure mania in bipolar patients. *Journal of Clinical Psychiatry, 59,* 151–158.

Goldman, S. J., D'Angelo, E. J., & DeMaso, D. R. (1993). Psychopathology in the families of children and adolescents with borderline personality disorder. *American Journal of Psychiatry, 150,* 1832–1835.

Goldman, S. J., D'Angelo, E. J., DeMaso, D. R., & Mezzacappa, E. (1992). Physical and sexual abuse histories among children with borderline personality disorder. *American Journal of Psychiatry, 149,* 1723–1726.

Golier, J., & Yehuda, R. (1999, November). The HPA axis in Gulf War veterans with PTSD: Preliminary findings. *Proceedings and Abstracts of the 1999 Meeting of Traumatic Stress and Studies* (Abstract No. 1662), Miami, FL.

Goodwin, J. M., Cheeves, K., & Connell, V. (1990). Borderline and other severe symptoms in adult survivors of incestuous abuse. *Psychiatric Annals, 20,* 22–32.

Gormley, G. J., Lowy, M. T., Reder, A. T., Hospelhorn, V. D., Antel J. P., & Meltzer, H. Y. (1985). Glucocorticoid receptors in depression: Relationship to the dexamethasone suppression test. *American Journal of Psychiatry, 142,* 1278–1284.

Grados, M. A., & Riddle, M. A. (1999). Obsessive–compulsive disorder in children and adolescents: Treatment guidelines. *CNS Drugs, 12,* 257–277.

Graham, P. (1999). Implementation of an outcomes management model of treatment. *Bulletin of The Menninger Clinic, 63,* 346–365.

Grant, K. A., Shively, C. A., Nader, M. A., Ehrenkaufer, R. L., Line, S. W., Morton, T. E., Gage, H. D., & Mach, R. H. (1998). Effect of social status on striatal dopamine D_2 receptor binding characteristics in cynomolgus monkeys assessed with positron emission tomography. *Synapse, 29,* 80–83.

Grcevich, S. J., Findling, R. L., Rowane, W. A., Friedman, L., & Schulz, S. C. (1996). Risperidone in the treatment of children and adolescents with schizophrenia: A retrospective study. *Journal of Child and Adolescent Psychopharmacology, 6,* 251–257.

Greenhill, L. L. (1998). Attention-deficit/hyperactivity disorder. In B. T. Walsh (Ed.), *Child psychopharmacology* (pp. 29–64). Washington, DC: American Psychiatric Press.

Greenhill, L. L., Halperin, J. M., & Abikoff, H. (1999). Stimulant medications. *Journal of the American Academy of Child and Adolescent Psychiatry, 38,* 503–512.

Greenhill, L. L., Swanson, J. M., Vitiello, B., Davies, M., Clevenger, W., Wu, M., Arnold, L. E., Abikoff, H. B., Bukstein, O. G., Conners, C. K., Elliott, G. R., Hechtman, L., Hinshaw, S. P., Hoza, B., Jensen, P. S., Kraemer, H. C., March, J. S., Newcorn, J. H., Severe, J. B., Wells, K., & Wigal, T. (2001). Impairment and deportment responses to different methylphenidate doses in children with ADHD: The MTA titration trial. *Journal of the American Academy of Child and Adolescent Psychiatry, 40,* 180–187.

Griest, D. L., & Forehand, R., Rogers, T., Breiner, J., Furey, W., & Williams, C. A. (1982). Effects of parent enhancement therapy on the treatment outcome and generalization of a parent training program. *Behaviour Research and Therapy, 20,* 429–436.

Gunderson, J. G. (1996). The borderline patient's intolerance of aloneness: Insecure attachments and therapist availability. *American Journal of Psychiatry, 153,* 752–758.

Gunderson, J. G. (2000). Psychodynamic psychotherapy for borderline personality disorder. In J. G. Gunderson & G. O. Gabbard (Eds.), *Psychotherapy for personality disorders* (pp. 33–64). Washington, DC: American Psychiatric Press.

Gunderson, J. G., Kolb, J. E., & Austin, V. (1981). The diagnostic interview for borderline patients. *American Journal of Psychiatry, 138,* 896–903.

Gunderson, J. G., & Links, P. (1995). Borderline personality disorder. In G. O. Gabbard (Ed.), *Treatments of psychiatric disorders, Vol. 2* (2nd ed., pp. 2291–2310). Washington, DC: American Psychiatric Press.

Gunderson, J. G., & Zanarini, M. C. (1989). Pathogenesis of borderline personality. In A. Tasman, R. E. Hales, & A. J. Frances (Eds.), *American Psychiatric Press review of psychiatry* (pp. 25–48). Washington, DC: American Psychiatric Press.

Gunderson, J. G., Zanarini, M. C., & Kisiel, C. L. (1991). Borderline personality disorder: A review of data on DSM-III-R descriptions. *Journal of Personality Disorders, 5,* 340–352.

Gunnar, M. R. (1992). Reactivity of the hypothalamic–pituitary–adrenocortical system to stressors in normal infants and children. *Pediatrics, 90,* 491–497.

Gurvits, T. V., Shenton, M. E., Hokama, H., Ohta, H., Lasko, N. B., Gilbertson, M. W., Orr, S. P., Kilkinis, R., Jolesz, F. A., McCarley, R. W., & Pitman, R. K.

(1996). Magnetic resonance imaging study of hippocampal volume in chronic, combat-related posttraumatic stress disorder. *Biological Psychiatry, 40,* 1091–1099.

Hagger, C., Buckley, P., Kenny, J. T., Friedman, L., Ubogy, D., & Meltzer, H. Y. (1993). Improvement in cognitive functions and psychiatric symptoms in treatment-refractory schizophrenic patients receiving clozapine. *Biological Psychiatry, 34,* 702–712.

Hare, R. D. (1996). Psychopathy: A clinical construct whose time has come. *Criminal Justice and Behavior, 23,* 25–54.

Harlow, H. F. (1958). The nature of love. *American Psychologist, 13,* 673–680.

Harlow, H. F., & Harlow, M. K. (1971). Psychopathology in monkeys. In H. D. Kimmel (Ed.), *Experimental psychopathology: Recent research and theory* (pp. 203–229). San Diego, CA: Academic Press.

Harris, J. R. (1998). *The nurture assumption: Why children turn out the way they do.* New York: Free Press.

Harris, P. L. (1994). The child's understanding of emotion: Developmental change and the family environment. *Journal of Child Psychology and Psychiatry and Allied Disciplines, 35,* 3–28.

Harris, P. L. (1996). Desires, beliefs, and language. In P. Carruthers & P. K. Smith (Eds.), *Theories of theories of mind* (pp. 200–221). Cambridge, UK: Cambridge University Press.

Hart, S. D., Hare, R. D., & Forth, A. E. (1994). Psychopathy as a risk marker for violence: Development and validation of a screening version of the revised Psychopathy Checklist. In J. Monahan & H. J. Steadman (Eds.), *Violence and mental disorder: Developments in risk assessment* (pp. 81–98). Chicago: University of Chicago Press.

Hartley, D. G., & Strupp, H. H. (1983). The therapeutic alliance: Its relationship to outcome in brief psychotherapy. In J. M. Masling (Ed.), *Empirical studies of psychoanalytical theories* (Vol. 1, pp. 7–11). Hillsdale, NJ: Analytic Press.

Hawkins, J. D., Catalano, R. F., Morrison, D. M., O'Donnell, J., Abbott, R. D., & Day, L. E. (1992). The Seattle Social Development Project: Effects of the first four years on protective factors and problem behaviors. In J. McCord & R. E. Tremblay (Eds.), *Preventing antisocial behavior: Interventions from birth through adolescence* (pp. 139–161). New York: Guilford Press.

Hay Group. (1999). *Health care plan design and cost trends: 1988 through 1998.* Arlington, VA: Author.

Heilman, K. M., Voeller, K. K., & Nadeau, S. E. (1991). A possible pathophysiologic substrate of attention deficit hyperactivity disorder. *Journal of Child Neurology, 6*(Suppl.), S76–S81.

Heinz, A., Higley, J. D., Gorey, J. G., Saunders, R. C., Jones, D. W., Hommer, D., Zajicek, K., Suomi, S. J., Lesch, K. P., Weinberger, D. R., & Linnoila, M. (1998). *In vivo* association between alcohol intoxication, aggression, and serotonin transporter availability in nonhuman primates. *American Journal of Psychiatry, 155,* 1023–1028.

Heinz, A., Ragan, P., Jones, D. W., Hommer, D., Williams, W., Knable, M. B., Gorey, J. G., Doty, L., Geyer, C., Lee, K. S., Coppola, R., Weinberger, D. R., &

Linnoila, M. (1998). Reduced central serotonin transporters in alcoholism. *American Journal of Psychiatry, 155,* 1544–1549.

Hendin, H. (1981). Psychotherapy and suicide. *American Journal of Psychotherapy, 35,* 469–480.

Henggeler, S. W., Rowland, M. D., Randall, J., Ward, D. M., Pickrel, S. G., Cunningham, P. B., Miller, S. L., Edwards, J., Zealberg, J. J., Hand, L. D., & Santos, A. B. (1999). Home-based multisystemic therapy as an alternative to the hospitalization of youths in psychiatric crisis: Clinical outcomes. *Journal of the American Academy of Child and Adolescent Psychiatry, 38,* 1331–1339.

Herman, J. L. (1992a). Complex PTSD: A syndrome in survivors of prolonged and repeated trauma. *Journal of Traumatic Stress, 5,* 377–391.

Herman, J. L. (1992b). *Trauma and recovery.* New York: Basic Books.

Herman, J. L., Perry, J. C., & van der Kolk, B. A. (1989). Childhood trauma in borderline personality disorder. *American Journal of Psychiatry, 146,* 490–495.

Higley, J. D., Hasert, M. F., Suomi, S. J., & Linnoila, M. (1991). Nonhuman primate model of alcohol abuse: Effects of early experience, personality, and stress on alcohol consumption. *Proceedings of the National Academy of Sciences of the United States of America, 88,* 7261–7265.

Higley, J. D., King, S. T., Jr., Hasert, M. F., Champoux, M., Suomi, S. J., & Linnoila, M. (1996). Stability of interindividual differences in serotonin function and its relationship to severe aggression and competent social behavior in rhesus macaque females. *Neuropsychopharmacology, 14,* 67–76.

Higley, J. D., Suomi, S. J., & Linnoila, M. (1996). A non-human primate model of Type II alcoholism? Part 2: Diminished social competence and excessive aggression correlates with low cerebrospinal fluid 5–hydroxyindoleacetic acid concentrations. *Alcoholism, Clinical and Experimental Research, 20,* 643–650.

Hinshaw, S. P., Heller, T., & McHale, J. P. (1992). Covert antisocial behavior in boys with attention-deficit hyperactivity disorder: External validation and effects of methylphenidate. *Journal of Consulting and Clinical Psychology, 60,* 274–281.

Hobson, R. P. (1993a). *Autism and the development of mind.* Hillsdale, NJ: Erlbaum.

Hobson, R. P. (1993b). The intersubjective domain: Approaches from developmental psychopathology. *Journal of the American Psychoanalytic Association, 41*(Suppl.), 167–192.

Holden, G. W., & Miller, P. C. (1999). Enduring and different: A meta-analysis of the similarity in parents' child rearing. *Psychological Bulletin, 125,* 223–254.

Hollander, E. (1999). Managing aggressive behavior in patients with obsessive–compulsive disorder and borderline personality disorder. *Journal of Clinical Psychiatry, 60*(Suppl. 15), 38–44.

Hollenbeck, A. R., Susman, E. J., Nannis, E. D., Strope, B. E., Hersh, S. P., Levine, A. S., & Pizzo, P. A. (1980). Children with serious illness: Behavioral correlates of separation and isolation. *Child Psychiatry and Human Development, 11,* 3–11.

Holsboer, F. (1999). The rationale for corticotropin-releasing hormone receptor (CRH-R) antagonists to treat depression and anxiety. *Journal of Psychiatric Research, 33,* 181–214.

Holsboer, F., von Bardeleben, U., Gerken, A., Stalla, G. K., & Muller, O. A. (1984).

Blunted corticotropin and normal cortisol response to human corticotropin-releasing factor in depression. *New England Journal of Medicine, 311,* 1127.

Horowitz, M. J. (1987). *States of mind: Configurational analysis of individual psychology* (2nd ed.). New York: Plenum Press.

Horrigan, J. P., & Barnhill, L. J. (1995). Guanfacine for treatment of attention-deficit hyperactivity disorder in boys. *Journal of Child and Adolescent Psychopharmacology, 5,* 215–223.

Horvath, A., Gaston, L., & Luborsky, L. (1993). The therapeutic alliance and its measures. In N. E. Miller, L. Luborsky, J. P. Barber, & J. P. Docherty (Eds.), *Psychodynamic treatment research: A handbook for clinical practice* (pp. 247–273). New York: Basic Books.

Horvath, A. O., & Symonds, B. D. (1991). Relation between working alliance and outcome in psychotherapy: A meta-analysis. *Journal of Counseling Psychology, 38,* 139–149.

Hsu, L. G. (1986). Lithium-resistant adolescent mania. *Journal of the American Academy of Child Psychiatry, 25,* 280–283.

Hughes, C. W., Emslie, G. J., Crismon, M. L., Wagner, K. D., Birmaher, B., Geller, B., Pliszka, S. R., Ryan, N. D., Strober, M., Trivedi, M. H., Toprac, M. G., Sedillo, A., Llana, M. E., Lopez, M., & Rush, A. J. (1999). The Texas Children's Medication Algorithm Project: Report of the Texas Consensus Conference Panel on medication treatment of childhood major depressive disorder. *Journal of the American Academy of Child and Adolescent Psychiatry, 38,* 1442–1454.

Hunt, R. D. (1987). Treatment effects of oral and transdermal clonidine in relation to methylphenidate: An open pilot study in ADD-H. *Psychopharmacology Bulletin, 23,* 111–114.

Hunt, R. D., Minderaa, R. B., & Cohen, D. J. (1985). Clonidine benefits children with attention deficit disorder and hyperactivity: Report of a double-blind placebo–crossover therapeutic trial. *Journal of the American Academy of Child Psychiatry, 24,* 617–629.

Ianni, F. A. J. (1989). *The search for structure: A report on American youth today.* New York: Free Press.

Iglehart, J. K. (1996). Managed care and mental health. *New England Journal of Medicine, 334,* 131–135.

Irwin, H. J. (1994). Proneness to dissociation and traumatic childhood events. *Journal of Nervous and Mental Disease, 182,* 456–460.

Isojarvi, J. I., Laatikainen, T. J., Pakarinen, A. J., Juntunen, K. T., & Myllyla, V. V. (1993). Polycystic ovaries and hyperandrogenism in women taking valproate for epilepsy. *New England Journal of Medicine, 329,* 1383–1388.

Jacobson, E. (1964). *The self and the object world.* New York: International Universities Press.

Jaffe, S. (1990). *Step workbook for adolescent chemical dependency recovery: A guide to the first five steps.* Washington, DC: American Psychiatric Press.

Jenkins, J. M., & Astington, J. W. (1996). Cognitive factors and family structure associated with theory of mind development in young children. *Developmental Psychology, 32,* 70–78.

Jenson, J. M., & Whittaker, J. K. (1989). Partners in care: Involving parents in chil-

dren's residential treatment. In R. D. Lyman, S. Prentice-Dunn, & S. Gabel (Eds.), *Residential and inpatient treatment of children and adolescents* (pp. 207–227). New York: Plenum Press.

Joffe, W. G., & Sandler, J. (1967). Some conceptual problems involved in the consideration of disorders of narcissism. *Journal of Child Psychotherapy, 2,* 56–66.

Johnson, A. M., & Szurek, S. A. (1952). The genesis of antisocial acting out in children and adults. *Psychoanalytic Quarterly, 21,* 323–343.

Johnson, C. (1996). Addressing parent cognitions in interventions with families of disruptive children. In K. S. Dobson & K. D. Craig (Eds.), *Advances in cognitive-behavioral therapy* (pp. 193–209). Thousand Oaks, CA: Sage.

Joseph, R. (1988). The right cerebral hemisphere: Emotion, music, visual–spatial skills, body–image, dreams, and awareness. *Journal of Clinical Psychology, 44,* 630–673.

Kafantaris, V., Campbell, M., Padron-Gayol, M. V., Small, A. M., Locascio, J. J., & Rosenberg, C. R. (1992). Carbamazepine in hospitalized aggressive conduct disorder children: An open pilot study. *Psychopharmacology Bulletin, 28,* 193–199.

Kagan, J. (with Snidman, N., Arcus, D., & Reznick, J. S.). (1994). *Galen's prophecy: Temperament in human nature.* New York: Basic Books.

Kagan, S., & Zentner, M. (1996). Early childhood predictors of adult psychopathology. *Harvard Review of Psychiatry, 3,* 341–350.

Kandel, E. R. (1983). From metapsychology to molecular biology: Explorations into the nature of anxiety. *American Journal of Psychiatry, 140,* 1277–1293.

Kandel, E. R. (1998). A new intellectual framework for psychiatry. *American Journal of Psychiatry, 155,* 457–469.

Kapfhammer, H. P., & Hippius, H. (1998). Pharmacotherapy in personality disorders. *Journal of Personality Disorders, 12,* 277–288.

Kastner, T., & Friedman, D. L. (1992). Verapamil and valproic acid treatment of prolonged mania. *Journal of the American Academy of Child and Adolescent Psychiatry, 31,* 271–275.

Kathol, R. G., Jaeckle, R. S., Lopez, J. F., & Meller, W. H. (1989). Pathophysiology of HPA axis abnormalities in patients with major depression: An update. *American Journal of Psychiatry, 146,* 311–317.

Kaufman, J., Birmaher, B., Perel, J., Dahl, R. E., Moreci, P., Nelson, B., Wells, W., & Ryan, N. D. (1997). The corticotropin-releasing hormone challenge in depressed abused, depressed nonabused, and normal control children. *Biological Psychiatry, 42,* 669–679.

Kavoussi, R. J., Liu, J., & Coccaro, E. F. (1994). An open trial of sertraline in personality disordered patients with impulsive aggression. *Journal of Clinical Psychiatry, 55,* 137–141.

Kaye, K. (1982). *The mental and social life of babies: How parents create persons.* Chicago: University of Chicago Press.

Kazdin, A. E. (1993). Psychotherapy for children and adolescents: Current progress and future research directions. *American Psychologist, 48,* 644–657.

Kazdin, A. E. (1996a). Problem solving and parent management in treating aggressive and antisocial behavior. In E. D. Hibbs & P. S. Jensen (Eds.), *Psychosocial treatments for child and adolescent disorders: Empirically based strategies for clinical practice* (pp. 377–408). Washington, DC: American Psychological Association.

Kazdin, A. E. (1996b). Dropping out of child psychotherapy: Issues for research and implications for practice. *Clinical Child Psychology and Psychiatry, 1,* 133–156.

Kazdin, A. E., Siegel, T. C., & Bass, D. (1992). Cognitive problem-solving skills training and parent management training in the treatment of antisocial behavior in children. *Journal of Consulting and Clinical Psychology, 60,* 733–747.

Keller, M. B., Gelenberg, A. J., Hirschfeld, R. M. A., Rush, A. J., Thase, M. E., Kocsis, J. H., Markowitz, J. C., Fawcett, J. A., Koran, L. M., Klein, D. N., Russell, J. M., Kornstein, S. G., McCullough, J. P., Davis, S. M., & Harrison, W. M. (1998). The treatment of chronic depression: Part 2. A double-blind, randomized trial of sertraline and imipramine. *Journal of Clinical Psychiatry, 59,* 598–607.

Kendall, P. C. (Ed.). (2000). *Child and adolescent therapy: Cognitive-behavioral procedures* (2nd ed.). New York: Guilford Press.

Kernberg, O. F. (1967). Borderline personality organization. *Journal of the American Psychoanalytic Association, 15,* 641–685.

Kernberg, O. F. (1970). Factors in the psychoanalytic treatment of narcissistic personalities. *Journal of the American Psychoanalytic Association, 18,* 51–85.

Kernberg, O. F. (1975). *Borderline conditions and pathological narcissism.* New York: Aronson.

Kernberg, O. F. (1976). *Object relations theory and clinical psychoanalysis.* New York: Aronson.

Kernberg, O. F. (1987). Projection and projective identification: Developmental and clinical aspects. *Journal of the American Psychoanalytic Association, 35,* 795–819.

Kernberg, O. F. (1992). *Aggression in personality disorders and perversions.* New Haven, CT: Yale University Press.

Kernberg, P. F. (1989). Narcissistic personality disorder in childhood. *Psychiatric Clinics of North America, 12*(3), 671–694.

Kernberg, P. F. (1990). Resolved: Borderline personality exists in children under twelve. *Journal of the American Academy of Child and Adolescent Psychiatry, 29,* 478–481, 482.

Kernberg, P. F., Weiner, A. S., & Bardenstein, K. K. (2000). *Personality disorders in children and adolescents.* New York: Basic Books.

Kierkegaard, S. (1938). *Purity of heart is to will one thing: Spiritual preparation for the office of confession* (D. V. Steere, Trans.). New York: Harper.

Kihlstrom, J. F., & Hoyt, I. P. (1995). Repression, dissociation, and hypnosis. In J. L. Singer (Ed.), *Repression and dissociation: Implications for personality theory, psychopathology, and health* (pp. 181–208). Chicago: University of Chicago Press.

Kirby, J. S., Chu, J. A., & Dill, D. I. (1993). Correlates of dissociative symptomatology in patients with physical and sexual abuse histories. *Comprehensive Psychiatry, 34,* 258–263.

Klein, D. F. (1977). Psychopharmacological treatment and delineation of borderline disorders. In P. Hartocollis (Ed.), *Borderline personality disorders: The concept, the syndrome, the patient* (pp. 365–383). New York: International Universities Press.

Klein, M. (1952a). Notes on some schizoid mechanisms. In M. Klein, P. Heimann, & S. Isaacs, *Developments in psycho-analysis* (J. Riviere, Ed.; pp. 292–320). London: Hogarth Press.

Klein, M. (1952b). Some theoretical conclusions regarding the emotional life of the infant. In M. Klein, P. Heimann, & S. Isaacs, *Developments in psycho-analysis* (J. Riviere, Ed.; pp. 198–236). London: Hogarth Press.

Klein, M. (1957). *Envy and gratitude: A study of unconscious sources.* New York: Basic Books.

Klein, M. (1958). On the development of mental functioning. *International Journal of Psycho-Analysis 39,* 84–90.

Kluft, R. P. (1984). An introduction to multiple personality disorder. *Psychiatric Annals, 14,* 19–24.

Kluft, R. P. (1992). A specialist's perspective on multiple personality disorder. *Psychoanalytic Inquiry, 12,* 139–171.

Kluft, R. P. (1998). Reflections on the traumatic memories of dissociative identity disorder patients. In S. J. Lynn & K. M. McConkey (Eds.), *Truth in memory* (pp. 304–322). New York: Guilford Press.

Koestler, A. (1945). *The yogi and the commissar and other essays.* New York: Macmillan.

Kohlberg, L. (1966). A cognitive-developmental analysis of children's sex-role concepts and attitudes. In E. E. Maccoby (Ed.), *The development of sex differences* (pp. 82–173). Stanford, CA: Stanford University Press.

Kohut, H. (1971). *The analysis of the self: A systematic approach to the psychoanalytic treatment of narcissistic personality disorder.* New York: International Universities Press.

Kohut, H. (1972). Thoughts on narcissism and narcissistic rage. *Psychoanalytic Study of the Child, 27,* 360–400.

Kohut, H. (1977). *The restoration of the self.* New York: International Universities Press.

Kovacs, M., Feinberg, T. L., Crouse-Novak, M. A., Paulauskas, S. L., & Finkelstein, R. (1984a). Depressive disorders in childhood: I. A longitudinal prospective study of characteristics and recovery. *Archives of General Psychiatry, 41,* 229–237.

Kovacs, M., Feinberg, T. L., Crouse-Novak, M. A., Paulauskas, S. L., Pollock, M., & Finkelstein, R. (1984b). Depressive disorders in childhood: II. A longitudinal study of the risk for a subsequent major depression. *Archives of General Psychiatry, 41,* 643–649.

Kowatch, R. A., Suppes, T., Carmody, T. J., Bucci, J. P., Hume, J. H., Kromelis, M., Emslie, G. J., Weinberg, W. A., & Rush, A. J. (2000). Effect size of lithium, divalproex sodium, and carbamazepine in children and adolescents with bipolar disorder. *Journal of the American Academy of Child and Adolescent Psychiatry, 39,* 713–720.

Kraemer, G. W. (1985). Effects of differences in early social experiences on primate neurobiological–behavioral development. In M. Reite & T. Field (Eds.), *The psychobiology of attachment and separation* (pp. 135–161). Orlando, FL: Academic Press.

Kumra, S. (2000). The diagnosis and treatment of children and adolescents with schizophrenia: "My mind is playing tricks on me." *Child and Adolescent Psychiatric Clinics of North America, 9,* 183–199.

Kumra, S., Jacobsen, L. K., Lenane, M., Karp, B. I., Frazier, J. A., Smith, A. K., Bedwell, J., Lee, P., Malanga, C. J., Hamburger, S., & Rapoport, J. L. (1998). Childhood-onset schizophrenia: An open-label study of olanzapine in adolescents. *Journal of the American Academy of Child and Adolescent Psychiatry, 37,* 377–385.

Kusumakar, V., & Yatham, L. N. (1997). An open study of lamotrigine in refractory bipolar depression. *Psychiatry Research, 72,* 145–148.

Kutcher, S. P. (1998). Affective disorders in children and adolescents: A critical clinically relevant review. In B. T. Walsh (Ed.), *Child psychopharmacology* (pp. 91–114). Washington, DC: American Psychiatric Press.

LaHoste, G. J., Swanson, J. M., Wigal, S. B., Glabe, C., Wigal, T., King, N., & Kennedy, J. L. (1996). Dopamine D_4 receptor gene polymorphism is associated with attention deficit hyperactivity disorder. *Molecular Psychiatry, 1,* 121–124.

Laible, D. J., & Thompson, R. A. (1998). Attachment and emotional understanding in preschool children. *Developmental Psychology, 34,* 1038–1045.

Larson, M. C., White, B. P., Cochran, A., Donzella, B., & Gunnar, M. (1998). *Developmental Psychobiology, 33,* 327–337.

LeDoux, J. E. (1996). *The emotional brain: The mysterious underpinnings of emotional life.* New York: Simon & Schuster.

Leichtman, M., & Leichtman, M. L. (1999). Facilitating the transition from residential treatment into the community: I. The problem. In C. Waller (Ed.), *Contributions to residential treatment 1999* (pp. 81–87). Washington, DC: American Association of Children's Residential Centers.

Leichtman, M., & Nathan, S. (1983). A clinical approach to the psychological testing of borderline children. In K. S. Robson (Ed.), *The borderline child: Approaches to etiology, diagnosis, and treatment* (pp. 121–170). New York: McGraw-Hill.

Leichtman, M. L., & Leichtman, M. (1996a). A model of psychodynamic short-term residential treatment: I. The nature of the challenge. In C. Waller (Ed.), *Contributions to residential treatment 1996* (pp. 85–92). Alexandria, VA: American Association of Children's Residential Centers.

Leichtman, M. L., & Leichtman, M. (1996b). A model of psychodynamic short-term residential treatment: II. General principles. In C. Waller (Ed.), *Contributions to residential treatment 1996* (pp. 93–102). Alexandria, VA: American Association of Children's Residential Centers.

Leichtman, M. L., & Leichtman, M. (1996c). A model of psychodynamic short-term residential treatment: III. Changing roles. In C. Waller (Ed.), *Contributions to residential treatment 1996* (pp. 103–109). Alexandria, VA: American Association of Children's Residential Centers.

Lenox, R. H., Manji, H. K., McElroy, S. L., Keck, P. E., & Dubovsky, S. L. (1995). Drugs for treatment of bipolar disorder. In A. F. Schatzberg & C. B. Nemeroff (Eds.), *The American Psychiatric Press textbook of psychopharmacology* (pp. 303–388). Washington, DC: American Psychiatric Press.

Leonard, H. L., March, J., Rickler, K. C., & Allen, A. J. (1997). Pharmacology of the selective serotonin reuptake inhibitors in children and adolescents. *Journal of the American Academy of Child and Adolescent Psychiatry, 36,* 725–736.

Lesch, K. P., Bengel, D., Heils, A., Sabol, S. Z., Greenberg, B. D., Petri, S., Benjamin, J., Muller, C. R., Hamer, D. H., & Murphy, D. L. (1996). Association of anxiety-related traits with a polymorphism in the serotonin transporter gene regulatory region. *Science, 274,* 1527–1531.

Levinson, A., & Fonagy, P. (1999). *Criminality and attachment: The relationship between interpersonal awareness and offending in a prison population with psychiatric disorder.* Unpublished manuscript, University College, London.

Lewinsohn, P. M., Klein, D. N., & Seeley, J. R. (1995). Bipolar disorders in a community sample of older adolescents: Prevalence, phenomenology, comorbidity, and course. *Journal of the American Academy of Child and Adolescent Psychiatry, 34,* 454–463.

Lewis, D. O. (1983). Neuropsychiatric vulnerabilities and violent juvenile delinquency. *Psychiatric Clinics of North America, 6,* 707–714.

Lewis, D. O., Shanok, S. S., & Balla, D. A. (1979). Perinatal difficulties, head and face trauma, and child abuse in the medical histories of seriously delinquent children. *American Journal of Psychiatry, 136,* 419–423.

Lewis, D. O., Yeager, C. A., Lovely, R., Stein, A., & Cobham-Portorreal, C. S. (1994). A clinical follow-up of delinquent males: Ignored vulnerabilities, unmet needs, and the perpetuation of violence. *Journal of the American Academy of Child and Adolescent Psychiatry, 33,* 518–528.

Lhuintre, J. P., Daoust, M., Moore, N. D., Chretien, P., Saligaut, C., Tran, G., Bosimare, F., & Hillemand, B. (1985). Ability of calcium bis acetyl homotaurine, a GABA agonist, to prevent relapse in weaned alcoholics. *Lancet, 1,* 1014–1016.

Lichtenberg, J. D. (1989). *Psychoanalysis and motivation.* Hillsdale, NJ: Analytic Press.

Liddle, H. A., & Hogue, A. (2000). A family-based, developmental–ecological preventive intervention for high-risk adolescents. *Journal of Marital and Family Therapy, 26,* 265–279.

Liebowitz, M. R., Quitkin, F. M., Stewart, J. W., McGrath, P. J., Harrison, W. M., Markowitz, J. S., Rabkin, J. G., Tricamo, E., Goetz, D. M., & Klein, D. F. (1988). Antidepressant specificity in atypical depression. *Archives of General Psychiatry, 45,* 129–137.

Linehan, M. M. (1993). *Skills training manual for treating borderline personality disorder.* New York: Guilford Press.

Linehan, M. M., Armstrong, H. E., Suarez, A., Allmon, D., & Heard, H. L. (1991). Cognitive-behavioral treatment of chronically parasuicidal borderline patients. *Archives of General Psychiatry, 48,* 1060–1064.

Linehan, M. M., Heard, H. L., & Armstrong, H. E. (1993). Naturalistic follow-up of a behavioral treatment for chronically parasuicidal borderline patients. *Archives of General Psychiatry, 50,* 971–974.

Linehan, M. M., Heard, H. L., & Armstong, H. E. (1994). "Naturalistic follow-up of a behavioral treatment for chronically parasuicidal borderline patients": Erratum. *Archives of General Psychiatry, 51,* 422.

Links, P. S., Heslegrave, R., & Villella, J. (1998). Psychopharmacological management of personality disorders: An outcome-focused model. In K. R. Silk (Ed.), *Biology of personality disorders* (pp. 93–127). Washington, DC: American Psychiatric Press.

Links, P. S., Steiner, M., Boiago, I., & Irwin, D. (1990). Lithium therapy for borderline patients: Preliminary findings. *Journal of Personality Disorders, 4,* 173–181.

Lochman, J. E., & Wells, K. C. (1996). A social–cognitive intervention with aggressive children: Prevention effects and contextual implementation issues. In R. D. Peters & R. J. McMahon (Eds.), *Preventing childhood disorders, substance abuse, and delinquency* (pp. 111–143). Thousand Oaks, CA: Sage.

Loewenstein, R. J., & Putnam, F. W. (1990). The clinical phenomenology of males with multiple personality disorder: A report of 21 cases. *Dissociation: Progress in the Dissociative Disorders, 3,* 135–143.

Long, P., Forehand, R., Wierson, M., & Morgan, A. (1994). Does parent training with young noncompliant children have long-term effects? *Behaviour Research and Therapy, 32,* 101–107.

Luborsky, L., Crits-Cristoph, P., Mintz, J., & Auerbach, A. (1981). *Who will benefit from psychotherapy? Predicting therapeutic outcomes.* New York: Basic Books.

Ludolph, P. S., Westen, D., Misle, B., Jackson, A., Wixom, J., & Wiss, F. C. (1990). The borderline diagnosis in adolescents: Symptoms and developmental history. *American Journal of Psychiatry, 147,* 470–476.

Lyons-Ruth, K., & Jacobvitz, D. (1999). Attachment disorganization: Unresolved loss, relational violence, and lapses in behavioral and attentional strategies. In J. Cassidy & P. R. Shaver (Eds.), *Handbook of attachment: Theory, research, and clinical applications* (pp. 520–554). New York: Guilford Press.

Mahler, M. S., Pine, F., & Bergman, A. (1975). *The psychological birth of the human infant: Symbiosis and individuation.* New York: Basic Books.

Mahler, M. S., Ross, J. R., & Defries, Z. (1949). Clinical studies in benign and malignant cases of childhood psychosis (schizophrenia-like). *American Journal of Orthopsychiatry, 19,* 295–305.

Main, M. (1991). Metacognitive knowledge, metacognitive monitoring, and singular (coherent) vs. multiple (incoherent) models of attachment: Findings and directions for future research. In C. M. Parkes, J. Stevenson-Hinde, & P. Marris (Eds.), *Attachment across the life cycle* (pp. 127–159). London: Tavistock/Routledge.

Main, M., & Goldwyn, R. (1984). *Adult attachment scoring and classification system.* Unpublished manuscript, University of California, Berkeley.

Main, M., & Goldwyn, R. (1998). *Adult attachment scoring and classification system (Version 6.3).* Unpublished manuscript, University of California, Berkeley.

Main, M., & Hesse, E. (1990). Parents' unresolved traumatic experiences are related to infant disorganized attachment status: Is frightened and/or frightening parental behavior the linking mechanism? In M. T. Greenberg, D. Cicchetti, & E. M. Cummings (Eds.), *Attachment in the preschool years: Theory, research, and intervention* (pp. 161–182). Chicago: University of Chicago Press.

Main, M., & Hesse, E. (1999). Second-generation effects of unresolved trauma in nonmaltreating parents: Dissociated, frightened, and threatening parental behavior. *Psychoanalytic Inquiry, 19,* 481–540.

Main, M., Kaplan, N., & Cassidy, J. (1985). Security in infancy, childhood, and adulthood: A move to the level of representation. *Monographs of the Society for Research in Child Development, 50,* 66–104.

Main, M., & Solomon, J. (1986). Discovery of an insecure–disorganized/disoriented attachment pattern. In T. B. Brazelton & M. W. Yogman (Eds.), *Affective development in infancy* (pp. 95–124). Norwood, NJ: Ablex.

Main, M., & Solomon, J. (1990). Procedures for identifying infants as disorganized/ disoriented during the Ainsworth Strange Situation. In M. T. Greenberg, D. Cicchetti, & E. M. Cummings (Eds.), *Attachment in the preschool years: Theory, research, and intervention* (pp. 121–160). Chicago: University of Chicago Press.

Maltsberger, J. T. (1999). Countertransference in the treatment of the suicidal borderline patient. In G. O. Gabbard (Ed.), *Countertransference issues in psychiatric treatment* (pp. 27–43). Washington, DC: American Psychiatric Press.

Mandelbaum, A. (1971). Family process in the diagnosis and treatment of children and adolescents. *Bulletin of the Menninger Clinic, 35,* 153–156.

March, J. S., Biederman, J., Wolkow, R., Safferman, A., Mardekian, J., Cook, E. H., Cutler, N. R., Dominguez, R., Ferguson, J., Muller, B., Riesenberg, R., Rosenthal, M., Sallee, F. R., Wagner, K. D., & Steiner, H. (1998). Sertraline in children and adolescents with obsessive–compulsive disorder: A multicenter randomized controlled trial. *Journal of the American Medical Association, 280,* 1752–1756.

Marcus, J. (1963). Borderline states in childhood. *Journal of Child Psychology and Psychiatry, 4,* 208–218.

Markovitz, P. J. (1995). Pharmacotherapy of impulsivity, aggression and related disorders. In E. Hollander & D. J. Stein (Eds.), *Impulsivity and aggression* (pp. 263–287). Chichester, UK: Wiley.

Marohn, R. C. (1991). Psychotherapy of adolescents with behavioral disorders. In M. Slomowitz (Ed.), *Adolescent psychotherapy* (pp. 145–161). Washington, DC: American Psychiatric Press.

Marohn, R. C., Offer, D., & Ostrov, E., & Trujillo, J. (1979). Four psychodynamic types of hospitalized juvenile delinquents. *Adolescent Psychiatry, 7,* 466–483.

Martin, A., Kaufman, J., & Charney, D. (2000). Pharmacotherapy of early-onset depression: Update and new directions. *Child and Adolescent Psychiatric Clinics of North America, 9,* 135–157.

Mason, B. J., Ritvo, E. C., Morgan, R. O., Salvato, F. R., Goldberg, G., Welch, B., & Mantero-Atienza, E. (1994). A double-blind, placebo-controlled pilot study to evaluate the efficacy and safety of oral nalmefene HCl for alcohol dependence. *Alcoholism, Clinical and Experimental Research, 18,* 1162–1167.

Mason, J. W., Giller, E. L., Kosten, T. R., Ostroff, R. B., & Podd, L. (1986). Urinary free-cortisol levels in posttraumatic stress disorder patients. *Journal of Nervous and Mental Disease, 174,* 145–149.

Masten, A. S., & Garmezy, N. (1985). Risk, vulnerability and protective factors in developmental psychopathology. In B. B. Lahey & A. E. Kazdin (Eds.), *Advances in clinical child psychology* (pp. 1–52). New York: Plenum Press.

Masten, A. S., Garmezy, N., Tellegen, A., Pellegrini, D. S., Larkin, K., & Larsen, A. (1988). Competence and stress in school children: The moderating effects of individual and family qualities. *Journal of Child Psychology and Psychiatry and Allied Disciplines, 29,* 745–764.

Masterson, J. F. (1972). *Treatment of the borderline adolescent: A developmental approach.* New York: Wiley.

Masterson, J. F. (1981). *The narcissistic and borderline disorders: An integrated developmental approach.* New York: Brunner/Mazel.

Masterson, J. F., & Rinsley, D. B. (1975). The borderline syndrome: The role of the mother in the genesis and psychic structure of the borderline personality. *International Journal of Psycho-Analysis, 56,* 163–177.

Matthys, W., Cuperus, J. M., & Van Engeland, H. (1999). Deficient social problem-solving in boys with ODD/CD, with ADHD, and with both disorders. *Journal of the American Academy of Child and Adolescent Psychiatry, 38,* 311–321.

Mayes, L. C., & Cohen, D. J. (1993). Playing and therapeutic action in child analysis. *International Journal of Psycho-Analysis, 74,* 1235–1244.

McDougall, J. (1989). *Theaters of the body: A psychoanalytic approach to psychosomatic illness.* New York: Norton.

McElroy, S. L., Keck, P. E., Jr., Pope, H. G., Jr., & Hudson, J. I. (1992). Valproate in the treatment of bipolar disorder: Literature review and clinical guidelines. *Journal of Clinical Psychopharmacology, 12*(Suppl. 1), S42–S52.

McEwen, B. S., & Magarinos, A. M. (1997). Stress effects on morphology and function of the hippocampus. *Annals of the New York Academy of Sciences, 821,* 271–284.

McFarlane, A. C., Weber, D. L., & Clark, C. R. (1993). Abnormal stimulus processing in posttraumatic stress disorder. *Biological Psychiatry, 34,* 311–320.

Meins, E., Fernyhough, C., Russell, J., & Clark-Carter, D. (1998). Security of attachment as a predictor of symbolic and mentalising abilities: A longitudinal study. *Social Development, 7,* 1–24.

Meloy, J. R. (1988). *The psychopathic mind: Origins, dynamics, and treatment.* Northvale, NJ: Aronson.

Meltzoff, A. N. (1990). Foundations for developing a concept of self: The role of imitation in relating self to other and the value of social mirroring, social modeling and self practice in infancy. In D. Cicchetti & M. Beeghly (Eds.), *The self in transition: Infancy to childhood* (pp. 139–164). Chicago: University of Chicago Press.

Meltzoff, A. N., & Moore, M. K. (1977). Imitation of facial and manual gestures by human neonates. *Science, 198,* 75–78.

Meltzoff, A. N., & Moore, M. K. (1983). Newborn infants imitate adult facial gestures. *Child Development, 54,* 702–709.

Meltzoff, A. N., & Moore, M. K. (1989). Imitation in newborn infants: Exploring the range of gestures imitated and the underlying mechanisms. *Developmental Psychology, 25,* 954–962.

Meltzoff, A. N., & Moore, M. K. (1994). Imitation, memory, and the representation of persons. *Infant Behavior and Development, 17,* 83–99.

Minuchin, S., & Fishman, H. C. (1981). *Family therapy techniques.* Cambridge, MA: Harvard University Press.

Mirsky, I. A. (1968). Communication of affects in monkeys. In D.C. Glass (Ed.), *Environmental influences: Proceedings of a conference under the auspices of Russell Sage Foundation and the Rockefeller University* (pp. 129–137). New York: Rockefeller University Press.

Mitchell, J. E., Raymond, N., & Specker, S. M. (1993). A review of the controlled trials of pharmacotherapy and psychotherapy in the treatment of bulimia nervosa. *International Journal of Eating Disorders, 14,* 229–247.

Moran, G. S. (1984). Psychoanalytic treatment of diabetic children. *Psychoanalytic Study of the Child, 38,* 407–447.

Moss, E., Parent, S., & Gosselin, C. (1995, March 30–April 1). *Attachment and theory of mind: Cognitive and metacognitive correlates of attachment during the preschool period.* Paper presented at the biennial meeting of the Society for Research in Child Development, Indianapolis, IN.

MTA Cooperative Group. (1999a). A 14–month randomized clinical trial of treatment strategies for attention-deficit/hyperactivity disorder: The Multimodal Treatment Study of Children with Attention-Deficit/Hyperactivity Disorder. *Archives of General Psychiatry, 56,* 1073–1086.

MTA Cooperative Group. (1999b). Moderators and mediators of treatment response for children with attention-deficit/hyperactivity disorder: The Multimodal Treatment Study of Children with Attention-Deficit/Hyperactivity Disorder. *Archives of General Psychiatry, 56,* 1088–1096.

Murburg, M. M. (Ed.). (1994). *Catecholamine function in posttraumatic stress disorder: Emerging concepts.* Washington, DC: American Psychiatric Press.

Murray, L. (1992). The impact of postnatal depression on infant development. *Journal of Child Psychology and Psychiatry and Allied Disciplines, 33,* 543–561.

Murray, L., Fiori-Cowley, A., Hooper, R., & Cooper, P. (1996). The impact of postnatal depression and associated adversity on early mother–infant interactions and later infant outcomes. *Child Development, 67,* 2512–2526.

Murray, L., & Trevarthen, C. (1985). Emotional regulation of interactions between two-month-olds and their mothers. In T. M. Field & N. A. Fox (Eds.), *Social perception in infants* (pp. 177–198). Norwood, NJ: Ablex.

Neisser, V. (1991). Two perceptually given aspects of the self and their development. *Developmental Review, 11,* 197–209.

Nichols, K., Gergely, G., & Fonagy, P. (2000, September). *Infant cognition, mother–infant interaction, affect regulation, and markers of stress responsiveness: Directions for the Menninger Infant Laboratory.* Presentation at the Menninger Symposium on Contingency, Perception, and Attachment in Infancy, Topeka, KS.

Noble, E. P. (1996). The gene that rewards alcoholism. *Scientific American, 2,* 52–61.

Noble, E. P. (1998). DRD_2 gene and alcoholism. *Science, 281,* 1287–1288.

Noshpitz, J. D. (1962). Notes on the theory of residential treatment. *Journal of the American Academy of Child Psychiatry, 1,* 284–296.

Noshpitz, J. D. (1975). Residential treatment of emotionally disturbed children. In

S. Arieti (Ed.), *American handbook of psychiatry* (Vol. 5, pp. 634–651). New York: Basic Books.

Noshpitz, J. D. (1984). Narcissism and aggression. *American Journal of Psychotherapy, 38,* 17–34.

Novick, J., & Novick, K. K. (1996). *Fearful symmetry: The development and treatment of sadomasochism.* Northvale, NJ: Aronson.

Offord, D. R., Boyle, M. H., Racine, Y. A., Fleming, J. E., Cadman, D. T., Blum, H. M., Byrne, C., Links, P. S., Lipman, E. L., MacMillan, H. L., Rae Grant, N. I., Sanford, M. N., Szatmari, P., Thomas, H., & Woodward, C. A. (1992). Outcome, prognosis, and risk in a longitudinal follow-up study. *Journal of the American Academy of Child and Adolescent Psychiatry, 31,* 916–923.

Ogden, T. H. (1979). On projective identification. *International Journal of Psycho-Analysis, 60,* 357–373.

Ogden, T. H. (1982). *Projective identification and psychotherapeutic technique.* New York: Aronson.

Ogden, T. H. (1989). *The primitive edge of experience.* Northvale, NJ: Aronson.

Ogden, T. H. (1994). *Subjects of analysis.* Northvale, NJ: Aronson.

Oliver, J. E. (1993). Intergenerational transmission of child abuse: Rates, research, and clinical implications. *American Journal of Psychiatry, 150,* 1315–1324.

O'Malley, S. S., Jaffe, A. J., Chang, G., Schottenfeld, R. S., Meyer, R. E., & Rounsaville, B. (1992). Naltrexone and coping skills therapy for alcohol dependence: A controlled study. *Archives of General Psychiatry, 49,* 881–887.

Ornstein, A. (1981). Self-pathology in childhood: Developmental and clinical considerations. *Psychiatric Clinics of North America, 4,* 435–453.

Panksepp, J., Meeker, R., & Bean, N. J. (1980). The neurochemical control of crying. *Pharmacology, Biochemistry and Behavior, 12,* 437–443.

Papatheodorou, G., Kutcher, S. P., Katic, M., & Szalai, J. P. (1995). The efficacy and safety of divalproex sodium in the treatment of acute mania in adolescents and young adults: An open clinical trial. *Journal of Clinical Psychopharmacology, 15,* 110–116.

Papousek, H., & Papousek, M. (1987). Intuitive parenting: A dialectic counterpart to the infant's integrative competence. In J. D. Osofsky (Ed.), *Handbook of infant development* (pp. 669–720). New York: Wiley.

Papousek, H., & Papousek, M. (1989). Forms and functions of vocal matching in interactions between mothers and their precanonical infants. *First Language, 9,* 137–157.

Paris, J., & Zweig-Frank, H. (1992). A critical review of the role of childhood sexual abuse in the etiology of borderline personality disorder. *Canadian Journal of Psychiatry, 37,* 125–128.

Paris, J., & Zweig-Frank, H. (1997). Parameters of childhood sexual abuse in female patients. In M.C. Zanarini (Ed.), *Role of sexual abuse in the etiology of borderline personality disorder* (pp. 15–28). Washington, DC: American Psychiatric Press.

Patterson, G. R. (1982). *Coercive family process.* Eugene, OR: Castalia.

Patterson, G. R., & Chamberlin, P. (1988). Treatment process: A problem at three levels. In L. C. Wynne (Ed.), *The state of the art in family therapy research: Con-*

troversies and recommendations (pp. 189–223). New York: Family Process Press.

Patterson, G. R., DeBaryshe, B. D., & Ramsey, E. (1989). A developmental perspective on antisocial behavior. *American Psychologist, 44,* 329–335.

Patterson, G. R., & Forgatch, M. S. (1995). Predicting future clinical adjustment from treatment outcome and process variables. *Psychological Assessment, 7,* 275–285.

Patterson, G. R., Reid, J. B., Jones, R. R., & Conger, R. E. (1975). *A social learning approach to family intervention: Vol. 1. Families with aggressive children.* Eugene, OR: Castalia.

Peet, M. (1994). Induction of mania with selective serotonin re-uptake inhibitors and tricyclic antidepressants. *British Journal of Psychiatry, 164,* 549–550.

Perner, J., & Ruffman, T. (1995). Episodic memory and autonoetic consciousness: Developmental evidence and a theory of childhood amnesia. *Journal of Experimental Child Psychology, 59,* 516–548.

Perry, B. (1997). Incubated in terror: Neurodevelopmental factors in the "cycle of violence." In J. D. Osofsky (Ed.), *Children in a violent society* (pp. 124–149). New York: Guilford Press.

Perry, B. D., & Pollard, R. (1998). Homeostasis, stress, trauma, and adaptation: A neurodevelopmental view of childhood trauma. *Child and Adolescent Psychiatric Clinics of North America, 7,* 33–51.

Perry, B. D., Pollard, R. A., Blakely, T. L., Baker, W. L., & Vigilante, D. (1995). Childhood trauma, the neurobiology of adaptation, and "use-dependent" development of the brain: How "states" become "traits." *Infant Mental Health Journal, 16,* 271–291.

Petti, T. A., & Vela, R. M. (1990). Borderline disorders of childhood: An overview. *Journal of the American Academy of Child and Adolescent Psychiatry, 29,* 327–337.

Pine, F. (1974). On the concept of "borderline" in children: A clinical essay. *Psychoanalytic Study of the Child, 29,* 341–368.

Pine, F. (1983). Borderline syndromes in childhood: A working nosology and its therapeutic implications. In K. S. Robson (Ed.), *The borderline child: Approaches to etiology, diagnosis, and treatment* (pp. 83–100). New York: McGraw-Hill.

Pinto, O. C., & Akiskal, H. S. (1998). Lamotrigine as a promising approach to borderline personality: An open case series without concurrent DSM-IV major mood disorder. *Journal of Affective Disorders, 51,* 333–343.

Plakun, E. M. (1999). Managed care discovers the talking cure. In H. Kaley, M. N. Eagle, & D. L. Wolitzky (Eds.), *Psychoanalytic therapy as health care: Effectiveness and economics in the 21st century* (pp. 239–255). Hillsdale, NJ: Analytic Press.

Pliszka, S. R., Greenhill, L. L., Crismon, M. L., Sedillo, A., Carlson, C., Conners, C. K., McCracken, J. T., Swanson, J. M., Hughes, C. W., Llana, M. E., Lopez, M., & Toprac, M. G. (2000a). The Texas Children's Medication Algorithm Project: Report of the Texas Consensus Conference Panel on medication treatment of childhood attention-deficit/hyperactivity disorder: Part II. Tactics. *Journal of the American Academy of Child and Adolescent Psychiatry, 39,* 920–927.

Pliszka, S. R., Greenhill, L. L., Crismon, M. L., Sedillo, A., Carlson, C., Conners, C. K., McCracken, J. T., Swanson, J. M., Hughes, C. W., Llana, M. E., Lopez, M., & Toprac, M. G. (2000b). The Texas Children's Medication Algorithm Project: Report of the Texas Consensus Conference Panel on medication treatment of childhood attention-deficit/hyperactivity disorder: Part I. *Journal of the American Academy of Child and Adolescent Psychiatry, 39,* 908–919.

Pliszka, S. R., McCracken, J. T., & Maas, J. W. (1996). Catecholamines in attention-deficit hyperactivity disorder: Current perspectives. *Journal of the American Academy of Child and Adolescent Psychiatry, 35,* 264–272.

Post, R. M., Ketter, T. A., Denicoff, K., Pazzaglia, P. J., Leverich, G. S., Marangell, L. B., Callahan, A. M., George, M. S., & Frye, M. A. (1996). The place of anticonvulsant therapy in bipolar illness. *Psychopharmacology, 128,* 115–129.

Post, R. M., Ketter, T. A., Pazzaglia, P. J., Denicoff, K., George, M. S., Callahan, A., Leverich, G., & Frye, M. (1996). Rational polypharmacy in the bipolar affective disorders. *Epilepsy Research Supplement, 11,* 153–180.

Post, R. M., Kramlinger, K. G., Altshuler, L. L., Ketter, T., & Denicoff, K. (1990). Treatment of rapid cycling bipolar illness. *Psychopharmacology Bulletin, 26,* 37–47.

Post, R. M., Weiss, S. R., Smith, M., Li, H., & McCann, U. (1997). Kindling versus quenching: Implications for the evolution and treatment of post-traumatic stress disorder. In R. Yehuda & A. C. McFarlane (Eds.), *Psychobiology of post-traumatic stress disorder* (pp. 285–295). New York: New York Academy of Sciences.

Prince, J. B., Wilens, T. E., Biederman, J., Spencer, T. J., & Wozniak, J. R. (1996). Clonidine for sleep disturbances associated with attention-deficit hyperactivity disorder: A systematic chart review of 62 cases. *Journal of the American Academy of Child and Adolescent Psychiatry, 35,* 599–605.

Prudic, J., Haskett, R. F., Mulsant, B., Malone, K. M., Pettinati, H. M., Stephens, S., Greenberg, R., Rifas, S. L., & Sackeim, H. A. (1996). Resistance to antidepressant medications and short-term clinical response to ECT. *American Journal of Psychiatry, 153,* 985–992.

Pulver, S. E. (1970). Narcissism: The term and the concept. *Journal of the American Psychoanalytic Association, 18,* 319–342.

Putnam, F. W., Jr. (1985). Dissociation as a response to extreme trauma. In R. P. Kluft (Ed.), *Childhood antecedents of multiple personality* (pp. 65–91). Washington, DC: American Psychiatric Press.

Putnam, F. W. (1996). Child development and dissociation. *Child and Adolescent Psychiatric Clinics of North America, 5,* 285–301.

Pynoos, R. S., Steinberg, A. M., & Wraith, R. (1995). A developmental model of childhood traumatic stress. In D. Cicchetti & D. J. Cohen (Eds.), *Developmental psychopathology: Vol. 2. Risk, disorder, and adaptation* (pp. 72–95). New York: Wiley.

Redl, F., & Wineman, D. (1951). *Children who hate: The disorganization and breakdown of behavior controls.* Glencoe, IL: Free Press.

Redl, F., & Wineman, D. (1957). *The aggressive child.* Glencoe, IL: Free Press.

Reeves, A. C. (1971). Children with surrogate parents: Cases seen in analytic therapy and an aetiological hypothesis. *British Journal of Medical Psychology, 44,* 155–171.

Riddle, M. A., Reeve, E. A., Yaryura-Tobias, J. A., Yang, H. M., Claghorn, J. L., Gaffney, G., Greist, J. H., Holland, D., McConville, B. J., Pigott, T., & Walkup, J. T. (2001). Fluvoxamine for children and adolescents with obsessive–compulsive disorder: A randomized, controlled, multicenter trial. *Journal of the American Academy of Child and Adolescent Psychiatry, 40,* 222–229.

Riggs, P. D., Baker, S., Mikulich, S. K., Young, S. E., & Crowley, T. J. (1995). Depression in substance-dependent delinquents. *Journal of the American Academy of Child and Adolescent Psychiatry, 34,* 764–771.

Rinsley, D. B. (1980a). The developmental etiology of borderline and narcissistic disorders. *Bulletin of the Menninger Clinic, 44,* 127–134.

Rinsley, D. B. (1980b). Principles of therapeutic milieu with children. In G. P. Sholevar, R. M. Benson, & B. J. Blinder (Eds.), *Emotional disorders in children and adolescents: Medical and psychological approaches to treatment* (pp. 191–208). New York: Spectrum.

Rinsley, D. B. (1984). A comparison of borderline and narcissistic personality disorders. *Bulletin of the Menninger Clinic, 48,* 1–9.

Rinsley, D. B. (1989). *Developmental pathogenesis and treatment of borderline and narcissistic personalities.* New York: Aronson.

Robins, L. N. (1981). Epidemiological approaches to natural history research: Antisocial disorders in children. *Journal of the American Academy of Child Psychiatry, 20,* 566–580.

Rochat, P. (1995). Early objectification of the self. In P. Rochat (Ed.), *The self in infancy: Theory and research* (pp. 53–71). Amsterdam: North-Holland/Elsevier.

Rosenfeld, S. K., & Sprince, M. P. (1963). An attempt to formulate the meaning of the concept "borderline." *Psychoanalytic Study of the Child, 18,* 603–635.

Roth, A. S., Ostroff, R. B., & Hoffman, R. E. (1996). Naltrexone as a treatment for repetitive self-injurious behavior: An open-label trial. *Journal of Clinical Psychiatry, 57,* 233–237.

Rounds-Bryant, J. L., Kristiansen, P. L., & Hubbard, R. L. (1999). Drug abuse treatment outcome study of adolescents: A comparison of client characteristics and pretreatment behaviors in three treatment modalities. *American Journal of Drug and Alcohol Abuse, 25,* 573–591.

Russell, G. F. M., Treasure, J., & Eisler, I. (1998). Mothers with anorexia nervosa who underfeed their children: Their recognition and management. *Psychological Medicine, 28,* 93–108.

Rutter, M. (1985). Resilience in the face of adversity: Protective factors and resistance to psychiatric disorder. *British Journal of Psychiatry, 147,* 598–611.

Rutter, M. (1987). Psychosocial resilience and protective mechanisms. *American Journal of Orthopsychiatry, 57,* 316–331.

Rutter, M. (1999). Resilience concepts and findings: Implications for family therapy. *Journal of Family Therapy, 21,* 119–144.

Rutter, M., & Giller, H. (1983). *Juvenile delinquency: Trends and perspectives.* New York: Guilford Press.

Rutter, M., Giller, H., & Hagell, A. (1998). *Antisocial behavior by young people.* Cambridge, UK: Cambridge University Press.

Rutter, M., & Quinton, D. (1984). Long-term follow-up of women institutionalized in childhood: Factors promoting good functioning in adult life. *British Journal of Developmental Psychology, 2,* 191–204.

Ryan, N. D., Meyer, V., Dachille, S., Mazzie, D., & Puig-Antich, J. (1988). Lithium antidepressant augmentation in TCA-refractory depression in adolescents. *Journal of the American Academy of Child and Adolescent Psychiatry, 27,* 371–376.

Sachar, E. J., Hellman, L., Roffwarg, H. P., Halpern, F. S., Fukushima, D. K., & Gallagher, T. F. (1973). Disrupted 24-hour patterns of cortisol secretion in psychotic depression. *Archives of General Psychiatry, 28,* 19–24.

Sackett, D. L., Rosenberg, W. M., Gray, J. A., Haynes, R. B., & Richardson, W. S. (1996). Evidence based medicine: What it is and what it isn't. *British Medical Journal, 312,* 71–72.

Safer, D. J., Zito, J. M., & Fine, E. M. (1996). Increased methylphenidate usage for attention deficit disorder in the 1990s. *Pediatrics, 98,* 1084–1088.

Safran, J. D., & Muran, J. C. (2000). *Negotiating the therapeutic alliance: A relational treatment guide.* New York: Guilford Press.

Salzman, C., Wolfson, A. N., Schatzberg, A., Looper, J., Henke, R., Albanese, M., Schwartz, J., & Miyawaki, E. (1995). Effect of fluoxetine on anger in symptomatic volunteers with borderline personality disorder. *Journal of Clinical Psychopharmacology, 15,* 23–29.

Sander, L. W. (1975). Infant and caretaking environment: Investigation and conceptualization of adaptive behavior in a system of increasing complexity. In E. J. Anthony (Ed.), *Explorations in child psychiatry* (pp. 129–166). New York: Holt, Rinehart & Winston.

Sanders, M. R., & Dadds, M. R. (1992). Children's and parents' cognitions about family interaction: An evaluation of video-mediated recall and thought listing procedures in the assessment of conduct-disordered children. *Journal of Clinical Child Psychology, 21,* 371–379.

Santiago, L. B., Jorge, S. M., & Moreira, A. C. (1996). Longitudinal evaluation of the development of salivary cortisol circadian rhythm in infancy. *Clinical Endocrinology, 44,* 157–161.

Sapolsky, R. M. (2000). Glucocorticoids and hippocampal atrophy in neuropsychiatric disorders. *Archives of General Psychiatry, 57,* 925–935.

Sass, H., Soyka, M., Mann, K., & Zieglgansberger, W. (1996). Relapse prevention by acamprosate: Results from a placebo-controlled study on alcohol dependence. *Archives of General Psychiatry, 53,* 673–680.

Schachtel, E. G. (1947). On memory and childhood amnesia. *Psychiatry: Journal for the Study of Interpersonal Processes, 10,* 1–26.

Schacter, D. L. (1992). Understanding implicit memory: A cognitive neuroscience approach. *American Psychologist, 47,* 559–569.

Schmidt, S. E., Liddle, H. A., & Dakof, G. A. (1996). Changes in parenting practices and adolescent drug abuse during multidimensional family therapy. *Journal of Family Psychology, 10,* 12–27.

Schmuckler, M. A. (1996). Visual–proprioceptive intermodal perception in infancy. *Infant Behavior and Development, 19,* 221–232.

Schneider-Rosen, K., & Cicchetti, D. (1991). Early self-knowledge and emotional development: Visual self-recognition and affective reactions to mirror self-image in maltreated and non-maltreated toddlers. *Developmental Psychology, 27,* 471–478.

Schneier, F. R., Liebowitz, M. R., Abi-Dargham, A., Zea-Ponce, Y., Lin, S., & Laruelle, M. (2000). Low dopamine D_2 receptor binding potential in social phobia. *American Journal of Psychiatry, 157,* 457–459.

Schulz, S. C., Camlin, K. L., Berry, S. A., & Jesberger, J. A. (1999). Olanzapine safety and efficacy in patients with borderline personality disorder and comorbid dysthymia. *Biological Psychiatry, 46,* 1429–1435.

Schwartz, C. E., Snidman, N., & Kagan, J. (1999). Adolescent social anxiety as an outcome of inhibited temperament in childhood. *Journal of the American Academy of Child and Adolescent Psychiatry, 38,* 1008–1015.

Schwartz, E. D., & Perry, B. D. (1999). The post-traumatic response in children and adolescents. *Psychiatric Clinics of North America, 17*(2), 311–321.

Schwartz, J. M., Stoessel, P. W., Baxter, L. R. J., Martin, K. M., & Phelps, M. E. (1996). Systematic changes in cerebral glucose metabolic rate after successful behavior modification treatment of obsessive–compulsive disorder. *Archives of General Psychiatry, 53,* 109–113.

Segal, H. (1981). Notes on symbol formation. In *The work of Hanna Segal* (pp. 49–65). New York: Aronson. (Original work published 1957)

Shalev, A. Y., Orr, S. P., Peri, T., Schreiber, S., & Pitman, R. K. (1992). Physiologic responses to loud tones in Israeli patients with posttraumatic stress disorder. *Archives of General Psychiatry, 49,* 870–875.

Shapiro, D. (1965). *Neurotic styles.* New York: Basic Books.

Shapiro, F. (1995). *Eye movement desensitization and reprocessing: Basic principles, protocols, and procedures.* New York: Guilford Press.

Shapiro, F., & Forrest, M. S. (1997). *EMDR: The breakthrough therapy for overcoming anxiety, stress, and trauma.* New York: Basic Books.

Shapiro, T. (1990). Resolved: Borderline personality exists in children under twelve: Negative [Debate forum]. *Journal of the American Academy of Child and Adolescent Psychiatry, 29,* 480–483.

Sharfstein, S. S., & Kent, J. J., Jr. (1997). Restructuring for survival: The Sheppard Pratt transformation. In R. K. Schreter, S. S. Sharfstein, & C. A. Schreter (Eds.), *Managing care, not dollars: The continuum of mental health services* (pp. 281–298). Washington, DC: American Psychiatric Press.

Sheard, M. H. (1975). Lithium in the treatment of aggression. *Journal of Nervous and Mental Disease, 160,* 108–118.

Sheard, M. H., Marini, J. L., Bridges, C. I., & Wagner, E. (1976). The effect of lithium on impulsive–aggressive behavior in man. *American Journal of Psychiatry, 133,* 1409–1413.

Shimamura, A. P. (1995). Memory and frontal lobe function. In M. S. Gazzaniga (Ed.), *The cognitive neurosciences* (pp. 803–813). Cambridge, MA: MIT Press.

Siegel, D. J. (1999). *The developing mind: Toward a neurobiology of interpersonal experience.* New York: Guilford Press.

Siever, L. J., Buchsbaum, M. S., New, A. S., Spiegel-Cohen, J., Wei, T., Hazlett, E. A., Sevin, E., Nunn, M., & Mitropoulou, V. (1999). d,1-fenfluramine response in impulsive personality disorder assessed with [18F] fluorodeoxyglucose positron emission tomography. *Neuropsychopharmacology, 20,* 413–423.

Siever, L. J., & Davis, K. L. (1991). A psychobiological perspective on the personality disorders. *American Journal of Psychiatry, 148,* 1647–1658.

Sifneos, P. E., Apfel-Savitz, R., & Frankel, F. H. (1977). The phenomenon of "alexithymia": Observations in neurotic and psychosomatic patients. *Psychotherapy and Psychosomatics, 28,* 47–57.

Smith, J., & Prior, M. (1995). Temperament and stress resilience in school-age children: A within-families study. *Journal of the American Academy of Child and Adolescent Psychiatry, 34,* 168–179.

Smith, P. K. (1996). Language and the evolution of mind-reading. In P. Carruthers & P. K. Smith (Eds.), *Theories of theories of mind* (pp. 344–354). Cambridge, UK: Cambridge University Press.

Soloff, P. H. (1998). Algorithms for pharmacological treatment of personality dimensions: Symptom-specific treatments for cognitive–perceptual, affective, and impulsive–behavioral dysregulation. *Bulletin of the Menninger Clinic, 62,* 195–214.

Solomon, J., & George, C. (1996). Defining the caregiving system: Toward a theory of caregiving. *Infant Mental Health Journal, 17,* 183–197.

Sorce, J. F., Emde, R. N., Campos, J. J., & Klinnert, M. D. (1985). Maternal emotional signaling: Its effect on the visual cliff behavior of 1-year-olds. *Developmental Psychology, 21,* 195–200.

Spelke, E. S. (1979). Perceiving bimodally specified events in infancy. *Developmental Psychology, 15,* 626–636.

Spelke, E. S., & Owsley, C. J. (1979). Intermodal exploration and knowledge in infancy. *Infant Behavior and Development, 2,* 13–27.

Spencer, T., Biederman, J., Kerman, K., Steingard, R., & Wilens, T. (1993). Desipramine treatment of children with attention-deficit hyperactivity disorder and tic disorder or Tourette's syndrome. *Journal of the American Academy of Child and Adolescent Psychiatry, 32,* 354–360.

Spencer, T., Biederman, J., & Wilens, T. (2000). Pharmacotherapy of attention deficit hyperactivity disorder. *Child and Adolescent Psychiatric Clinics of North America, 9,* 77–97.

Spencer, T., Biederman, J., Wilens, T., Harding, M., O'Donnell, D., & Griffin, S. (1996). Pharmacotherapy of attention-deficit hyperactivity disorder across the life cycle. *Journal of the American Academy of Child and Adolescent Psychiatry, 35,* 409–432.

Spencer, T., Biederman, J., Wilens, T., Steingard, R., & Geist. D. (1993). Nortriptyline treatment of children with attention-deficit hyperactivity disorder and tic disorder or Tourette's syndrome. *Journal of the American Academy of Child and Adolescent Psychiatry, 32,* 205–210.

Spillius, E. B. (1992). Clinical experiences of projective identification. In R. Anderson (Ed.), *Clinical lectures on Klein and Bion* (pp. 59–73). London: Tavistock/ Routledge.

Spillius, E. B. (1994). Developments in Kleinian thought: Overview and personal view. *Psychoanalytic Inquiry, 14,* 324–364.

Spitz, R. A. (1945). Hospitalism: An inquiry into the genesis of psychiatric conditions in early childhood. *Psychoanalytic Study of the Child, 1,* 53–74.

Spitz, R., & Wolf, K. M. (1946). Anaclitic depression: An inquiry into the genesis of psychiatric conditions in early childhood. *Psychoanalytic Study of the Child, 2,* 313–342.

Spivak, G., & Shure, M. B. (1978). *Problem solving techniques in child-rearing.* San Francisco: Jossey-Bass.

Squire, L. R. (1987). *Memory and brain.* New York: Oxford University Press.

Squire, L. R. (1992). Declarative and non-declarative memory: Multiple brain systems supporting learning and memory. *Journal of Cognitive Neuroscience, 4,* 232–243.

Squire, L. R., Knowlton, B., & Musen, G. (1993). The structure and organization of memory. *Annual Review of Psychology, 44,* 453–495.

Squire, L. R., & Zola-Morgan, S. (1991). The medial temporal lobe memory system. *Science, 253,* 1380–1386.

Sroufe, L. A. (1983). Infant–caregiver attachment and patterns of adaptation in preschool: The roots of maladaptation and competence. In M. Perlmutter (Ed.), *Development and policy concerning children with special needs* (pp. 41–81). Hillsdale, NJ: Erlbaum.

Sroufe, L. A. (1989). Relationships, self, and individual adaptation. In A. J. Sameroff & R. N. Emde (Eds.), *Relationship disturbances in early childhood: A developmental approach* (pp. 70–94). New York: Basic Books.

Sroufe, L. A. (1990). An organizational perspective on the self. In D. Cicchetti & M. Beeghly (Eds.), *The self in transition: Infancy to childhood* (pp. 281–307). Chicago: University of Chicago Press.

Sroufe, L. A. (1996). *Emotional development: The organization of emotional life in the early years.* New York: Cambridge University Press.

Sroufe, L. A. (1997). Psychopathology as an outcome of development. *Development and Psychopathology, 9,* 251–268.

Stanley, M., & Mann, J. J. (1983). Increased serotonin-2 binding sites in frontal cortex of suicide victims. *Lancet, 1,* 214–216.

Steele, H., Steele, M., & Fonagy, P. (1996). Associations among attachment classifications of mothers, fathers, and their infants. *Child Development, 67,* 541–555.

Stein, H., Fonagy, P., Ferguson, K. S., & Wisman, M. (2000). Lives through time: An ideographic approach to the study of resilience. *Bulletin of the Menninger Clinic, 64,* 281–305.

Stein, M. B., Hanna, C., Koverola, C., Torchia, M., & McClarty, B. (1997). Structural brain changes in PTSD: Does trauma alter neuroanatomy? *Annals of the New York Academy of Sciences, 821,* 76–82.

Stein, M. B., Yehuda, R., Koverola, C., & Hanna, C. (1997). Enhanced dexamethasone suppression of plasma cortisol in adult women traumatized by childhood sexual abuse. *Biological Psychiatry, 42,* 680–686.

Steiner, H., Cauffman, E., & Duxbury, E. (1999). Personality traits in juvenile delinquents: Relation to criminal behavior and recidivism. *Journal of the American Academy of Child and Adolescent Psychiatry, 38,* 256–262.

Steingard, R., Biederman, J., Spencer, T., Wilens, T., & Gonzalez, A. (1993). Comparison of clonidine response in the treatment of attention-deficit hyperactivity disorder with and without comorbid tic disorders. *Journal of the American Academy of Child and Adolescent Psychiatry, 32,* 350–353.

Stern, D. N. (1985). *The interpersonal world of the infant: A view from psychoanalysis and developmental psychology.* New York: Basic Books.

Stern, D. N. (1990). *Diary of a baby.* New York: Basic Books.

Stern, D. N. (1995). *The motherhood constellation: A unified view of parent–infant psychotherapy.* New York: Basic Books.

Stern, D. N. (1998). The process of therapeutic change involving implicit knowledge: Some implications of developmental observations for adult psychotherapy. *Infant Mental Health Journal, 19,* 300–308.

Stern, D. N., Hofer, L., Haft, W., & Dore, J. (1985). Affect attunement: The sharing of feeling states between mother and infant by means of inter-modal fluency. In T. M. Fields & N. A. Fox (Eds.), *Social perception in infants* (pp. 249–268). Norwood, NJ: Ablex.

Stern, D. N., Sander, L. W., Nahum, J. P., Harrison, A. M., Lyons-Ruth, K., Morgan, A. C., Bruschweiler-Stern, N., & Tronick, E. Z. (1998). Non-interpretive mechanisms in psychoanalytic therapy: The "something more" than interpretation. *International Journal of Psycho-Analysis, 79,* 903–921.

Stokes, P. E., & Sikes, C. R. (1987). Hypothalamic–pituitary–adrenal axis in affective disorders. In H. Y. Meltzer (Ed.), *Psychopharmacology: The third generation of progress* (pp. 589–607). New York: Raven Press.

Stolorow, R. (1975). Toward a functional definition of narcissism. *International Journal of Psycho-Analysis, 56,* 179–185.

Stone, M. H. (1979). Contemporary shift of the borderline concept from a subschizophrenic disorder to a subaffective disorder. *Psychiatric Clinics of North America, 2,* 577–594.

Stone, M. H. (2000). Gradations of antisociality and responsivity to psychosocial therapies. In J. G. Gunderson & G. O. Gabbard (Eds.), *Psychotherapy for personality disorders* (pp. 95–130). Washington, DC: American Psychiatric Press.

Stone, M. H., Kahn, E., & Flye, B. (1981). Psychiatrically ill relatives of borderline patients: A family study. *Psychiatric Quarterly, 53,* 71–84.

Strauss, G., Chassin, M., & Lock, J. (1995). Can experts agree when to hospitalize adolescents? *Journal of the American Academy of Child and Adolescent Psychiatry, 34,* 418–424.

Strayhorn, J. M., & Weidman, C. S. (1989). Reduction of attention deficit and internalizing symptoms in preschoolers through parent–child interaction training. *Journal of the American Academy of Child and Adolescent Psychiatry, 28,* 886–896.

Strober, M., DeAntonio, M., Schmidt-Lackner, S., Pataki, C., Freeman, R., Rigali, J., & Rao, U. (1999). The pharmacotherapy of depressive illness in adolescents:

An open-label comparison of fluoxetine with imipramine-treated historical controls. *Journal of Clinical Psychiatry, 60,* 164–169.

Strober, M., Freeman, R., Rigali, J., Schmidt, S., & Diamond, R. (1992). The pharmacotherapy of depressive illness in adolescence: II. Effects of lithium augmentation in nonresponders to imipramine. *Journal of the American Academy of Child and Adolescent Psychiatry, 31,* 16–20.

Strober, M., Morrell, W., Burroughs, J., Lampert, C., Danforth, H., & Freeman, R. (1988). A family study of bipolar I disorder in adolescence: Early onset of symptoms linked to increased familial loading and lithium resistance. *Journal of Affective Disorders, 15,* 255–268.

Strober, M., Morrell, W., Lampert, C., & Burroughs, J. (1990). Relapse following discontinuation of lithium maintenance therapy in adolescents with bipolar I illness: A naturalistic study. *American Journal of Psychiatry, 147,* 457–461.

Stroul, B. A., & Friedman, R. M. (1988). Caring for severely emotionally disturbed children and youth: Principles for a system of care. *Child Today, 17,* 11–15.

Suomi, S. J. (1984). The development of affect in rhesus monkeys. In N. A. Fox & R. J. Davidson (Eds.), *The psychobiology of affective development* (pp. 119–159). Hillsdale, NJ: Erlbaum.

Suomi, S. J. (1997). Early determinants of behaviour: Evidence from primate studies. *British Medical Bulletin, 53,* 170–184.

Suomi, S. J., & Harlow, H. F. (1972). Social rehabilitation of isolate-reared monkeys. *Developmental Psychology, 6,* 487–496.

Suomi, S. J., Harlow, H. F., & Novak, M. A. (1974). Reversal of social deficits produced by isolation rearing in monkeys. *Journal of Human Evolution, 3,* 527–534.

Swanson, J. M., Sunohara, G. A., Kennedy, J. L., Regino, R., Fineberg, E., Wigal, T., Lerner, M., Williams, L., LaHoste, G. J., & Wigal, S. (1998). Association of the dopamine receptor D_4 (DRD_4) gene with a refined phenotype of attention deficit hyperactivity disorder (ADHD): A family-based approach. *Molecular Psychiatry, 3,* 38–41.

Terr, L. C. (1991). Childhood traumas: An outline and overview. *American Journal of Psychiatry, 148,* 10–20.

Thompson, J. W., Rosenstein, M. J., Milazzo-Sayre, L. J., & MacAskill, R. L. (1986). Psychiatric services to adolescents: 1970–1980. *Hospital and Community Psychiatry, 37,* 584–590.

Thompson, R. A. (1999). Early attachment and later development. In J. Cassidy & P. R. Shaver (Eds.), *Handbook of attachment: Theory, research and clinical applications* (pp. 265–286). New York: Guilford Press.

Tohen, M., Sanger, T. M., McElroy, S. L., Tollefson, G. D., Chengappa, K. N. R., Daniel, D. G., Petty, F., Centorrino, F., Wang, R., Grundy, S. L., Greaney, M. G., Jacobs, T. G., David, S. R., Toma, V., & the Olanzapine HGEH Study Group. (1999). Olanzapine versus placebo in the treatment of acute mania. *American Journal of Psychiatry, 156,* 702–709.

Tollefson, G. D., Sanger, T. M., Lu, Y., & Thieme, M. E. (1998). Depressive signs and symptoms in schizophrenia: A prospective blinded trial of olanzapine and haloperidol. *Archives of General Psychiatry, 55,* 250–258.

Tooley, K. (1973). Playing it right: A technique for the treatment of borderline children. *Journal of the American Academy of Child Psychiatry, 12,* 615–631.

Tooley, K. (1975). The small assassins: Clinical notes on a subgroup of murderous children. *Journal of the American Academy of Child Psychiatry, 14,* 306–318.

Trevarthen, C. (1979). Communication and cooperation in early infancy: A description of primary intersubjectivity. In M. Bullowa (Ed.), *Before speech: The beginning of interpersonal communication* (pp. 321–347). New York: Cambridge University Press.

Trevarthen, C., & Hubley, P. (1978). A secondary inter-subjectivity: Confiding, confiders, and acts of meaning in the first year. In A. Lock (Ed.), *Action, gesture, and symbol: The emergence of language* (pp. 183–229). New York: Academic Press.

Tronick, E. Z. (1989). Emotions and emotional communication in infants. *American Psychologist, 44,* 112–119.

Tuma, J. M. (1989). Mental health services for children: The state of the art. *American Psychologist, 44,* 188–199.

Twemlow, S. W., Fonagy, P., Sacco, F. C., Gies, M. L., Evans, R., & Ewbank, R. (2001). Creating a peaceful school learning environment: A controlled study of an elementary school intervention to reduce violence. *American Journal of Psychiatry, 158,* 808–810.

Tyson, P. (1982). A developmental line of gender identity, gender role, and choice of love object. *Journal of the American Psychoanalytic Association, 30,* 61–86.

Vaidya, C. J., Austin, G., Kirkorian, G., Ridlehuber, H. W., Desmond, J. E., Glover, G. H., & Gabrieli, J. D. (1998). Selective effects of methylphenidate in attention deficit hyperactivity disorder: A functional magnetic resonance study. *Proceedings of the National Academy of Sciences of the United States of America, 95,* 14494–14499.

van der Kolk, B. A., Burbridge, J. A., & Suzuki, J. (1997). The psychobiology of traumatic memory. In R. Yehuda & A. C. McFarlane (Eds.), *Psychobiology of posttraumatic stress disorder* (pp. 99–113). New York: New York Academy of Sciences.

van der Kolk, B. A., & Fisler, R. E. (1994). Childhood abuse and neglect and loss of self-regulation. *Bulletin of the Menninger Clinic, 58,* 145–168.

van der Kolk, B. A., & Fisler, R. E. (1995). Dissociation and the fragmentary nature of traumatic memories: Overview and exploratory study. *Journal of Traumatic Stress, 8,* 505–525.

van der Kolk, B. A., & van der Hart, O. (1989). Pierre Janet and the breakdown of adaptation in psychological trauma. *American Journal of Psychiatry, 146,* 1530–1540.

van der Meere, J., Gunning, B., & Stemerdink, N. (1999). The effect of methylphenidate and clonidine on response inhibition and state regulation in children with ADHD. *Journal of Child Psychology and Psychiatry and Allied Disciplines, 40,* 291–298.

Vela, R. M., Gottlieb, E. H., & Gottlieb, H. P. (1983). Borderline syndromes in childhood: A critical review. In K. S. Robson (Ed.), *The borderline child: Approaches to etiology, diagnosis, and treatment* (pp. 31–48). New York: McGraw-Hill.

Vitiello, B., & Stoff, D. M. (1997). Subtypes of aggression and their relevance to child psychiatry. *Journal of the American Academy of Child and Adolescent Psychiatry, 36,* 307–315.

Volkow, N. D., Wang, G. J., Fowler, J. S., Gatley, S. J., Logan, J., Ding, Y. S., Hitzemann, R., & Pappas, N. (1998). Dopamine transporter occupancies in the human brain induced by therapeutic doses of oral methylphenidate. *American Journal of Psychiatry, 155,* 1325–1331.

Volpicelli, J. R., Davis, M. A., & Olgin, J. E. (1986). Naltrexone blocks the postshock increase of ethanol consumption. *Life Sciences, 38,* 841–847.

Volpicelli, J. R., Volpicelli, L. A., & O'Brien, C. P. (1995). Medical management of alcohol dependence: Clinical use and limitations of naltrexone treatment. *Alcohol and Alcoholism, 30,* 789–798.

Vygotsky, L. S. (1962). *Thought and language* (E. Hanfmann & G. Vakar, Eds. & Trans.). Cambridge, MA: MIT Press.

Vygotsky, L. S. (1978). *Mind in society: The development of higher psychological processes.* Cambridge, MA: Harvard University Press.

Waldinger, R. J., & Frank, A. F. (1989a). Transference and the vicissitudes of medication use by borderline patients. *Psychiatry, 52,* 416–427.

Waldinger, R. J., & Frank, A. F. (1989b). Clinicians' experiences in combining medication and psychotherapy in the treatment of borderline patients. *Hospital and Community Psychiatry, 40,* 712–718.

Waldinger, R. J., & Gunderson, J. G. (1984). Completed psychotherapies with borderline patients. *American Journal of Psychotherapy, 38,* 190–202.

Wasman, M., & Flynn, J. P. (1962). Directed attack elicited from hypothalamus. *Archives of Neurology, 6,* 208–219.

Watson, J. S. (1972). Smiling, cooing, and "the game." *Merrill–Palmer Quarterly, 18,* 323–339.

Watson, J. S. (1979). Perception of contingency as a determinant of social responsiveness. In E. Thoman (Ed.), *Origins of the infant's social responsiveness* (pp. 33–64). Hillsdale, NJ: Erlbaum.

Watson, J. S. (1985). Contingency perception in early social development. In T. M. Field & N. A. Fox (Eds.), *Social perception in infants* (pp. 157–176). Norwood, NJ: Ablex.

Watson, J. S. (1994). Detection of self: The perfect algorithm. In S. T. Parker, R. W. Mitchell, & M. L. Boccia (Eds.), *Self-awareness in animals and humans: Developmental perspectives* (pp. 131–148). New York: Cambridge University Press.

Watson, J. S. (1995). Mother–infant interaction: Dispositional properties and mutual designs. In N. S. Thompson (Ed.), *Perspectives in ethology* (Vol. 11, pp. 189–210). New York: Plenum Press.

Webster-Stratton, C. (1996). Early intervention with videotape modeling: Programs for families of children with oppositional defiant disorder or conduct disorder. In E. D. Hibbs & P. S. Jensen (Eds.), *Psychosocial treatments for child and adolescent disorders: Empirically based strategies for clinical practice* (pp. 435–474). Washington, DC: American Psychological Association.

Webster-Stratton, C., & Hammond, M. (1997). Treating children with early-onset conduct problems: A comparison of child and parenttraining interventions. *Journal of Consulting and Clinical Psychology, 65,* 93–109.

Webster-Stratton, C., & Herbert, M. (1994). *Troubled families—problem children: Working with parents: A collaborative process.* New York: Wiley.

Weil, A. P. (1954). Certain severe disturbances of ego development in childhood. *Psychoanalytic Study of the Child, 8,* 271–287.

Weithorn, L. A. (1988). Mental hospitalization of troublesome youth: An analysis of skyrocketing admission rates. *Stanford Law Review, 40,* 773–838.

Werner, E. E., & Smith, R. S. (1982). *Vulnerable but invincible: A longitudinal study of resilient children and youth.* New York: McGraw-Hill.

Weston, J. (1968). The pathology of child abuse. In R. E. Helfer & C. H. Kempe (Eds.), *The battered child* (pp. 77–100). Chicago: University of Chicago Press.

Whalen, C. K., & Henker, B. (1992). The social profile of attention-deficit hyperactivity disorder: Five fundamental facets. *Child and Adolescent Psychiatric Clinics of North America, 1,* 395–410.

Whalen, C. K., Henker, B., & Granger, D. A. (1990). Social judgment processes in hyperactive boys: Effects of methylphenidate and comparisons with normal peers. *Journal of Abnormal Child Psychology, 18,* 297–316.

Whalen, P. J., Rauch, S. L., Etcoff, N. L., McInerney, S. C., Lee, M. B., & Jenike, M. A. (1998). Masked presentations of emotional facial expressions modulate amygdala activity without explicit knowledge. *Journal of Neuroscience, 18,* 411–418.

Wichstrom, L., Skogen, K., & Oia, T. (1996). Increased rate of conduct problems in urban areas: What is the mechanism? *Journal of the American Academy of Child and Adolescent Psychiatry, 35,* 471–479.

Wilens, T. E., & Biederman, J. (1993). Psychopathology in preadolescent children at high risk for substance abuse: A review of the literature. *Harvard Review of Psychiatry, 1,* 207–218.

Winnicott, D. W. (1953). Transitional objects and transitional phenomena: A study of the first not-me possession. *International Journal of Psycho-Analysis, 34,* 89–97.

Winnicott, D. W. (1958). *Collected papers: Through paediatrics to psycho-analysis.* New York: Basic Books.

Winnicott, D. W. (1965). *The maturational processes and the facilitating environment: Studies in the theory of emotional development.* New York: International Universities Press.

Winnicott, D. W. (1967). Mirror role of mother and family in child development. In P. Lomas (Ed.), *The predicament of the family: A psycho-analytical symposium* (pp. 26–33). London: Hogarth Press and the Institute of Psychoanalysis.

Wolf, E. S., Gedo, J. E., & Terman, D. M. (1972). On the adolescent process as a transformation of the self. *Journal of Youth and Adolescence, 1,* 257–272.

Wolfgang, M. E., Figlio, R. M., & Sellin, J. T. (1972). *Delinquency in a birth cohort.* Chicago: University of Chicago Press.

Woody, G. E., McLellan, A. T., Luborsky, L. & O'Brien, C. P. (1985). Sociopathy and psychotherapy outcome. *Archives of General Psychiatry, 42,* 1081–1086.

Wyman, P. A., Cowen, E. L., Work, W. C., Hoyt-Meyers, L., Magnus, K. B., & Fagen, D. B. (1999). Caregiving and developmental factors differentiating young at-risk urban children showing resilient versus stress-affected outcomes: A replication and extension. *Child Development, 70,* 645–659.

Yehuda, R. (1997). Stress and glucocorticoid. *Science, 275,* 1662–1663.

Yehuda, R. (1998). Neuroendocrinology of trauma and posttraumatic stress disorder. In R. Yehuda (Ed.), *Psychological trauma* (pp. 97–131). Washington, DC: American Psychiatric Press.

Yehuda, R., Kahana, B., Binder-Brynes, K., Southwick, S. M., Mason, J. W., & Giller, E. L. (1995). Low urinary cortisol excretion in Holocaust survivors with posttraumatic stress disorder. *American Journal of Psychiatry, 152,* 982–986.

Yehuda, R., & McFarlane, A. C. (1995). Conflict between current knowledge about posttraumatic stress disorder and its original conceptual basis. *American Journal of Psychiatry, 152,* 1705–1713.

Yeomans, F. E., Selzer, M. A., & Clarkin, J. F. (1992). *Treating the borderline patient: A contract-based approach.* New York: Basic Books.

Youngblade, L. M., & Dunn, J. (1995). Individual differences in young children's pretend play with mother and sibling: Links to relationships and understanding of other people's feelings and beliefs. *Child Development, 66,* 1472–1492.

Zanarini, M. C., & Frankenburg, F. R. (1997). Pathways to the development of borderline personality disorder. *Journal of Personality Disorders, 11,* 93–104.

Zanarini, M. C., Frankenburg, F. R., Reich, D. B., Marino, M. F., Haynes, M. C., & Gunderson, J. G. (1999). Violence in the lives of adult borderline patients. *Journal of Nervous and Mental Disease, 187,* 65–71.

Zanarini, M. C., Gunderson, J. G., Marino, M. F., Schwartz, E. O., & Frankenburg, F. R. (1989). Childhood experiences of borderline patients. *Comprehensive Psychiatry, 30,* 18–25.

Index